Pronatalism

Pronatalism

The Myth of Mom & Apple Pie

EDITED BY

Ellen Peck

AND

Judith Senderowitz

THOMAS Y. CROWELL COMPANY

Established 1834 New York

Designed by ABIGAIL MOSELEY

Manufactured in the United States of America

Library of Congress Cataloging in Publication Data

Peck, Ellen, 1942– comp.
Pronatalism: the myth of mom and apple pie.

Includes bibliographical references.
1. Childlessness—United States—Addresses, essays, lectures. I. Senderowitz, Judith, joint comp. II. Title.
HQ536.P4 301.42'7 74–6087
ISBN 0–690–00498–2 (hardcover) / 0–8152–0355–1 (Apollo edition)

1 2 3 4 5 6 7 8 9 10

ACKNOWLEDGMENTS

"Social Devices for Impelling Women to Bear and Rear Children," by Leta S. Hollingworth, reprinted from *American Journal of Sociology*, 1916.
"Coercive Pronatalism and American Population Policy," by Judith Blake, for the Commission on Population Growth and the American Future, with permission of the author.
"Pronatalism in Women's Magazine Fiction," by Helen H. Franzwa, by arrangement with the author.
"Pronatal Influences in Home Economics Texts in a Junior High School," by Nancy Cox, by arrangement with the author.
"Is There a Relationship Between Childlessness and Marriage Breakdown?" by

Robert Chester, reprinted from *Journal of Biosocial Science,* 1972, v. 4, © 1972 by Galton Foundation.

"Burgess and Cottrell Data on 'Desire for Children': An Example of Distortion in Marriage and Family Textbooks?" by Edward Pohlman, reprinted from *Journal of Marriage and the Family* (30), © 1968 by National Council on Family Relations.

"Motherhood: Myth or Need?", by Betty Rollin, originally published as "Motherhood: Who Needs It?" reprinted from *Look* Magazine (September 22, 1970), © 1970 by Cowles Communications, Inc.

"Motivations in Wanting Conceptions," by Edward Pohlman, from *Psychology of Birth Planning,* © 1969 by Schenkman Publishing Company, Inc., Cambridge, Mass., reprinted by permission.

"Wrong Reasons," with permission of Planned Parenthood-World Population.

"The Wrong Reasons to Have Children," by Robert E. Gould, reprinted from *New York Times Magazine* (May 3, 1970), © 1970 The New York Times Company.

"Parenthood as Crisis," by E. E. LeMasters, reprinted from *Marriage and Family Living,* v. 19, no. 4, © 1957 by National Council on Family Relations.

"Changes in Marriage and Parenthood: A Methodological Design," by Harold Feldman, with permission of the author.

"The Implications of Motherhood for Political Participation," by Naomi B. Lynn and Cornelia B. Flora, © 1972 by American Political Science Association.

"Why We Don't Want Children," by Lynnell Michels, reprinted from *Redbook* Magazine (January, 1970), © 1969 by The Redbook Publishing Company.

"A Vote Against Motherhood," by Gael Greene, reprinted from *Saturday Evening Post* (January 26, 1963), © 1963 by Gael Greene.

"The Future Is a Cruel Hoax," by Stephanie Mills, with permission of the author.

"Reflections of a Non-Parent," by Stewart R. Mott, with permission of the author.

"Changes in Views Toward Childlessness, 1965–1970," by Edward Pohlman, with permission of the author.

"Motivations of Childless Marriages," by Paul Popenoe, reprinted with permission from the *Journal of Heredity,* v. 27, 1936.

"Correlates of Voluntary Childlessness in a Select Population," by Susan O. Gustavus and James R. Henley, Jr., reprinted from *Social Biology,* 1971, v. 18, no. 3, © 1971 by American Eugenics Society.

"Voluntarily Childless Wives: An Exploratory Study," by J. E. Veevers, from *Sociology and Social Research,* 1973, reprinted with permission.

"Voluntary Childlessness: A Neglected Area of Family Study," by J. E. Veevers, reprinted from *The Family Coordinator* (April, 1973), © 1973 by National Council on Family Relations.

To
Ethel Senderowitz and Bill Peck

Personal Acknowledgments

For their help and advice in making this book a reality, we wish to express thanks to Dr. Jessie Bernard, Dr. Paul Ehrlich, Mr. Robin Elliott, Dr. Robert Gould and Lois Gould, Dr. E. James Lieberman, Dr. Margaret Mead, Ms. Vicki Pellegrino, Dr. Edward Pohlman, the Population Reference Bureau of Washington, D.C., Dr. Michael Potegal, Mr. Bob Rothenberg, Dr. Norman Ryder, Mr. John Simon, Ms. Joyce Snyder, Professor Jean E. Veevers, and Dr. Charles Westoff.

We wish to express special thanks to Sherry Barnes of Zero Population Growth and to Audrey Bertolet of the National Organization for Non-Parents; their willingness to take over organizational responsibilities for us enabled us to spend the time necessary to prepare this manuscript.

Finally, thanks to those close to us during the preparation of this book, who had faith in its worth and patience with its authors: Jay Harris, Margaret Miner, Stewart R. Mott, and Bill Peck.

Ellen Peck
Judith Senderowitz

Contents

Pronatalism

Introduction

As electronic monitoring, hidden persuaders, and other invisible devices of the modern age confront us, we realize that what we don't see and don't know *can* hurt us, more than a recognized enemy.

Pronatalism falls within this category of invisible devices. It exists. It affects the lives of all of us. But practically nobody knows it's there. In fact, the word itself has only recently received attention, although it refers to ancient beliefs and practices.

We are here attempting to add that word—*pronatalism*—to the general vocabulary, so that its implications may be recognized, understood, and acted upon.

Pronatalism is not a comfortable word. Like several other isms with which it might be compared, pronatalism connotes inequalities, biases, and discriminations within a rigid social value system. And full comprehension of its pervasiveness in our thought, actions, and institutions will not be painless.

Perceiving the extent of racism in our society was not an easy knowledge to assume. Those who first maintained that we were a sexist society were similarly met with disbelief, skepticism, hostility. Suggesting that we are a pronatalist society is perhaps the most sensitive task of all, since reproduction in all cultures has been accepted as central to identity, immortality, or survival. In challenging pronatalism, we challenge as well central concepts of myth and folklore, custom and belief, along with formal institutions —and must directly confront what might be termed the "reproductive ethic."

Simply and literally, pronatalism refers to any attitude or policy that is "pro-birth," that encourages reproduction, that exalts the role of parenthood.

A key element in pronatalist thought is the age-old idea that woman's role must involve maternity—that woman's destiny and fulfillment are closely wedded to the *natal,* or birth, experience.

At its extreme, such thinking results in a view of woman as essentially a reproducing machine. One physician, in fact, has publicly suggested that woman be thought of as "a uterus surrounded by a supporting organism and a directing personality"—thus succintly providing a pronatalist definition of the female of the human species: *woman as womb*.

Pronatalism has previously been used mainly by demographers, with reference to policies that affect national or world population trends. We are employing it here in a new context, and considering its implications for the lives of individuals. This is not intended to slight the significance of over-all population growth; indeed the fact of overpopulation reinforces the need to examine the nature of pronatalism at this time.

Pronatalism is dangerous because it denies or at the least limits free choice to individuals: there usually cannot be free choice in a prejudiced cultural context.

Pronatalist prejudice, or bias, exists at all stages of life.

Little girls who are encouraged to play with dolls—to play *at* motherhood—are already experiencing pronatalist conditioning, particularly if their choice of available playthings is otherwise limited. (We are *not* suggesting that young female children be denied dolls—only that they be given, perhaps, toy violins, building blocks, and doctors' kits with equal emphasis. Even then, the attitude accompanying the various playthings is important. Author Anna Silverman has noted, for example, that mothers enter more eagerly into daughter's play if the play object is a doll rather than a truck.)

"*When* you grow up and have children of your own . . ." is a litany repeated throughout childhood, creating an early impression of the inevitability of parenthood.

Reinforcing this are children's reading texts, which present women mainly in nurturing roles—mother, nurse, school-crossing guard (or, in a feminist-approved text, as *Mommies at Work*).

Later, in high school and college texts, the pronatalist orientation continues: here, in most cases, homage is paid to theories of maternal instinct; the inevitability of marriage and/or parenthood is assumed; the growing trend toward single and childfree lifestyles is unmentioned; and even statistical data in secondary sources are sometimes misrepresented so as to support pronatalist assumptions.

Meanwhile, from the Madonna theme in art to the covers of popular women's magazines, young women growing up are presented with idealized visual images of maternity.

If a young woman goes to a family-planning clinic, she'll find brochures in the reception room that say *"when"* not *"if"* in referring to childbearing.

The single woman is urged to marry; the married woman is urged to have children. The anxious in-laws, the would-be grandparents, must be faced—as must many other "pressures to bear." An employer may ask a wife when she plans to start her family—or use her assumed parental predisposition as an excuse not to advance her beyond the typing pool. "We can't train you for management; soon you'll want to quit and have children, and we can't waste the training" is a sexist rationale which is apt to have a pronatalist result. Kept from a challenging job because of her sex, a young woman is apt to deem childbearing and -rearing more creative than typing—and have a child. Would her choice have been the same if the available options had been different?

Men experience pronatalist pressures as well. In large corporations, men without children face a subtle handicap of not having the right executive "image" as a family man: an account manager or staff assistant who talks about Little League games and has pictures of his children on his desk is regarded benevolently, considered a "stable guy." Men without children must cope with senseless wisecracks about their virility, or lack of it. And in the Army, pronatalist pressures on adult males are codified in the *Officer's Guide,* which specifically instructs what gifts and rewards are to be given to officers of various ranks on the birth of children to them.

The pressure on men to produce *sons* crosses all social strata, from the poverty-stricken minority male to the wealthy scion who is expected to provide a son to inherit the fortune, carry on the family name.

Many group-insurance plans carry a pronatalist presumption. Maternity benefits are a required component of medical policies even though this benefit presumably covers a choice not exercised by all who share in the payments. At the same time, termination of pregnancy is often not covered; thus economic discrimination persists in favor of those who will bear children. Group-insurance plans also tend to favor producers of large families. It is not unheard of for group plans to assess families of two members and twelve members *identical payments* for health or life policies (though the larger family will cost the insurance company more in terms of benefits).

Our tax laws are pronatalist: the $750 deduction allowed to parents for each dependent child means, in effect, that those without children must pay a premium every year for the privilege of not reproducing. Though it might well be argued that tax deductions for progeny have little real power as incentives for parenthood, the symbolic message is important enough and may be interpreted as "approval" for parenthood, there being no comparable benefits for those without children.

At social gatherings, it's acceptable to ask a childfree man or woman, "Why don't you have children?" But it would be considered rude—indeed unthinkable—to ask a parent, "Why *did* you have a child?"

Multiply these small social and economic harassments and discriminations by the many occasions on which they occur, and the result is a powerful social force indeed: the social force we call pronatalism.

Pronatalism is not always so easily defined or exemplified, however. It exists as an undercurrent to the mainstream of the way of life we know as "the American way": the way of motherhood and the family; the nostalgia of Norman Rockwell and the homeyness of apple pie.

This idealized way of life, which was fading even as Norman Rockwell depicted it, seems almost a myth in today's world in which crisis, alienation, and distrust have become bywords. Yet it retains a certain power: the power of any illusion to outlive the forces that created it, the power of any myth to evoke sentiment as a defense against reasoned critique or objective examination.

In the oft-repeated phrase "as American as apple pie," apple pie has become a code reference to an illusion—an illusion of the romance and rightness of all our past traditions. Reactions to such words as *motherhood* and *apple pie* are not intellectual responses to what is denoted, but emotional yearnings for what the words have come to symbolize: America as we were told it was; life as we wish it were.

Thus, criticism of any part of the traditional pattern faces emotional resistance. One is not supposed to question religion or patriotism, for example: it is difficult even to suggest a difference between rational patriotic feeling and that sort expressed by such phrases as "My country right or wrong." Patriotism is protected by the myth.

So also, one is not supposed to question motherhood or traditional sex-role divisions, both of which protect the sanctity of our most revered institution—the family. (One may be regarded suspiciously even when presenting objective evidence of familial dissatisfactions. Here again, the myth proves protective—the illusion of family life is cherished even as the reality presents malaise to many.)

The high cultural esteem in which the family is held is surely evidenced by the wealth of ceremony which accompanies the initiation of a formal family unit. Premarital rites, such as teen-age customs of going steady and exchanging rings, are socially approved "dress rehearsals" for future engagements. China, silver, diamond rings, and hope chests are lures that encourage young women to yearn toward the gala showers and parties associated with betrothal and marriage. Final touches include the bachelor dinner for him; the starring role in the long walk down the aisle for her; the champagne reception and the tossing of the bouquet; community recognition through the newspaper wedding photographs. (For the single adults of our society, there are no such ceremonies.) The ceremonies signify social expectations: one is expected to marry.

One is expected not only to marry, but also to follow certain other guidelines afterward. A steady job is a prerequisite to social respect; material acquisitions are an announcement of normality, as are certain lifestyle hallmarks: the station wagon and the house in the suburbs, the two-week vacation in the camper with the children, membership in the PTA, and token appearances at church on Christmas and Easter, and more. All are "as American as apple pie."

To be considered a *true* family, a married couple must have children. Again, were one to examine ceremonies, one would find those surrounding childbearing numerous indeed; and here too these ceremonies provide an index to social expectation and valuation.

A final notable aspect of traditional American life is the character of expected loyalties. Though one is encouraged to care about the well-being of the community and nation, highest loyalties are supposed to be given to those of one's "own" family unit—and particularly to one's children. Though writers of various persuasions have criticized the insularity of this value system (labeling the family a "greedy institution that consumes its members" or "peculiarly chauvinistic"), it remains true that the man who is seen as a "good family man" or a "good provider" for his children can expect to be excused from a good many faults of character in other areas.

All these values and lifestyle guidelines serve pronatalism.

(For example, concern for the proper financial support and the right religious upbringing for children provides at least one rationale for the "work hard and get ahead" syndrome, the "pray together and stay together" ethic.)

But these guidelines do more than function as adjuncts to pronatalism: like pronatalism itself, they also serve as aids to maintain a society that is constant and predictable; stable and well-ordered; and above all, manageable.

Conformity of life-style facilitates manageability; nonconformity threatens it. Were many self-determined citizens to replace well-conditioned ones, the effects on social order might be considerable. Particularly, were many individuals to become freed from pronatalist conditioning, a greater degree of citizen independence might result. (It is in fact possible to wonder whether a historical treatment of pronatalism might disclose childbearing to have been especially encouraged, in some instances, by governments intent on citizen control; simply put, having children *can* "disarm" an individual.)

In the future, perhaps the myriad social energies now applied to encourage a conforming way of life can be devoted instead to a search for ways to make social stability compatible with life-style diversity. For, as controlling influences on our lives such as pronatalism are increasingly recognized and challenged, their power to enforce conformity will surely lessen.

Our present work is a collection of writings intended to explicate both hidden and overt pronatalist influences and to present issues that must be widely recognized, and more fully researched, if our pronatalist social orientation is to change.

Selections were made with the assumption that at least four prominent issues which relate to our central theme have begun to emerge. These issues include:

1. *The existence of pronatalism per se.* Our first selections consider what this force is, how it works, and the various guises in which it appears.

2. *The increasing recognition that motives for parenthood are individual, not universal.* The fact that experts have now begun to examine and analyze *individual* dynamics of reproduction weakens such pronatalist presumptions as "reproduction is natural and instinctive" or "children must inevitably be part of life."

3. *The effects that parenthood can have on personality and identity.* The past strength of pronatalism has meant that negative life changes which can result from parenthood have not been given attention. Our presentation of selections which highlight problems

that parenthood can bring is an attempt to counterbalance a biased cultural perception of the meaning of childbearing.

4. *The emergence of a "child-free by choice" alternative life-style.* The emergence of a small vanguard of child-free individuals (about 4 percent of adults now are without children by choice) is a direct affront to pronatalist sentiment; thus childfree men and women who proclaim themselves so by intention often serve as a "lightning rod" for concentrated and direct personal criticism. An examination of the childfree alternative is therefore relevant to an understanding of the strength of pronatalism.

An important factor regarding our selections must be noted: the field we deal with here is quite new. Whereas many editors of anthologies are able judiciously to review and select those articles and papers most precisely relevant to their purpose, we, in some instances, had no such luxury: we are often in the position of presenting the *only* writings available on a specific aspect within our scope of inquiry.

This in no way reflects ill on our selections, which we feel are excellent and which we present with no small degree of pride. It *does* mean that the style, length, approach, and perspective of our selections vary a good deal—from the highly personal to the highly academic, from general overviews to extremely specific "close-ups" of subjects.

Again, this is because recognition of pronatalism as a controlling social force has barely begun. In fact, the vocabulary of the field has not yet become standardized: in these selections, for example, *childless* alternates with the newer term *childfree; pronatal, pro-natalist,* and *pronatalist* variously appear as the adjectival form of pronatalism; and one researcher employs *pronatality* rather than *pronatalism.* For the time being, we have made no effort to standardize these variations in terminology. The important thing, to us, is that significant research and writings available at this time be presented, as a beginning and as a call for *further* research into vital questions of pronatalism and society.

It is undoubtedly more than coincidental that the social dimensions of pronatalism have come to initial scrutiny at a time when continued population growth clearly courts disaster. It may be that when investigators became aware of population's impact on social systems and ecosystems, more than a few of them began to ask *why* the universality of childbearing prevailed. The search for answers to that question *Why?* may have brought about initial perceptions of pronatalism.

We personally are not writing here, however, from our roles as proponents of population stabilization. Here our concern for the personal, rather than the planetary, dangers of pronatalism predominates.

We write, first of all, as two women who have violated a social norm by remaining without children beyond our thirtieth year. As individuals, we are no strangers to pronatalist pressures.

We write, also, in recognition of the fact that it is not *only* the childfree who are harmed by pronatalism. Child or adult, man or woman, parent or nonparent—we are all affected. Parents have often been denied free choice in their childbearing decisions, due to lack of contraception or subtle social coercions; child-free men and women must make their choice against great social odds and face lack of understanding which threatens their contentment; children growing up today are still exposed, as their parents were, to the various forms that social pronatalist conditioning can take.

We write especially out of concern for these children growing up now and for the children of tomorrow (who are, in a sense, the children of all of us). We do not say this to establish our credentials as women who care about children; nor to reassure those who may be nervous about the ideas we are presenting; but because the statement is deeply felt and true.

It is both a social statement, and one made with an ecological concern. Pronatalist pressures compromise opportunities for individual freedom of reproductive choice. They also serve as prime aggravators of population problems. Thus, if pronatalist pressures are not abated, the future of children is doubly jeopardized.

We write, finally, as feminists—with the view that pronatalism, as that part of sexism not yet confronted, poses a threat to true self-determination for women.

Feminism has developed as a movement with the goal of removing past restraints on women's roles, image, and identity. The drive for full equality for women, however, has not emphasized pronatalist constraints. (Several writers within this volume speak somewhat critically on this point.) Yet there are reasons why the women's movement has not challenged the childbearing role aggressively. Feminism's concerns must of necessity be directed to the realities that exist today, and today it is the norm for virtually all women to have or to expect to have children.

To meet present needs, feminists must attempt to liberate the mother from usual nurturing chores and to allow the rearing of children *along with* a career.

But a probable forthcoming feminist development will be an increased emphasis on freedom to choose *not* to bear children, along with a continuing interest in facilities for caring for children already born. The newer generation of feminists, who have not yet become mothers, are most fully aware of increased opportunities in the world outside the home—the world of business, science, and the arts. Most will probably still combine motherhood with an outside career of some sort. And some, as always, will find their careers *in* motherhood. But tomorrow's feminists will increasingly include those who desire to devote themselves exclusively to interests outside the domestic sphere, and who will choose not to have children. Even today the trend is beginning. The women who are beginning the trend are those who now sense pronatalist pressures.

In the introduction to her anthology of feminist writings, *Sisterhood Is Powerful,* Robin Morgan wrote, "This book is an action." And, indeed, more than the personalities or statements, more than the social theories rejected and new abstracts advanced, her book reflected the high energy and impressive organization of women which had resulted from the *action* of the contemporary feminist movement over a few short years.

In preparing this work, we foresee a similar "action" and movement, which now seems to be taking shape.

But if, indeed, there is to be a new dimension to feminism (or a new movement of women—and men) which rises up to question the centrality of childbearing to the experience of all of us—this movement has not yet fully coalesced around certain writings presented here. Though such a movement seems to be forming, the area of concern which prompts us to present this anthology is still uncharted, its vocabulary and concepts not well known, its spokespersons somewhat isolated from one another.

This work is, therefore, an introduction, a beginning. The collected writings which follow harbor several innovative suggestions:

That parenthood is neither an inevitability, nor a universally desirable condition nor a prerequisite to a full life—but a vocation for which only some of us are suited, by aptitude or choice

That serious biases exist at all levels of society against those who choose not to become parents

That there is a strong and heretofore unquestioned social force which has produced both the universal-parenthood ideal and its attendant discriminations. This social force is called pronatalism.

PART I

Pronatalism

> The drudgery, the monotonous labor, and other disagreeable features of child-rearing are minimized by the "social guardians." On the other hand, the joys and compensations of motherhood are magnified and presented to consciousness at every hand. . . .

> Yes, having a baby did upset our lives. But Lisa has also enriched them beyond anything I could have imagined. . . .

The first quotation above was written by early feminist Leta S. Hollingworth in 1916. The second is from the October 1973 issue of *Good Housekeeping* magazine. Are the "social guardians" whom Leta Hollingworth mentioned still around?

> Not only have the "social guardians" used education as a negative means of control, by failing to provide any real enlightenment for women, but education has been made a positive instrument for control. This was accomplished by drilling into the young and unformed mind, while it was yet too immature to reason independently, such facts and notions as would give a girl a conception of herself only as future wife and mother. . . .

> The job of parenthood is, in a sense, the most responsible job a person ever accepts. . . . The mother's role usually includes the major responsibility for the smooth running of the household, whether or not she works outside the home. . . . Many women find fulfillment in working roles as well as in their roles as wives and mothers. . . .

Again, the first quotation is from Leta Hollingworth. The second is from a modern textbook, *Teen Guide to Homemaking* (McGraw-Hill, 1972). Are our "social guardians" still intent on protecting woman's role as wife-and-mother, even if they must now acknowledge the possibility of an outside role as well? And—who *are* the social guardians to whom Hollingworth alludes?

Leta S. Hollingworth wished to see women's social roles expanded, and argued fervently for this development. Her physician-husband, Harry Hollingworth, supported her desire to attend medical school, and she became a leading clinical psychologist. The couple had no children.

As a woman without children, Leta Hollingworth became keenly sensitive to social influences that attempted to shape women for motherhood and for that role alone. When she wrote "Social Devices for Impelling Women to Bear and Rear Children" in 1916, she was, perhaps for the first time, explaining what pronatalism is. (Her title, in fact, might constitute a definition.) Further, she postulated that pronatalism was enforced by "social guardians": these included highly regarded social thinkers, men of medicine and law, teachers, ministers, and politicians—in short, the most influential and powerful members of our basic social and cultural institutions.

Hollingworth explains society's long-standing need to encourage childbearing as "necessary for tribal or national existence." Historically, high fertility was required to aid chances for survival; once survival was assured, high fertility continued to be favored by governments interested in militarism and aggrandizement. (Governments too, Hollingworth implies, were "social guardians" of fertility.) But insistence on childbearing meant sacrifices, suffering, and sometimes death for those who gave birth. Thus, Hollingworth explains, it was necessary to institute social devices which encouraged the bearing of children, which brought pressure on women from as many sources as possible: among these sources were public opinion, law, education, custom, and art, and the tendency to value women on the basis of their fulfilling the maternal role.

Mentioned by Hollingworth are a "fervid insistence on maternal instinct"; an idealization of maternity in art, song, and poetry; and selective education for women. These and other controlling factors created a *personal ideal* (a *maternal* ideal) of the "womanly woman" to which all women were expected to conform. Just as strong as the ideals were the taboos—unalluring aspects of maternity were proscribed as topics of conversation or public attention.

The aim of the "social guardians" was to protect the formation of families and to assure population growth. (Hollingworth mentions two objections to nineteenth-century feminism: "The family will decay," and, "The birth rate will fall.")

The emphasis on high fertility, virtually unquestioned in Hollingworth's time, has now reversed itself. The danger has clearly become over—not under—population.

The population movement has changed our notion that universal reproduction is a *need* of nations. And to some extent the feminist movement has broken the old taboos and disclosed disagreeable features of motherhood. Yet have the "social controls" impelling women to bear children changed so very much since Leta Hollingworth described them? Perhaps the social controls went so deep that they became indistinguishable elements within the entire system of social customs and belief—and are only now, as Hollingworth had hoped, being "raised to consciousness."

Since Hollingworth's time, the expectation that all women should bear children has lessened only somewhat; today, for example, it is praiseworthy for a woman to want to limit her family.

Certain social controls have abated (laws against birth control, for example) but others—such as the idealization of maternity—have strengthened with the development of the mass media. The net result is pretty much the same.

At the end of her paper, Leta Hollingworth forecasts, "The time is coming, and is indeed almost at hand, when all the most intelligent women of the community . . . will become conscious of the methods of social control." Now, decades later, this prediction may finally be coming true: though the available literature on pronatalist social controls is presently meager, selections presented here show that the problem is no longer totally unrecognized.

In the opinion of demographer and author Judith Blake, who reviewed present-day pronatalist influences for the Commission on Population Growth and the American Future, these influences (or controls) are sufficiently strong to merit her title "Coercive Pronatalism. . . ."

Coercion obviously limits choice. Thus, Blake claims, voluntarism as a family-planning policy cannot exist until coercive pronatalism ceases. When she speaks of the desirability of "anti-natalist" policies, she is concerned not only with general overpopulation problems but especially with the need to establish individuals' rights to reproductive freedom. But she sees instituting this missing half of social normative influences (i.e., antinatalist forces to counter existing pronatalist ones) as an undesirable means to a wider spectrum of choice for each person: a better approach would be to remove existing pronatalist constraints.

Far from threatening freedom of reproductive decision, Blake states firmly that eliminating or countering pronatalism would mean true reproductive voluntarism (which, she stresses, *does not exist at this time*).

Blake underscores the significance of pronatalism as part of the sexist tradition that has kept women from attaining equal opportunity in the job market. In her view, the opposition to women working grew out of a concern not only for the diminution of male supremacy, but concern as well that this threatened family formation.

Challenges to pronatalism, in careers and other fields, would seem a logical evolution of feminist action—and can be expected, perhaps, to obviate what Blake perceives as pronatalism even *within* the women's movement.

Blake's overview of pronatalism provides useful background for the several more specialized discussions that follow, the first of which is written by Helen H. Franzwa, Ph.D., of the Communications Department at Hunter College, City University of New York.

In "Pronatalism in Women's Magazine Fiction," Franzwa turns to an exploration of pro-motherhood influences found in short-story themes created for a wide audience of women.

Results of a content analysis of 122 stories appearing in popular women's magazines during the years 1940 to 1970 provide support for Franzwa's contention that fiction in these periodicals is pronatalist—in fact, strongly so.

The themes of these stories, she explains, as well as the number of children portrayed per family, serve to communicate pronatalist ideals and attitudes. Typical themes she notes include "The Housewife-Mother Career Is Best of All" and "To Solve Your Problems Have Another Baby."

The possibility that pronatalist themes in fiction affect readers' attitudes is explored insofar as available data to test such influences permits. Though only anecdotal information bears directly on readers' psychological response to the women's magazines studied, Franzwa introduces scholarly opinions which hold that recipients of *similar* media influences (confession magazines and soap operas) do indeed find these media situations "believable and real." Thus it seems likely that some readers of women's magazines will, similarly, regard their fictional fertile sisters as role models to be copied in real behavior.

A related possibility is that pronatalist stories help gloss over any conflict a reader might feel if she has already chosen the role of mother.

In describing pronatalist television programming and commercial content, Ellen Peck was speaking directly to those who prepare such images: members of the National Academy of Television Arts and Sciences. But her examples of the "Romance with Reproduction" carried on by our most powerful medium provide scenes which should be familiar to almost anyone who has ever tuned to a typical daytime drama or game show.

The blatant nature of pronatalist messages is conveyed in a mood at once amused and indignant. The hysterical desire to experience childbirth, the use of pregnancy as a competitive device between wife and mistress ("whoever conceives, wins"), the seeming need to have children by the right man, the wrong man, any man, or even as a result of rape—all these pronatalist plot lines would indeed be amusing did not the ominous possibility exist that they are taken seriously by many!

Though this report concentrates mainly on daytime dramas, the author also notes a preoccupation with reproduction on game and talk shows—viewing the predictable audience applause which follows a game show guest's statement "I have seven children . . ." as a conditioned response, almost Pavlovian in nature.

The many pregnancies and childbirths which form the dramatic focus for TV shows are seen as palliatives, substitutes for active and self-determined roles for women—and worse, as role models for millions of women viewing at home, taking time off from their routine chores to gain a bit of vicarious excitement. Conceiving a child, these viewers are told, can serve to attract the attention of men, distract one from unresolved conflicts, or at least fill an otherwise empty life.

Pregnancy and maternity, when used as product sales tools in commercials, serve to "sell" pregnancy along with the product —and more deeply to reinforce reproductive illusions by the necessarily simple thirty-second blast.

One might expect the motherhood message to be more responsibly presented in schools. Yet a strong pronatalist orientation was found in a study of the eighteen home economics texts used in a typical, suburban junior high school.

Nancy Cox, Commissioner on the Status of Women for the State of Maryland, begins her paper "Pronatalism in Home Economics Texts in a Junior High School" with a statement of her own personal feminist orientation and her reasons for choosing this particular group of texts for a pilot study.

Although the women's movement has placed a high priority on the analysis of textbooks, Cox notes that this traditional bastion of sex-role distinction has nevertheless been neglected because the "solution" to bias in home ec was to insist that girls be given a chance to take shop!

She notes, however, that for the next few years, many girls

will continue to enroll in a home ec course, whether the course is required or elective. (And even when a better balance is achieved in these previously sex-segregated courses, will the same pronatalist acculturization be present?) With such thoughts in mind, Cox is unwilling to dismiss this area of study as unimportant.

A quality commonly found in the books examined was a certain rosy optimism regarding traditional marriage-and-family ("apple pie") values. Appealing photographs combined with "most marriages are happy" messages offer an easy recipe for future life.

And it must be remembered that in many school systems home ec courses are unaccompanied by any course content in sex education or birth control. *This situation in itself* lends a pro-birth influence to the education of many adolescents. In no text cited by Cox was mention given to the well-documented dangers of teen-age childbearing for both the child and the mother; instead, several times, implicit encouragements of youthful childbearing were found!

Thus this specialized branch of education offers (a) glorification of a family life "ideal" for women, and (b) concealment of risks involved when very young women bear children. It is perhaps worth referring once more to Leta Hollingworth, who pointed out the existence of such "glorification" and such "concealment" more than half a century ago.

It might seem surprising that social scientists could be conveyors of pronatalist bias. Yet Robert Chester, a professor in the Department of Social Administration at the University of Hull, points out in "Is There a Relationship Between Childlessness and Marriage Breakdown?" that studies seeking a correlation between the two actually start out with the *assumption* that divorces are more common among childfree couples. He points to typical errors in studies of this subject, such as neglecting to take into account duration of marriage or cohabitation and failing to control for remarriage (where the incidence of progency would be less).

Though Chester is a British author, it is fair to assume that comparable biases exist on this side of the Atlantic. A disquieting example is presented by a noted authority on studies of family life, Edward W. Pohlman of the University of the Pacific, in "Burgess and Cottrell Data on 'Desire for Children': An Example of Distortion in Marriage and Family Textbooks?"

A study by researchers Burgess and Cottrell in 1939 concerned "desire for children" and "marital adjustment." The Burgess-Cottrell data per se was insufficient to suggest a positive correlation between these two factors. Yet Pohlman demonstrates that the data have been *incorrectly presented* over the years by marriage and family textbooks so as to imply, *"Procreate for a happy marriage."*

This "distortion" may simply be due to lack of academic scrupulousness in handling research. It is also possible that the misinterpretations result from a generalized pronatalist bias on the part of marriage and family textbook writers. (An author cited by Pohlman, in fact, suggests that this could be the case.)

Pohlman's report here must raise a serious question: *How many other studies have been similarly mishandled, in how many other textbooks?*

It indeed seems possible that pronatalism has a hold even in academia. We feel the need for more investigation in this area to be critical.

Our final selection should serve to discredit any idea that pronatalism is a mere academic abstraction, suitable for discussion at seminars but without much relevance to average American citizens—for this selection reaches into what may be the most quintessentially "American" of all our institutions: the Army.

The Armed Forces might be seen as a repository for many traditional values: adherence to authority, capacity for leadership, bravery and aggressiveness, idealism and loyalty. American virtues such as hard work and discipline predominate here within a framework that is perhaps more rigidly authoritative than that of any other American institution. The army does not merely admire such virtues—it *requires* them.

Pronatalism can perhaps be seen in clear focus here—for the Army has codified it. In civilian society gifts and congratulations to new parents are customary; in the Army, they are explicitly prescribed by *The Officers' Guide.*

Society at large gives parents token economic benefits (tax breaks, motel "family plans"), but the Army magnifies the benefits allowed to parents to the point where a clearly definable disparity is created. The author of "Pronatalism in the Army" interprets this disparity as discrimination—discrimination against those Army personnel who do not have children—and considers subtler, psychological discriminations which exist as well.

The author of "Pronatalism in the Army" is a career officer stationed in the West who has been married eight years and has no children by choice. He has requested that this piece be published anonymously.

1

Social Devices for Impelling Women to Bear and Rear Children

LETA S. HOLLINGWORTH

Early feminist and clinical psychologist

> Again, the breeding function of the family would be better discharged if public opinion and religion conspired, as they have until recently, to crush the aspirations of woman for a life of her own. But the gain would not be worth the price.—E. A. Ross, *Social Control* (1904).

In this quotation from Ross we have suggested to us an exceedingly important and interesting phase of social control, namely, the control by those in social power over those individuals who alone can bring forth the human young, and thus perpetuate society. It is necessary that at the very outset of this discussion we should consent to clear our minds of the sentimental conception of motherhood and to look at facts. W. G. Sumner [*Folkways,* 1906] states these facts as well as they have ever been stated, in his consideration of the natural burdens of society. He says:

> Children add to the weight of the struggle for existence of their parents. The relation of parent to child is one of sacrifice. The interests of parents and children are antagonistic. The fact that there are or may be compensations does not affect the primary relation between the two. It may well be believed that, if procreation had not been put under the dominion of a great passion, it would have been caused to cease by the burdens it entails.

This is especially true in the case of the mothers.

The fact is that child-bearing is in many respects analogous to the work of soldiers: it is necessary for tribal or national exis-

From *The American Journal of Sociology,* 1916

tence; it means great sacrifice of personal advantage; it involves danger and suffering, and, in a certain percentage of cases, the actual loss of life. Thus we should expect that there would be a continuous social effort to insure the group-interest in respect to population, just as there is a continuous social effort to insure the defense of the nation in time of war. It is clear, indeed, that the social devices employed to get children born, and to get soldiers slain, are in many respects similar.

But once the young are brought into the world they still must be reared, if society's ends are to be served, and here again the need for and exercise of social control may be seen. Since the period of helpless infancy is very prolonged in the human species, and since the care of infants is an onerous and exacting labor, it would be natural for all persons not biologically attached to infants to use all possible devices for fastening the whole burden of infant-tending upon those who are so attached. We should expect this to happen, and we shall see, in fact, that there has been consistent social effort to establish as a norm the woman whose vocational proclivities are completely and "naturally" satisfied by child-bearing and child-rearing, with the related domestic activities.

There is, to be sure, a strong and fervid insistence on the "maternal instinct," which is popularly supposed to characterize all women equally, and to furnish them with an all-consuming desire for parenthood, regardless of the personal pain, sacrifice, and disadvantage involved. In the absence of all verifiable data, however, it is only common-sense to guard against accepting as a fact of human nature a doctrine which we might well expect to find in use as a means of social control. Since we possess no scientific data at all on this phase of human psychology, the most reasonable assumption is that if it were possible to obtain a quantitative measurement of maternal instinct, we should find this trait distributed among women, just as we have found all other traits distributed which have yielded to quantitative measurement. It is most reasonable to assume that we should obtain a curve of distribution, varying from an extreme where individuals have a zero or negative interest in caring for infants, through a mode where there is a moderate amount of impulse to such duties, to an extreme where the only vocational or personal interest lies in maternal activities.

The facts, shorn of sentiment, then, are: (1) The bearing and rearing of children is necessary for tribal or national existence and aggrandizement. (2) The bearing and rearing of children is painful, dangerous to life, and involves long years of exacting labor and self-sacrifice. (3) There is no verifiable evidence to show that a maternal instinct exists in women of such all-consuming strength and fervor as to impel them voluntarily to seek the pain, danger, and exacting labor involved in maintaining a high birth rate.

We should expect, therefore, that those in control of society would invent and employ devices for impelling women to maintain a birth rate sufficient to insure enough increase in the population to offset the wastage of war and disease. It is the purpose of this paper to cite specific illustrations to show just how the various social institutions have been brought to bear on women to this end. Ross has classified the means which society takes and has taken to secure order, and insure that individuals will act in such a way as to promote the interests of the group, *as those interests are conceived by those who form "the radiant points of social control."* These means, according to the analysis of Ross, are public opinion, law, belief, social suggestion, education, custom, social religion, personal ideals (the type), art, personality, enlightenment, illusion, and social valuation. Let us see how some of these means have been applied in the control of women.

Personal ideals (the type).—The first means of control to which I wish to call attention in the present connection is that which Ross calls "personal ideals." It is pointed out that "a developed society presents itself as a system of unlike individuals, strenuously pursuing their personal ends." Now, for each person there is a "certain zone of requirement," and since "altruism is quite incompetent to hold each unswervingly to the particular activities and forbearances belonging to his place in the social system," the development of such allegiance must be—

> effected by means of types or patterns, which society induces its members to adopt as their guiding ideals. . . . To this end are elaborated various patterns of conduct and of character, which may be termed social types. These types may become in the course of time personal ideals, each for that category of persons for which it is intended.

For women, obviously enough, the first and most primitive "zone of requirement" is and has been to produce and rear families large enough to admit of national warfare being carried on, and of colonization.

Thus has been evolved the social type of the "womanly woman," "the normal woman," the chief criterion of normality being a willingness to engage enthusiastically in maternal and allied activities. All those classes and professions which form "the radiant points of social control" unite upon this criterion. Men of science announce it with calm assurance (though failing to say on what kind or amount of scientific data they base their remarks). For instance, W. McDougall [*Social Psychology,* 1908] writes:

> The highest stage is reached by those species in which each female produces at birth but one or two young, and protects them so efficiently that most of the young born reach maturity; the maintenance of the species thus becomes in the main the work of the parental instinct. In such species the protection and cherishing of the young is the constant and all-absorbing occupation of the mother, to which she devotes all her energies, and in the course of which she will at any time undergo privation, pain, and death. The instinct (maternal instinct) becomes more powerful than any other, and can override any other, even fear itself.

Professor J. Jastrow [*Character and Temperament,* 1915] writes:

> . . . *charm* is the technique of the maiden, and *sacrifice* the passion of the mother. One set of feminine interests expresses more distinctly the issues of courtship and attraction; the other of qualities of motherhood and devotion.

The medical profession insistently proclaims desire for numerous children as the criterion of normality for women, scornfully branding those so ill-advised as to deny such desires as "abnormal." As one example among thousands of such attempts at social control let me quote the following, which appeared in a New York newspaper on November 29, 1915:

> Only abnormal women want no babies. Trenchant criticism of modern life was made by Dr. Max G. Schlapp, internationally known as a neurologist. Dr. Schlapp addressed his remarks to the congregation of the Park Avenue M.E. Church. He said, "The birth rate is falling off. Rich people are the ones who have no children, and the poor have the greatest number of offspring. Any woman who does not desire offspring is abnormal. We have a large number, particularly among the women, who do not want children. Our social society is becoming intensely unstable."

And this from *The New York Times,* September 5, 1915:

> Normally woman lives through her children; man lives through his work.

Scores of such implicit attempts to determine and present the type or norm meet us on every hand. This norm has the sanction of authority, being announced by men of greatest prestige in the community. No one wishes to be regarded by her fellow-creatures as "abnormal" or "decayed." The stream of suggestions playing from all points inevitably has its influence, so that it is or was, until recently, well-nigh impossible to find a married woman who would admit any conflicting interests equal or paramount to the interest of caring for children. There is a universal refusal to admit that the maternal instinct, like every other trait of human nature, might be distributed according to the probability curve.

Public opinion.—Let us turn next to public opinion as a means of control over women in relation to the birth rate. In speaking of public opinion Ross says:

> Haman is at the mercy of Mordecai. Rarely can one regard his deed as fair when others find it foul, or count himself a hero when the world deems him a wretch. . . . For the mass of men the blame and the praise of the community are the very lords of life.

If we inquire now what are the organs or media of expression of public opinion we shall see how it is brought to bear on women. The newspapers are perhaps the chief agents, in modern times, in the formation of public opinion, and their columns abound in interviews with the eminent, deploring the decay of the population. Magazines print articles based on statistics of depopulation, appealing to the patriotism of women. In the year just passed fifty-five articles on the birth rate have chanced to come to the notice of the present writer. Fifty-four were written by men, including editors, statesmen, educators, ex-presidents, etc. Only one was written by a woman. The following quotation is illustrative of the trend of all of them:

> M. Emil Reymond has made this melancholy announcement in the Senate: "We are living in an age when women have pronounced upon themselves a judgment that is dangerous in the highest degree to the development of the population. . . . We have the right to do what we will with the life that is in us, say they."

Thus the desire for the development of interests and aptitudes other than the maternal is stigmatized as "dangerous," "melancholy," "degrading," "abnormal," "indicative of decay." On the other hand, excessive maternity receives many cheap but effective rewards. For example, the Jesuit priests hold special meetings to laud maternity. The German Kaiser announces that he will now be godfather to seventh, eighth, and ninth sons, even if daughters intervene. The ex-President has written a letter of congratulation to the mother of nine.

Law.—Since its beginning as a human institution law has been a powerful instrument for the control of women. The subjection of women was originally an irrational consequence of sex differences in reproductive function. It was not *intended* by either men or women, but simply resulted from the natural physiological handicaps of women, and the attempts of humanity to adapt itself to physiological nature through the crude methods of trial and error. When law was formulated, this subjection was defined, and thus furthered. It would take too long to cite all the legal provisions that contribute, indirectly, to keep women from developing individualistic interests and capacities. Among the most important indirect forces in law which affect women to keep them child-bearers and child-rearers only are those provisions that tend to restrain them from possessing and controlling property. Such provisions have made of women a comparatively possessionless class, and have thus deprived them of the fundamentals of power. While affirming the essential nature of woman to be satisfied with maternity and with maternal duties only, society has always taken every precaution to close the avenues to ways of escape therefrom.

Two legal provisions which bear directly on women to compel them to keep up the birth rate may be mentioned here. The first of these is the provision whereby sterility in the wife may be made a cause of divorce. This would be a powerful inducement to women who loved their husbands to bear children if they could. The second provision is that which forbids the communication of the data of science in the matter of the means of birth control. The American laws are very drastic on this point. Recently in New York City a man was sentenced to prison for violating this law. The more advanced democratic nations have ceased to practice military conscription. They no longer conscript their men to bear arms, depending on the volunteer army. But they conscript their women to bear children by legally prohibiting the publication or communication of the knowledge which would make child-bearing voluntary.

Child-rearing is also legally insured by those provisions which forbid and punish abortion, infanticide, and infant desertion. There could be no better proof of the insufficiency of maternal instinct as a guaranty of population than the drastic laws which we have against birth control, abortion, infanticide, and infant desertion.

Belief.—Belief, "which controls the hidden portions of life," has been used powerfully in the interests of population. Orthodox women, for example, regard family limitation as a sin, punishable in the hereafter. Few explicit exhortations concerning the birth rate are discoverable in the various "Words" of God. The belief that family limitation will be punished in the hereafter seems to have been evolved mainly by priests out of the slender materials of a few quotations from Holy Writ, such as "God said unto them, 'Multiply and replenish the earth,' " and from the scriptural allusion to children as the gifts of God. Being gifts from God, it follows that they may not be refused except at the peril of incurring God's displeasure.

Education.—The education of women has always, until the end of the nineteenth century, been limited to such matters as would become a creature who could and should have no aspirations for a life of her own. We find the proper education for girls outlined in the writings of such educators as Rousseau, Fénelon, St. Jerome, and in Godey's *Lady's Book.* Not only have the "social guardians" used education as a negative means of control, by failing to provide any real enlightenment for women, but education has been made a positive instrument for control. This was accomplished by drilling into the young and unformed mind, while yet it was too immature to reason independently, such facts and notions as would give the girl a conception of herself only as future wife and mother. Rousseau, for instance, demanded freedom and individual liberty of development for everybody except Sophia, who was to be deliberately trained up as a means to an end. In the latter half of the nineteenth century when the hard battle for the real enlightenment of women was being fought, one of the most frequently recurring objections to admitting women to knowledge was that "the population would suffer," "the essential nature of woman would be changed," "the family would decay," and "the birth rate would fall." Those in control of society yielded up the old prescribed education of women only after a stubborn struggle, realizing that with the passing of the old training an important means of social control was slipping out of their hands.

Art.—A very long paper might be written to describe the various uses to which art has been put in holding up the ideal of motherhood. The mother, with children at her breast, is the favorite theme of artists. The galleries of Europe are hung full of Madonnas of every age and degree. Poetry abounds in allusions to the sacredness and charm of motherhood, depicting the yearning of the adult for his mother's knee. Fiction is replete with happy and adoring mothers. Thousands of songs are written and sung concerning the ideal relation which exists between mother and child. In pursuing the mother-child theme through art one would not be led to suspect that society finds it necessary to make laws against contraception, infanticide, abortion, and infant desertion. Art holds up to view only the compensations of motherhood, leaving the other half of the theme in obscurity, and thus acting as a subtle ally of population.

Illusion.—This is the last of Ross's categories to which I wish to refer. Ross says:

> In the taming of men there must be provided coil after coil to entangle the unruly one. Mankind must use snares as well as leading-strings, will-o-the-wisps as well as lanterns. The truth by all means if it will promote obedience, but in any case obedience! We shall examine not creeds now, but the films, veils, hidden mirrors, and half lights by which men are duped as to that which lies nearest them, their own experience. This time we shall see men led captive, not by dogmas concerning a world beyond experience, but by artfully fostered misconceptions of the pains, satisfactions, and values lying under their very noses.

One of the most effective ways of creating the desired illusion about any matter is by concealing and tabooing the mention of all the painful and disagreeable circumstances connected with it. Thus there is a very stern social taboo on conversation about the processes of birth. The utmost care is taken to conceal the agonies and risks of child-birth from the young. Announcement is rarely made of the true cause of deaths from child-birth. The statistics of maternal mortality have been neglected by departments of health, and the few compilations which have been made have not achieved any wide publicity or popular discussion. Says Katherine Anthony, in her recent book on *Feminism in Germany and Scandinavia* (1915):

> There is no evidence that the death rate of women from child-birth has caused the governing classes many sleepless nights.

Anthony gives some statistics from Prussia (where the figures have been calculated), showing that

> between 1891 and 1900 11 percent of the deaths of all women between the ages of twenty-five and forty years occurred in child-birth. . . . During forty years of peace Germany lost 400,000 mothers' lives, that is, ten times what she lost in soldiers' lives in the campaign of 1870 and 1871.

Such facts would be of wide public interest, especially to women, yet there is no tendency at all to spread them broadcast or to make propaganda of them. Public attention is constantly being called to the statistics of infant mortality, but the statistics of maternal mortality are neglected and suppressed.

The pains, the dangers, and risks of child-bearing are tabooed as subjects of conversation. The drudgery, the monotonous labor, and other disagreeable features of child-rearing are minimized by "the social guardians." On the other hand, the joys and compensations of motherhood are magnified and presented to consciousness on every hand. Thus the tendency is to create an illusion whereby motherhood will appear to consist of compensations only, and thus come to be desired by those for whom the illusion is intended.

There is one further class of devices for controlling women that does not seem to fit any of the categories mentioned by Ross. I refer to threats of evil consequence to those who refrain from child-bearing. This class of social devices I shall call "bugaboos." Medical men have done much to help population (and at the same time to increase obstetrical practice!) by inventing bugaboos. For example, it is frequently stated by medical men, and is quite generally believed by women, that if first child-birth is delayed until the age of thirty years the pains and dangers of the process will be very gravely increased, and that therefore women will find it advantageous to begin bearing children early in life. It is added that the younger the woman begins to bear the less suffering will be experienced. One looks in vain, however, for any objective evidence that such is the case. The statements appear to be founded on no array of facts whatever, and until they are so founded, they lie under the suspicion of being merely devices for social control.

One also reads that women who bear children live longer on the average than those who do not, which is taken to mean that child-bearing has a favorable influence on longevity. It may well be that women who bear many children live longer than those who do not, but the only implication probably is that those women who could not endure the strain of repeated births died young, and thus naturally did not have many children. The facts may indeed be as above stated, and yet child-bearing may be distinctly prejudicial to longevity.

A third bugaboo is that if a child is reared alone, without brothers and sisters, he will grow up selfish, egoistic, and an undesirable citizen. Figures are, however, so far lacking to show the disastrous consequences of being an only child.

From these brief instances it seems very clear that "the social guardians" have not really believed that maternal instinct is alone a sufficient guaranty of population. They have made use of all possible social devices to insure not only child-bearing, but child-rearing. Belief, law, public opinion, illusion, education, art, and bugaboos have all been used to re-enforce maternal instinct. We shall never know just how much maternal instinct alone will do for population until all the forces and influences exemplified above have become inoperative. As soon as women become fully conscious of the fact that they have been and are controlled by these devices, the latter will become useless, and we shall get a truer measure of maternal feeling.

> One who learns why society is urging him into the straight and narrow way will resist its pressure. One who sees clearly how he is controlled will thenceforth be emancipated. To betray the secrets of ascendancy is to forearm the individual in his struggle with society.

The time is coming, and is indeed almost at hand, when all the most intelligent women of the community, who are the most desirable child-bearers, will become conscious of the methods of social control. The type of normality will be questioned; the laws will be repealed and changed; enlightenment will prevail; belief will be seen to rest upon dogmas; illusion will fade away and give place to clearness of view; the bugaboos will lose their power to frighten. How will "the social guardians" induce women to bear a surplus population when all these cheap, effective methods no longer work?

The natural desire for children may, and probably will, always guarantee a stationary population, even if child-bearing should become a voluntary matter. But if a surplus population is desired for national aggrandizement, it would seem that there will remain but one effective social device whereby this can be secured, namely, *adequate compensation,* either in money or in fame. If it were possible to become rich or famous by bearing numerous fine children, many a woman would no doubt be eager to bring up eight or ten, though if acting at the dictation of maternal instinct only, she would have brought up but one or two. When the cheap devices no longer work, we shall expect expensive devices to replace them, if the same result is still desired by the governors of society.

If these matters could be clearly raised to consciousness, so that this aspect of human life could be managed rationally, instead of irrationally as at present, the social gain would be enormous—assuming always that the increased happiness and usefulness of women would, in general, be regarded as social gain.

2

Coercive Pronatalism and American Population Policy

JUDITH BLAKE

Graduate School of Public Policy and International Population and Urban Research, University of California, Berkeley

The achievement of zero population growth implies that American childbearing be limited to an average of approximately 2 children per woman. Since women who are currently approaching the end of the reproductive age span have borne an average of 3 children, advocates of population stabilization are concerned about the mechanisms for achieving a two-child average.[1] The search for measures to insure us a reproductive level that is both low and nonfluctuating is intensified by a growing recognition of the lead-time required to achieve zero population growth. For example, the two-child average will afford us zero growth only *after* the age structure of the population has become less favorable to reproduction than is currently the case. Until the baby-boom babies, who have grown up to be mothers and potential mothers, move out of the reproductive ages, the achievement of zero growth implies fewer than two children per woman.[2] It is clear, therefore, that long-run population stability will require either that Americans, in general, restrict themselves to micro-families, or that a substantial share of the population remain childless (and/or have only one child) while others have the moderate-sized families to which we are now accustomed.

It is perhaps not surprising that such a major change in our reproductive behavior would seem to call for the introduction of state-imposed coercions on individuals—an abrogation of the "voluntary" character of child-bearing decisions.[3] This popular view of what must be done in order to achieve population stability is, of

Prepared for the Commission on Population Growth and the American Future, 1972

course, both shocking and frightening to government officials. In the face of suggestions regarding state "control" over reproduction, programs that promise population stability through the elimination of "unwanted" fertility alone seem reassuringly inoffensive. Understandably, they are embraced with relief regardless of how unlikely it is that they will be effective. Their selling point is "the right to choose" one's family size and this "right" is celebrated as an ultimate end. In the words of Frank Notestein: [4]

> . . . Family planning represents a new and important freedom in the world. It will surely be a happy day when parents can have and can avoid having children, as they see fit. . . . It is a matter of major importance that this kind of new freedom to choose, now existing for the bulk of the population, be extended to its most disadvantaged parts. If it were extended, reproduction would be brought fairly close to the replacement level. However, I would advocate the right to choose even if I thought the demographic consequences would be highly adverse, because it will always be possible to manipulate the environment in which the choice is made.

However, both the coercion approach and the laissez-faire approach ("the right to choose") suffer from a serious empirical flaw. They each assume that free choice and voluntarism now exist and that they are marred only by incomplete distribution of contraceptives. One approach says that voluntarism must be curtailed, the other claims that it must be preserved at all cost. Neither recognizes that it does not exist right now. Neither takes into account that at present, reproductive behavior is under stringent institutional control and that this control constitutes, in many respects, a coercive pronatalist policy. Hence, an effective anti-natalist policy will not necessarily involve an increase in coercion or a reduction in the "voluntary" element in reproduction, because individuals are under pronatalist constraints right now. People make their "voluntary" reproductive choices in an institutional context that severely constrains them not to choose non-marriage, not to choose childlessness, not to choose only one child, and even not to limit themselves solely to two children. If we can gain insight into the coercions and restraints under which we currently operate, it may become more obvious that an anti-natalist policy can be one that is *more* voluntary—allows a wider spectrum of individual choice—than is presently the case. Let us first examine why individuals may be said to be under constraint and suffer coercion, in any society, regarding reproduction. We may then turn to the main body of our paper—the actual nature of some important existing reproductive coercions in American society.

The Sociology of the Family and the Reproductive Function

In order to understand the long-run determinants of birth rates, in so far as these relate to motivational and not conditional factors, one must translate birth rates into the operational context of reproduction.[5] People do not have birth rates, they have children. Their willingness to bear and rear children—to expend their human and material resources in this manner—cannot be taken for granted. Rather, childbearing and childrearing take place in an organizational content which influences people strongly to do one set of things—reproduce, and not do other sets of things—activities that would conflict or compete with reproduction. The bearing and rearing of children thus represents one kind of allocation and organization of human and material resources. In all viable societies social control has operated to organize human beings into childbearing and childrearing groups—families—that, by definition, have proven to be highly efficient reproductive machines. Reproductively inefficient societies have not survived for historical man to study.

As with other forms of social control, that responsible for the support of the family as an institution rests on informal and formal (legal) rules of behavior. These will range from behavior that must be performed—prescribed, to behavior that is forbidden—proscribed. Large areas of behavior are simply permitted or preferred. What leads us to abide by these rules? Clearly, the same mechanisms of social control that lead us to abide by any rules. First of all, we are socialized from the beginning both to learn the rules and to believe they are right. Second, the everyday process of interaction with others puts us in constant contact with the norm-enforcement process, since other people have a stake in how we behave. They can reward us with approval, or punish us with rejection. If these informal sanctions are not effective, then formal ones may be invoked such as, for example, the law. Finally, the master control of all is what might be called the "sociological predicament." This is that any existing social organization represents a selection of possible roles and statuses, goals and activities, etc., available to individuals. Not only are persons with certain characteristics allocated to particular roles and statuses and proscribed from others, but all individuals in a given society typically have available to them, as the outer perimeter of their expectations, what the society has to offer from a role and status point of view. Such limitation of role alternatives obviates the need for many more direct coercions.

Individuals are usually not afforded role options that might be deviant. This fact is abundantly documented by the social sciences. An illustration of particular relevance to this paper is Burgess and Wallin's criticism of Waller's well-known theory of the function of romantic love. Waller presupposed that the idealization and euphoria of being "in love" are necessary to propel people into marriage. He reasoned that a powerful force is needed to overcome the attractions of alternative ways of life. Burgess and Wallin's point is simple—such attractive alternatives do not exist.[6]

> . . . The woman who does not marry is likely to be judged a failure, the implication generally being that she was not chosen, she was not desired. Apart from the injury to her self-esteem, nonmarriage imposes difficulties and frustrations. Adult social life tends to be organized around married couples. Sexual satisfaction is not easily obtained without risk by the unmarried female who desires it, and the experience of motherhood is denied her. . . .
>
> [As for men,] . . . to marry is to be normal, and from childhood on we are exposed to the idea of marriage as something to be desired, the risk of divorce notwithstanding. Although some men can secure their sexual satisfaction outside the matrimonial relationship, most of them are strongly attracted by the promise of sexual gratification with the regularity, convenience and comfort which marriage affords.

In sum, reproduction and replacement, like other societal functions, require an organized allocation of human and material resources. Societies have resolved this problem of resource allocation by means of diffused control mechanisms (rather than a government planning board, for example), but the mechanisms are nonetheless quite palpably there. And they involve the individual in an articulated and coercive set of constraints. He has some choice among fixed alternatives, but, as we shall see, even his "choices" are deeply influenced by his past social experience and the kind of person he has been influenced to become. His behavior is "voluntary" only in a restricted sense—not in the sense of being unpatterned, uncontrolled, or unrestrained. In effect, regardless of whether a typical birth cohort of individuals contains a large proportion of persons who might be unsuited to family life, human societies are so organized as to attempt to make individuals as suited as possible, to motivate them to want to be suited, and to provide them with little or no alternative to being suited as they mature. By fiction and by fiat, parenthood is the "natural" human condition, and to live one's life as a family member is the desideratum. In this context, individuals make their reproductive "choices."

The present paper will concentrate on two such diffused and implicit pronatalist coercions in modern American society—the prescribed primacy of parenthood in the definition of adult sex roles and the prescribed congruence of personality traits with the demands of the sex roles as defined. I believe it can be shown that there is, in American society, not only an absence of legitimate alternatives to sex roles having parenthood as a primacy focus, but that change is particularly difficult to effect because those individuals who might aspire to such alternatives are suppressed and neutralized. My thesis is that unless we realize that we have been locking pronatalism into both the structure of society and the structure of personality, the problem of fertility control will appear to be the reverse of what it actually is. We will continue to believe that our principal policy problem is one of *instituting* antinatalist coercions instead of *lifting* pronatalist ones. We will see fertility reduction as involving *more* regimentation than presently exists, when, in fact, it should involve *less,* since individuals will no longer be universally constrained to forsake other possible interests and goals in order to devote themselves to the reproductive function.

Role Differentiation by Sex and the Primacy of Parenthood

Role differentiation by sex in American society makes actual or anticipated parenthood a pre-condition for all other aspects of men's and women's roles. The content of sex roles—men's and women's "spheres"—uses as a bench mark the sexually differentiated relation to childbearing and rearing. The feminine role is normatively maternal and, hence, intra-familial, "integrative," emotionally supportive, and "expressive." The masculine role is normatively paternal and, as a result, primarily the complement of the maternal role—extra-familial, protective, economically supportive, and "instrumental" (or "task-oriented"). By according primacy to the kinship statuses of "mother" and "father" these role expectations thus assume that parenthood is implicit in the very definition of masculinity and femininity. Moreover, not only does the identification of masculinity and femininity with parenthood mean that reproduction is implicitly prescribed for everyone but, as might be expected, it means that alternative role definitions for the sexes are, at best, tolerated, and, at worst, proscribed.

Since we have been speaking of the United States, it is worth asking whether the identification of gender with parenthood is unusual in human societies. Are Americans odd? The answer is, of course, negative. We share this linkage of sex roles and parenthood functions with a large number of primitive and technologically backward peoples, as well as with some more modern ones.[7] Indeed, it is probably true that, insofar as men and women engage in reproduction in families, this division of labor will be subject to only minor modifications. What is open to question, however, is the demographic appropriateness for a low-mortality society of rigidly identifying, for *everyone,* the sexual with the parental role. Since sex is an aspect of a person's identity that begins its influence from birth, we appear to be locking ourselves into reproduction through sex-role expectations that ceased to be demographically necessary for our entire population before most of us were born.

What is the evidence for the identification of sex roles with traditional parental functions in American society? Is such an identification really normative? One significant way of answering this question is to see what happens when the norm is challenged, or when there is some large-scale defection from the sex-role expectations as defined. If the norm is operative, we would expect to discover that a variety of sanctions are invoked to bring behavior back into line. Additionally, we might expect to see an effort to label the deviation as not merely contranormative but pathological as well.

In the remainder of this section on sex roles, we shall examine a number of challenges to the traditional expectations for the sexes in American society. These challenges are: the labor force participation of women, higher education for women, feminism, and male homosexuality. We shall find, in all cases, widespread opposition to the recognized threat to sex-role expectations. Furthermore, in the case of the first three, we shall see that adjustment to this opposition has taken place so effectively as to substantially neutralize these sources of change in sex-role expectations. In the case of the last example, the deviancy is regarded as an aberration (a pathology) for which diverse causes and cures are sought. There is systematic refusal to recognize that *intra*-sex variability in temperament, personality traits, and physical and mental capability may, in actuality, be fully as important as *inter*-sex variation, if one but excludes the difference in reproductive capacity.

The Working Woman and the Primacy of Parenthood for Both Sexes

Nothing better illustrates the absence of genuine options to parental roles in our society than the nature of the opposition to having women work outside the home. The most salient and enduring objections to a genuine career role for women—a commitment to outside work—have been two: First, that no women—even unmarried women—should be allowed to challenge men's prior claim on jobs since men must support families; and second, that outside work is unsuited to women physically and mentally since their natural fulfillment lies in another sphere entirely—motherhood. In effect, the opposition to work-commitment by women has reaffirmed *both* the male's role as father and family supporter and the female's role as mother and housewife. Smuts documents legal and public concern along these lines since the 1870's.[8] Although, as he shows, the emphasis on the physical inappropriateness of outside work for women has disappeared, the "psychological" and temperamental uniqueness of women is still emphasized strongly. Hence, jobs are sex-typed, women are "protected" by legislation, and both hiring and firing take advantage of the typical women's marginal commitment to full-time, long-term employment. Through an analysis of articles on women's labor force participation in major American popular magazines since 1900, Betty Stirling has shown that the dual considerations of concern for protecting the man's family-supporting job and concern for protecting the woman's motherhood role has characterized opposition to female employment outside the home from the beginning.[9] Public opinion polls have demonstrated the same anxieties.[10] Religious opposition to women working has been particularly vocal in the Catholic press and marriage manuals—specifically on the bases of threats to the supporting role of men and the motherhood role of women.[11]

In effect, although economic opportunities might have led us to expect the emergence of a career role for a numerically important group of unmarried, and married but childless, women, in actual fact the immense increase in labor force participation by women took a different tack entirely. Women's labor in the market has been utilized and tolerated only on condition that it supported and enhanced the traditional parental roles for both sexes. In the words of the National Manpower Council: [12]

> . . . Americans view the man in the family as the primary breadwinner and, when jobs are scarce, are inclined to believe that women workers should not compete with men who have families to support. Americans also believe that mothers should personally care for their children during their early formative years. Consequently, even though there are today over 2.5 million mothers in the labor force whose children are under six, there is still little sympathy with the idea of mothers holding full-time jobs when their children

> are of preschool age, unless they are compelled to do so by economic necessity . . .

The difficulties women experienced who wished to challenge the identity of sexual and parental roles have not been simply "male dominance" or "male power," but rather the intense societal supports for the *family roles* of mother and father. The opposition to women working thus stemmed fully as much from the obligatory nature of family formation (and the sex differentiation of parents), as from a fear of the dimunition of male authority generally. We shall see, moreover, in a later section, that, after World War II, when women's educational and economic opportunities could, objectively, have provided some challenge to the primacy of the parental role, the unmarried, and married but childless, women came under attack from "scientific" sources. In the face of declining religious influence, a breakdown of Victorian "traditions," and expanding career opportunities for women, "science" stepped in, in the guise of psychoanalysis, to provide an authoritative prescription of parenthood, and severe condemnation of the career women. Not surprisingly, few unmarried or childless females were available to re-define the role of the working woman along career lines. Women's labor force participation evolved as an adjunct, not an alternative, to motherhood.[13] The peculiar character of this participation—low wages, dead-end jobs, and sex-typing—tends moreover, to be self-perpetuating. Each generation of girls views the market and finds few realistic career options therein. The primacy of men's and women's family roles has successfully absorbed what might have been a genuine alternative to reproduction for a number of women. As Smuts says: [14]

> . . . the woman who urgently wants to develop and utilize her abilities in work still has barriers to overcome. Employers tend to judge all working women on the basis of their experience with the majority who are content with modest rewards for modest efforts . . .

Higher Education for Women: The Mother's Helper

Theoretically, the provision of higher education to women constituted a major challenge to the primacy of motherhood as *the* sex role for American females. Far more than the franchise, higher education seemed to imply that women *should* be given career avenues equal in all respects to the channels afforded to men. In this sense, it cast into doubt the norm that motherhood is the primary role for all but the unhappy few.

The initial efforts in the United States to provide higher education for women were met with much explicit verbalization concerning the possible undermining of the wife-mother role—the only proper feminine role. This history is well known and need not concern us here.[15] More important is the mounting evidence that genuine educational opportunities for women have been subtly infused by an implicit (occasionally even explicit) premise—the unchallenged assumption that the wife-mother role is a pre-condition for all other roles women might wish to play. As Mabel Newcomer has said: [16]

> The fact that homemaking is woman's most important role has never been seriously questioned either by those arguing in favor of college education for women or by those opposing it. Those opposing higher education for women have usually expressed the fear that it will encourage them to pursue independent careers, foregoing marriage; or if they marry, that it will make them dissatisfied with the homemaker's lot. Those promoting higher education have, on the contrary, insisted that college women make better wives and mothers than their less educated sisters. Even those who have been concerned with the rights and interests of unmarried women have never argued that higher education might encourage women to remain single, except as it occasionally offered a reasonably satisfactory alternative when the only available young men were not entirely acceptable.

Indeed, the women's colleges—in the vanguard of higher education for women—early learned to stress that their effect on diverting their charges from the path of wifehood and motherhood would be nonexistent. Defensively, they assured their trustees, their backers, the prospective parents of their tuition-paying student bodies that higher education for women would leave unchallenged woman's *role* and women's *expectations*.[17]

The stated "aims" of the colleges, as reviewed by Newcomer in the late 1950's, were sufficiently vague concerning the purposes for which young girls were attending as to leave unthreatened either the classical feminine role definition, or the intellectual fantasies of the students.[18] Clearly, the educators of young women had learned the hard way that the uncomfortable resolution between the promise of "equality"—even for some—and the reality of motherhood for all was best left to each individual girl to resolve as best she could. The college was not to be the champion of the "odd-ball" girl.

The most obvious deviant among the college presidents and promoters of women's education was Lynn White, Jr. (then President of Mills College), who attempted to clarify and make explicit the hidden agenda behind women's education in America. Almost all women do marry, few women pursue systematic careers, and even these careers are typically "feminine" rather than masculine. Why not face it? Why not educate our daughters in the light of definitively sex-linked capabilities and the appropriate social roles that express these capabilities? [19] So eager was White to clinch his point, that he fell into the familiar position adopted by some of the feminists—the moral *superiority* of the traditional female virtues over the crasser male qualities. Thus, if women were constitutionally debarred from the more highly regarded cultural pursuits, they should not feel badly. These pursuits have been overrated anyway.[20] White thus invoked the position that helped legitimate the downfall of feminism—women's battles were to be on higher ground as befits their universally more civilized, sensitive, and gentle natures. Of similar sentiments expressed by the feminists, O'Neill has written, "Definitions like this left men with few virtues anyone was bound to admire, and inspired women to think of themselves as a kind of super race condemned by historical accident and otiose convention to serve their natural inferiors." [21] In keeping with his effort to legitimate separate and unequal education for women, White celebrated motherhood as women's noblest pursuit.[22] He even deplored the anti-family bias that, he alleged, was being transmitted to men by the "celibate tradition" in higher education. For men as well as women, the family should come first, ". . . unless men as well as women can be given the conviction that personal cultivation and career are secondary to making a success of the family, and indeed that both are bleak satisfactions apart from a warm hearth, we shall not have found wisdom." [23] In a significant chapter that constitutes a paean to motherhood, he claimed that the American population was not replacing itself, that "the best" people were particularly remiss in their reproductive obligation, and that it was the duty of high-minded American women to devote themselves to maternity.[24] Repeatedly he emphasized the hopelessness of combining a genuine career with a family of sufficient size, and enjoined college women not to be inhibited by a college education from "flinging themselves with complete enthusiasm and abandon" into family life.[25]

Is the aim-inhibition that has suffused higher education for women, its absorption into the anticipated motherhood role, merely an intellectual preoccupation of the educators, or have young college women themselves received the message that their college experience must be adapted to their future role as mothers? Two studies of American college girls, one done by Komarovsky in the 1940's, and another done by Goldsen and others in the 1950's, show clearly that the pressures on women to remain undiverted from motherhood followed them into college.

Komarovsky, writing in 1953, expressed the concern of the educator over holding out to women impossible and contradictory goals.[26]

> . . . The very education which is to make the college housewife a cultural leaven of her family and her community may develop in her interests which are frustrated by other phases of housewifery. We are urged to train women for positions of leadership in civic affairs when, at the same time, we define capacity for decisive action, executive ability, hardihood in the face of opposition as "unfeminine" traits. We want our daughters to be able, if the need arises, to earn a living at some worth-while occupation. In doing so, we run the risk of awakening interests and abilities which, again, run counter to the present definition of femininity.

Her case studies of women students seemed to indicate to her that these young women were presented with "equally compelling" but "contradictory" pressures. Actually, the data seem to trace a temporal change in parental and peer pressure concerning academic and occupational achievement and the traditional female role. Parents and peers were encouraging of achievement until it seemed to stand in the way of marriage and motherhood. Then, for the girl who had not already received "the message" by means of less obvious cues, sanctions came into play. She was effectively told that she should not allow academic or professional achievement "to get in her way." [27] For example:

> All through grammar school and high school my parents led me to feel that to do well in school was my chief responsibility. A good report card, an election to student office, these were the news Mother bragged about in telephone conversations with her friends. *But recently they suddenly got worried about me: I don't pay enough attention to social life, a woman needs* some *education but not that much.* They are disturbed by my determination to go to the School of Social Work. Why my ambitions should surprise them after they have exposed me for four years to some of the most inspired and stimulating social scientists in the country, I can't imagine. They have some mighty strong arguments on their side. What is the use, they say, of investing years in training for a profession, only to drop it in a few years? Chances of meeting men are slim in this profession. Besides, I may become so preoccupied with it as to sacrifice social life. The next few years are, after all, the proper time to find

a mate. But the urge to apply what I have learned, and the challenge of this profession is so strong that I shall go on despite the family opposition.

I . . . work for a big metropolitan daily as a correspondent in the city room. I am well liked there and may possibly stay as a reporter after graduation in February. I have had several spreads (stories running to more than eight or ten inches of space), and this is considered pretty good for a college correspondent. Naturally, I was elated and pleased at such breaks, and as far as the city room is concerned I'm off to a very good start on a career that is hard for a man to achieve and even harder for a woman. General reporting is still a man's work in the opinion of most people. *I have a lot of acclaim but also criticism, and I find it difficult to be praised for being clever and working hard and then, when my efforts promise to be successful, to be condemned and criticized for being unfeminine and ambitious.*

The 1952 study of both male and female Cornell students by Goldsen, Rosenberg, Williams, and Suchman shows that the co-eds had almost universally accepted motherhood as a pre-condition for any other activity.[28]

A traditional middle-class idea that a woman's only career should be her family is rejected by almost all the students. Instead, they are neither unequivocally for nor unequivocally against the idea of women having careers. The attitude seems to be, "It's okay providing. . . ." Providing she is not married, or providing she has no children, or providing her children are "old enough"—a notion about which there is a wide range of opinion. Let the women have careers, indeed encourage them, but be sure it does not interfere with her main job of bearing and rearing children.

Interestingly, the young women in the Cornell study had adjusted their ideas of the proper jobs for women to the demands of their motherhood role. Unlike the new feminists of the 1960's and 1970's, these women assumed that their labor market activity would not be equal in demands or prestige with that of men.[29]

. . . Our data indicate that just about every college girl wants to marry and have children, and that she fully expects to do so. . . . Most of them see no essential conflict between family life and a career—the sort of career, that is, that they consider "suitable" for a woman. . . . The occupations women choose to go into are quite different from those chosen by men. They overwhelmingly select the traditional "women's occupations."

Why did they want to work at all? One reason was to keep occupied before marriage. Another was insurance—against the remote possibility of remaining single, and against adversity in their marriage. More significant, however, was ambivalence about the suitability of homemaking and motherhood to their interests and temperaments. A striking feature of these data is that these young women did not appear to be overwhelmingly *attracted* to maternity, they simply did not see any alternative role as realistic.[30]

> There is no question that college girls count on building up equity in family life, not in professional work. A dedicated career-girl is a deviant: in a real sense she is unwilling to conform to her sex-role as American society defines it. For professional work among women in this country (and the college-trained women agree) is viewed as an interlude, at best a part-time excursion away from full-time family life which the coeds yearn for, impatiently look forward to . . . and define as largely monotony, tedium, and routine.

The intention to work, the vision of personal realization through the use of the talents and capabilities they had come, through their college training, to know they possessed, represented the psychological life-preserver they promised themselves to keep at hand.[31]

By what mechanisms was the "career girl" role rendered so deviant? One mechanism was clearly the girls' perception of what men wanted in a woman. The Cornell study found, for example, that other than the condition that an ideal mate love her spouse, two-thirds of all college men in the sample cited "interested in having a family" as highly important in a mate.[32] To the young college woman, a way of life as deviant as a genuine and demanding career represented a journey toward an unknown, inappropriate, and potentially tragic destination. She might never meet *any* man who was interested in such a freak. Half of the Cornell men were quite clear in stating that they either did not approve of women having careers, or approved only if the woman was unmarried or, if married, had no children. Only 22 percent of the men approved of a woman having a career regardless of the age of her children, and most of the remainder approved only if the children were of high school age or older.[33] Finally, the young women's sense of constraint concerning pre-marital sexual relations made an indefinite postponement of marriage appear lonely and sexless. Even among girls who were interested in careers, sexual relationships were defined only in romantic, emotional terms, and close to 40 percent felt that pre-marital sex relations were "never justified" for women. Among young women who ranked low on careerism, half felt that pre-marital relations were "never justified." [34]

Has it all changed by 1971? Obviously, there have been many external changes. The development of contraception—especially the pill—has greatly altered the conditions under which young college men and women may consider non-marital relationships. Public policy is increasingly concerned with equal educational and occupational opportunity for women, and the country has been literally deluged by anti-natalist and neo-feminist propaganda. How have college women reacted? And what reactions must they cope with in college men? Is there yet a perceived alternative to marriage and a family, or simply a scaling down of family size desires? In an attempt to clarify this and other issues, I inserted a set of ques-

TABLE 1

Family-Size Preferences and Attitudes Toward Age at Marriage and Non-Marriage Among a National Sample of White American College Students, June 1971. Percentages.*

	College Men	*College Women*
How many children would you like to have?		
None	7	9
1	3	4
2	56	49
3 or more	33	38
Total	100	100
(N)	(548)	(348)
According to your personal tastes and preferences, what size family do you think is too small—a husband, wife, and how many children?		
No children	36	31
One child	53	58
Two children	7	6
Three or more	4	5
Total	100	100
(N)	(529)	(331)
And what size family do you think is too large—a husband, wife, and how many children?		
One child	1	0
Two children	1	1
Three children	19	16
Four children	25	21
Five children	25	23
Six children	11	15
Seven or more children	17	25
Total	100	100
(N)	(548)	(350)

*The difference between N's shown under the various questions and the total number of respondents (562 males and 355 females) constitutes the NA/DK [No Answer/Don't Know] category in each case.

tions on family size preferences, preferred age at marriage, nonmarriage, attitudes toward the pill and abortion in a special youth study conducted by the Gallup Poll in June 1971. The study included two samples of young people aged 18–24—one a college sample and one a representative national sample of persons in this age group. Table 1 presents some relevant data for the college sample.

The results indicate clearly that few men or women in this

TABLE 1 (Cont.)

	College Men	*College Women*
What do you think is the best age for a girl to marry.		
Under 18	1	0
18–19	5	2
20	14	12
21	21	16
22	23	20
23–25	31	44
Over 25	5	6
Total	100	100
(N)	(529)	(343)
What do you think is the best age for a man to marry?		
Under 21	5	3
21–22	22	20
23–24	26	26
25	24	27
26–30	21	24
Over 30	2	1
Total	100	100
(N)	(533)	(344)
Do you think a woman can have a happy life even if she never marries?		
Yes	81	82
No	16	15
DK	3	3
Total	100	100
(N)	(562)	(355)
What about a man—do you think he can have a happy life if he never marries?		
Yes	87	84
No	12	13
DK	1	3
Total	100	100
(N)	(562)	(355)
Total Respondents	(562)	(355)

college sample would like to be childless, or have only one child. More than half of the men, and approximately half of the women would like to have a two-child family. A third of the men and almost 40 percent of the women want three or more children. Although these results show that family-size preferences are smaller than those expressed in the 1950's and 1960's, the desire for at least two children is clear and apparently firm. A question on the family size considered "too small" demonstrates that an acceptable family size begins with two children. On the other hand, there seems to be no clear proscription against even a relatively large family. A question concerning the size family the respondent would consider "too large" shows that three children are tolerated by all but a minority of respondents—20 percent. Even at the level of five children, 27 percent of the men and 40 percent of the women have not yet designated the family as "too large."

Turning to age at marriage we see that, according to both men and women, women should definitely be married by age 25. Men believe that women should marry earlier than do women themselves, but there is consensus that age 25 is the upper limit. Although the best age at marriage for men is clearly older than for women, there is remarkable consensus between men and women concerning what this age should be. Not before age 21, not after age 30. Preferably between ages 21 and 25. However, although marrying and having a family are clearly the norm, the college men and women in this sample do not deny that either a man or a woman can have a happy life in the unmarried state. There is a clear recognition that at least *some* people can do this. Unfortunately, we do not know, from this single question, whether respondents believe the "average" or "normal" person can be happy unmarried, or whether they believe only an unusual person can so exist.

These results may seem surprising in today's context. Has neo-feminism had no effect? Why is there no clear break with the family role altogether among a substantial number of the college elite?[35] In order to understand their position, one must realize that no call has come to make such a break, no models have been presented, no champion of a genuinely alternative role has appeared. "Women's liberation," like higher education for women and women's labor force activity, has absorbed, in its turn, the norm that the American woman's adult role *includes* motherhood. To have done otherwise would have been to sacrifice its principal constituency, as we shall see. It, like higher education for women and jobs for women, has *accommodated* itself to maternity and even become its militant champion. Motherhood, is, after all, one of "women's rights."

Feminism and the "Do Both" Syndrome

It is often assumed that the present-day "woman's liberation" movement is essentially anti-natalist in ideology and that its effects will be anti-natalist as well. Actually, however, the main thrust of the movement's stand is supportive of motherhood for all; what is decried is the relative disadvantage that women experience because of childbearing and rearing. In effect, women's liberation is concerned with lowering the exclusionary barriers for women in the labor force, opening up educational channels, elevating women's awareness of subtle forms of discrimination against them in the outside world *and* supporting women's right to have families as well. Rather than concerning itself with the atypical spinster, or childless woman, the movement has gained popularity through its recognition of the problems of women who already have made a choice to be mothers and who then are dissatisfied with their impaired occupational chances, or who find motherhood less than they expected it to be and wish to switch gears. Betty Friedan's book, *The Feminine Mystique,* was addressed primarily to this group of women—those suffering from "the problem that has no name." However, although the movement has pitched its appeal to women who have already made their reproductive choices and urged them to seek out an alternative identity as well, its general philosophy for *all* women is one of *combining* marriage and motherhood, on the one hand, with a non-familial role, on the other. Indeed, it is this militant statement that women should not *have* to make a choice that gives the movement wide appeal. For example, Friedan says,[36]

> When enough women make life plans geared to their real abilities, and speak out for maternity leaves or even maternity sabbaticals, professionally run nurseries, and other changes in the rules that may be necessary, they will not have to sacrifice the right to honorable competition and contribution *any more than they will have to sacrifice marriage and motherhood.*

The movement sees the major injustice toward women as inhering in the expenditure of time and effort on child-rearing, together with the loss of seniority and skills in the labor market due to interrupted career patterns. This philosophy is embodied in the Statement of Purpose of the National Organization for Women.

The modern liberationist position, which requires that women generally be enabled to forego choice in their dominant career roles and shift child-rearing onto outside agencies, has been elaborated by a number of sociologists.

Wring in 1964, Alice Rossi claims that: [37]

> . . . There is no sex equality until women participate on an equal basis with men in politics, occupations, and the family. . . . In politics and the occupational world, to be able to participate depends primarily on whether home responsibilities can be managed simultaneously with work or political commitments. Since women have had, and probably will continue to have, primary responsibility for child-rearing, their participation in politics, professions or the arts cannot be equal to that of men unless ways are devised to ease the combination of home and work responsibilities.

Rossi goes on to outline the need for mother-substitutes, child-care centers, less sexual demarcation in personal traits, and a less demanding definition of the mother's role in socialization. However, she accepts the parental roles for both sexes. Rather than recognizing that men and women may be variably suited to parenthood, she assumes that all are suited and all could be androgynous. Thus they could reconcile the demands of child-care and the desire of the woman to excel outside the home by having both parents play the "inside" and "outside" roles.[38]

Epstein sees the primacy of motherhood obligations for women as the principal barrier to occupational commitment and success. Yet, like Rossi, she does not question the basic premise of the universal desirability of motherhood. As she notes, being single or childless is being a "nonconformist." Thus, the basic inequality lies in the fact that although women are normatively held to child care and the home, men can ignore their families with impunity. She says [39]

> The man who spends too much time with his family is considered something of a loafer . . . In extreme cases of neglect, wives may be permitted to complain, but clearly the absorption of the man in his work is not considered intolerable. Professors who prefer their work to their wives or children are usually "understood" and forgiven. A similar absorption in work was reported by Stanley Talbot in *Time* magazine; he found that the business tycoon (not surprisingly) clearly preferred his work to his family. There is no comparable "lady tycoon" with a husband and children to neglect; and the lady professional who gives an indication of being more absorbed in work than in her husband and family is neither understood nor forgiven. The woman, unlike the man, cannot spend "too much time" with her family; her role demands as mother and wife

are such that they intrude on all other activities. She remains on call during any time spent away from the family and, if she works, many of her family tasks must be fitted into what usually would be working time.

We thus see that, far from questioning the basic premise that all women *should* be mothers, or for that matter that all men should be fathers, the woman's liberation movement accepts the goal of reproduction for all as a basic "good." Childlessness is regarded as an inherent deprivation for all, rather than a socially induced deprivation for some (perhaps even many). Women who cannot share equally with men in ignoring and neglecting their children are "disadvantaged." Unquestioned is the notion of why persons of *either* sex who have such a marginal commitment to child-rearing should be pressed into having children. If a man wishes to spend virtually his entire time on occupational achievement, travel, and golf, why should the parental status be socially supported as obligatory, or his way of life condemned as self-centered and hedonistic? At present, he has to buy his way out of censure by having a family as "window-dressing" even though he may not change his way of life as a result.[40] Similarly, if a woman wishes to enjoy an externally oriented way of life, it is intensely pronatalist to specify that nominal parenthood—shored up by maids, nurseries, and child-care centers—be required as a badge of respectability, normality, or conformity.

The woman's liberation movement thus parts company with anti-natalism by failing to recognize that it is not in society's interest to encourage the emergence of families in which *neither* parent is committed to parenthood. Rather, a genuine anti-natalist policy would be aimed at the *indiscriminate* nature of the family-building vortex that now exists. At present, marriage and parenthood are almost ascribed statuses. They are not really chosen, they happen to people, as the Burgess and Wallin quotation cited earlier states admirably. Moreover, the state takes an essentially frivolous attitude toward the *contracting* of the marital obligation, far more carefree than the attitude it takes toward business contracts. This point is well made by Robert Kingsley in an article on the grounds for granting annulments in the United States.[41]

A few courts have said that the issue was whether or not the party was mentally capable of entering into an ordinary commercial contract; but the later cases have held that there is no necessary connection between the capacity to make commercial contracts and the capacity to become married. The test today is usually put as requiring the mental ability to "understand the nature of the marriage-relation and the duties and obligations involved therein." So put, it is clear that the capacity to enter into business relations has no bearing on the capacity to marry. . . . For the numerically considerable group of mentally weak persons, whose estates are controlled by guardians but who are permitted to go at large in the community, a legal prohibition on marriage would simply result in fornication, temporary liaisons, and similar socially undesirable practices. Consequently, the law wisely has permitted such persons to marry if it appeared that, concerning that particular kind of relationship, they had a reasonably intelligent attitude.

Clearly, the state has, as a matter of public policy, viewed marriage not as the licensing of parental responsibility, but as a sop to Mrs. Grundy. Yet, the modern interest of the state concerning a marriage lies in the quality of the children produced, not in the prevention of pre-marital fornication. Nonetheless, the law of marriage is still geared to a time when it was important to use sex as a means of enticing people into marriage and childbearing. In this regard we may suggest that a significant control over reproductive motivation in the future could be the further development of the legal personality of the child, and a diminution of his being treated, at law, as the property of his parents. The "rights" of parents to "choose" parenthood, and the number of offspring they will have could be tempered by the rights of children to certain legal guarantees from their parents.[42] If fathers have already been "liberated" from many parental obligations, and mothers are on the way to "liberation," then obviously the rights and welfare of children must come under far more detailed legal and social scrutiny.

It is of some interest that the origins of the acceptance of (even insistence on) universal motherhood were clearly visible in the suffragette movement. As O'Neill points out: [43]

. . . Having already taken the economic context of American life as essentially given, feminists went on to do the same thing for the marital and domestic system, accepting, for the most part, Victorian marriage as a desirable necessity. In so doing they assured the success of woman suffrage while guaranteeing that when women did get the vote and enter the labor market in large numbers, the results would be bitterly disappointing.

. . . while feminism was born out of a revolt against stifling domesticity . . . by the end of the century most feminists had succumbed to what Charlotte Perkins Gilman called the "domestic mythology." . . . The original feminists had demanded freedom in the name of humanity; the second generation asked for it in the name of maternity. What bound women into selfless sisterhood, it was now maintained, was their reproductive capacity.

> . . . So the effort to escape domesticity was accompanied by an invocation of the domestic ideal—woman's freedom road circled back to the home from which feminism was supposed to liberate her. In this manner feminism was made respectable by accommodating it to the Victorian ethos which had originally forced it into being.

Charlotte Perkins Gilman, however, recognized the logical problems inherent in the motherhood emphasis and presaged the feminist movement of the 1960's and 1970's by a formula that is now familiar to us: Women, generically, should both have families *and* take an equal place with men, in the non-familial world. In order to enable them to do this, the society must provide mechanisms to relieve them of their homemaking burdens.[44]

The assumption was made then, as it is now, that men—most or all men—find self-expression and fulfillment in the labor market, and that parenthood (and the economic obligations it involves) essentially leaves men's, but not women's, life chances untouched. Since the movement is a special pleading device, it could not be expected to recognize that those differential social and economic advantages that men experience as patriarchs have constituted an incentive for them to undertake the economic obligations of domesticity and parenthood. In many cases, men's chances for social and personal mobility, for education, for promotion, etc., may be impaired by parenthood, although these personal losses may be concealed or dulled by the satisfactions of conforming and the lesser social approval attached to bachelors and the childless. As with women, so with men, the society has many mechanisms for obscuring the costs of parenthood. The fact that men's story of frustration and despair has found expression in a context different from women's—that of liberation from external economic exploitation—should not obscure the relevance of this story for our concern with pro-natalist coercions. . . .

Social Science and the Law: The Reaffirmation and Legitimation of Pronatalist Sex Roles

Implicit in our description of how challenges to traditional sex roles have been neutralized is the existence of powerful sources of legitimation for the identity of masculinity and femininity with parental functions. Meeting the challenges required reaffirmation and revalidation of the norm. However, the traditional legitimations would not do for moderns who had rejected a fundamentalist interpretation of Genesis, on the one hand, and a blind faith in natural law, on the other. What did it mean that women were working under the same conditions as men, competing with men in universities, demanding the right to vote? What did the psychiatric cases in World War I, the ineffective soldiers of World War II, the increasingly obvious manifestation of "effeminacy" in men portend? Where were we going? Where was there a model of society—a successful, functioning society (not, like Rome, on the road to ruin)—in which the obligations and rights of the sexes were in such a muddle? Were there other principles of organization more suited to modern life? If so, what were they?

To such questions no novel answers were forthcoming. Yet people had to make decisions, to act, to see themselves and their children as living in and moving toward some way of life that was predictable and socially validated. The answers they found reconnected them with the past. The answers came primarily from the social sciences—from psychology, sociology, and anthropology. They came directly, through the popularization of social science, and, indirectly, through the educational system, social welfare, the ministry, clinical medicine and psychology, and the courts. With few exceptions, the social sciences served to reaffirm the validity of identifying sex roles with parental functions. In the case of psychoanalysis this legitimation involved an elaborate biologistic psychology. With regard to sociology and anthropology the legitimation came about not because the research itself was necessarily biased or contaminated, but because the questions that were asked virtually assumed the consequence. Rather than regarding the identity of sex role with parental role as an *object* for research, sociology and anthropology have, by and large, taken this identity as given. The research questions that have been raised related to possible differences in sex role definitions *given* the assumption of almost universal parenthood, and to an investigation of child-rearing by means alternative to the nuclear family. There has been a notable lack of interest in, even recognition of, sex roles apart from the family and kinship. With tradition seemingly validated by scientific expertise, it is hardly surprising that legal re-affirmations of the identity of sexual and parental roles should seem legitimate as well. Let us look at the record.

Psychoanalysis and Prescriptive Parenthood

One of the strongest sources of legitimation for parenthood as the only "normal" adult sexual role comes from psychoanalytic psychology. Psychoanalysis views parenthood as the natural culmination of "normal" development to adulthood and insists that sex role differentiation should be congruent with the basic psycho-biological substratum. The natural predispositions should not be thwarted or by-passed by inappropriate social demands, activities, or expectations. Indeed, it is regarded as mandatory that the sex *roles* properly *express* what is believed to be the normal psycho-biological given. The only "normal" woman is heterosexual and a mother, the only "normal" man is heterosexual and a father.

Freud's writings on the diverse characters of the sexes, particularly his unabashed denigration of women under the guise of "scientific" description, have already been criticized in a voluminous literature.[45] Our concern here, however, is not with Freud's misogyny, but with the pronatalism which the psychoanalytic view of female psycho-biology has prescribed.

As is well known, in the Freudian scheme the basic determination of female psychology is negative. Freud believed that women were highly motivated to compensate for the lack of a penis by having children. Indeed, in Freudian psychology, the only way for women to achieve a "normal" (i.e., not cripplingly neurotic) existence is to accept their passive and denuded condition and seek their fulfillment in childbearing. Freudian psychology, from Freud to Deutsch to Erikson, is invariant in its insistence that the reproductive capacity must be actualized for the woman to approach mental health. Motherhood is what women do and they should not be encouraged to embark on social roles that conflict with the realization of their basic psycho-biological needs.[46]

One might, of course, argue that Freudian psychology has had little popular influence, that Freud's depiction of the "normal" feminine role (updated by Erikson and others) has exerted no moral pressure on women to pursue reproduction as a career, and to eschew social roles that might label them as neurotic "masculine protesters." I believe, however, that the burden of such an argument rests with its proponent. Not only has Freudian psychology been popularly absorbed throughout the Western world, but its influence on mediating agencies of society—on schools, welfare agencies, the medical profession, and the arts and mass media, to say nothing of the social sciences—has been demonstrably profound.[47] In the words of Philip Rieff: [48]

> In America today, Freud's intellectual influence is greater than that of any other modern thinker. He presides over the mass media, the college classroom, the chatter at parties, the playgrounds of the middle classes where child-rearing is a prominent and somewhat anxious topic of conversation; he has bequeathed to many couples a new self-consciousness about their marriages and the temperature of their social enthusiasms.

Indeed, as will be readily apparent, the Freudian influence on other social sciences has contributed what might be called "back up" legitimation for the emphasis on motherhood as the primary lifetime role for women. For example, Parsons says: [49]

> . . . By and large a "good" marriage from the point of view of the personality of the participants, is likely to be one with children; the functions as parents reinforce the functions in relation to each other as spouses. . . . The most important part . . . is the contingency of sexual love on the assumption of fully adult responsibilities in roles other than that of marriage directly. Put very schematically, a mature woman can love, sexually, only a man who takes his full place in the masculine world, above all its occupational aspects, and who takes responsibility for a family; conversely, the mature man can only love a woman who is really an adult, a full wife to him and mother to his children. . . .

The "experts" thus appear to agree. And, indeed, the more the dogma is paraphrased and embellished by sources at some remove from psychoanalysis, the more pervasively "right" it seems to be.

Perhaps the best evidence of the normative influence of psychoanalytic thinking concerning sex-role differentiation is the allegedly disastrous effect on child-rearing if the parents do not adhere to traditional, polarized sex roles. In effect, a person who does not exemplify the Freudian sex role definitions will not only suffer himself but, if he has children, will warp their personalities as well. The following quotation exemplifies the psychoanalytic belief in the overriding importance of the early years; the emphasis on parents playing highly differentiated, traditional sex roles; and the attribution to parental "failure" of diseases of unknown etiology like schizophrenia (that is, the clear formulation of a terrible punishment for non-conformity).[50]

> The maintenance of the appropriate sexual roles by parents in their coalition plays a major role in guiding the child's development as a male or female. Security of sexual identity is a cardinal factor in the achievement of a stable ego identity. *Of all factors entering into the formation of personality characteristics, the sex of the child is the most decisive.* Confusions and dissatisfactions concerning sexual identity can contribute to the etiology of many neuroses and character defects as well as perversions. Probably all schizophrenic patients are seriously confused in this area. . . .
>
> Clear-cut role reversals in parents can obviously distort the child's development, both when they are marked in the sexual sphere, as when the father or mother is an overt homosexual, or when they concern the task divisions in maintaining the family. A child whose

> father performs the mothering functions both tangibly and emotionally while the mother is preoccupied with her career can easily gain a distorted image of masculinity and femininity. . . . While the sharing of role tasks has become more necessary and acceptable in the contemporary family, there is still need for the parents to maintain and support one another in their primary sex roles.

Not only has psychoanalysis provided a "scientific" rationalization for prescriptive motherhood, it has attempted to consign to the realm of abnormality and mental illness any deviation from patriarchal masculinity for men. Thus psychoanalysis views male homosexuality as axiomatically indicating mental illness. In Bieber's words: [51]

> All *psychoanalytic* theories assume that adult homosexuality is pathologic and assign differing weights to constitutional and experiential determinants. All agree that the experiential determinants are in the main rooted in childhood and are primarily related to the family.

Indeed, psychoanalytic studies of homosexuals, based invariably on those who have psychological problems serious enough to bring them to an analyst, turn up pathological syndromes.[52] Data such as these are used to question controlled studies of homosexuals and heterosexuals who are functioning adequately in the community without psychoanalytic help.[53]

It may be noted that the psychoanalytic view of homosexuality, which equates deviation from a social norm as equivalent to mental illness, is not shared by biologically oriented students of sexual behavior. Both the Kinsey study and the study by Ford and Beach present evidence indicating that human beings, like other animals, are normally capable of indiscriminate sexual responsiveness. In their view, the rejection of homosexuality is culturally conditioned rather than indicative of the only "normal" psychological development for the human male.[54]

Finally, we must emphasize that the doctrine of the libidinal causes of neurosis promulgated by psychoanalysis has rendered a sexually active way of life prescriptive for all. Within this framework there is no place, except as a deviant, for the person of relatively low-keyed sexual interests. Thus, the social role of the unattached bachelor or spinster has been denigrated as psychologically abnormal.

In sum, in a century of massive social change (and accompanying personal uncertainty and anxiety), Freud reaffirmed for modern man the family roles of a people whose customs long antedated the Christian era. Freudianism, whether applied to women or to men, decreed that any deviation from the ideal of the tribal Jewish patriarch be an object of clinical contempt. At best, psychoanalysis could guide human beings who did not measure up to the idea from "hysterical misery" to "common unhappiness" as a way of life.

The Reproductive Function and Sex Role Differentiation in Sociology

Psychoanalysis has viewed traditional role differentiation by sex—differentiation in terms of wife-mother and husband-father roles—as a reflection of human psycho-biology in its "normal" form. By contrast, sociology has studied masculinity and femininity in cross-cultural perspective and come to the conclusion that the relative invariance in sex role definitions among human societies relates to the functionality of these definitions for the family—that is, for reproductive efficiency. The conclusion reached by sociology is, however, essentially very similar to that of psychoanalysis—there is not much variability possible in the masculine and feminine roles. Why? Not because of a psycho-biological substratum but because of the need for role differentiation within the family (as with other small groups) along the lines of internally versus externally oriented activities and functions, "task-oriented" as against "emotionally supportive" behavior.[55] The internal, familially oriented role goes to women because of their biological connection with childbearing and child-rearing (particularly nursing and feeding), the external role goes to men pretty much *faute de mieux*.[56] It is frequently noted that efforts to vary this pattern of sex differentiation within the reproducing family have not, to date, proven very successful.[57] In the United States, Parsons now believes that American women no longer suffer from the "role conflict" he once postulated as resulting from the option to work outside the home. They have adjusted to the "functional demands" of their wife-mother role—adjusted better than he believed they would when he first started writing about American women.[58] Recently, he has said: [59]

> It seems quite safe in general to say that the adult feminine role has not ceased to be anchored primarily in the internal affairs of the family, as wife, mother and manager of the household, while the role of the adult male is primarily anchored in the occupational world, in his job and through it by his status-giving and income-earning functions for the family. Even if, as seems possible, it should come about that the average married woman had some kind of job,

> it seems most unlikely that this relative balance would be upset; that either the roles would be reversed, or their qualitative differentiation in these respects completely erased.

In a footnote to the passage just quoted, Parsons makes the point that, even when women do attain "higher-level jobs," the latter typically mirror the "expressive" components of the "normal" female role.[60]

> The distribution of women in the labor force clearly confirms this general view of the balance of the sex roles. Thus, on higher levels typical feminine occupations are those of teacher, social worker, nurse, private secretary and entertainer. Such roles tend to have prominent expressive components, and often to be "supportive" to masculine roles. Within the occupational organization they are analogous to the wife-mother role in the family. It is much less common to find women in the "top executive" roles and the more specialized and "impersonal" technical roles. Even within professions we find comparable differentiations, e.g., in medicine women are heavily concentrated in the two branches of pediatrics and psychiatry, while there are few women surgeons.

Consequently, in interpreting the relevance of sociological thinking to possible changes in sex roles, we must be aware that such thinking is about men and women viewed as actual and potential parents. The sociological questions that have been asked about sex roles have never strayed far from the basic presupposition that most, or all, persons will and should form families of procreation. Indeed, modern sociology has typically assumed that no structural deviations from parentally defined sex roles can be tolerated (except perhaps in pariah form), since they detract from individual motivation to marry and have children.

Yet, this definition of sex roles is "functional" for the society only in so far as the number of children so produced is actually needed. If the society needs fewer children, far fewer, than will be forthcoming from sex role differentiation on the basis of parenthood, then such differentiation, in its traditional form, is no longer functional. The logic of sociological analysis concerning sex roles may well be correct. However, the conclusions are based on a long-outdated demographic assumption—that the country's problem is to secure itself an abundance of children. If the same logic is applied to our current demographic needs, the conclusion is that role differentiation by sex must be released from its total dependency on kinship, if the country is to achieve fertility low enough to match its highly favorable mortality.

The Legal Identification of Sex Roles with Parental Functions

In a recent review of sex discrimination and the law in the United States, Kanowitz traces the ways in which the law explicitly and implicitly considers issues of sex differentiation in terms of parental roles.[61] Although his study was undertaken to expose the "injustice" of sex-based legal discrimination and its presumed reinforcement of male dominance, Kanowitz acknowledges that it would be a mistake to assume that all (or even most) sex-based legal differentiation disadvantages women in the sense of restricting their rights or elaborating their obligations. On the contrary, such discrimination in many cases defines the obligations of men as husbands and fathers.[62] Indeed, what comes through most consistently in Kanowitz's presentation of American sex-discrimination laws and the philosophy behind them is not a dimension of social stratification, of "advantage" or "disadvantage" of one sex over the other, as much as an explicit legal affirmation of and concern for the differential *family* roles of the sexes, particularly their *parental* roles. The law sees men and women primarily in terms of the reproductive arrangement, and draws its conclusions accordingly. Given the assumption, the conclusions cannot be regarded as affording one sex an advantage—the assumption is that the sex roles are incommensurable and complementary. There is also the assumption that *intra*-sex variability in physique, temperament, or actual achievement of the ideal sex role in society is negligible. Hence, the application to all men and all women of a legal philosophy that assumes universal parenthood seems to be only logical.

However, from a demographic point of view, such a legal philosophy clearly represents a strong pronatalist coercion since the basic assumptions are applied to cases in which role *alternatives* might emerge were it not for the precedent of reaffirming the primacy of marital and parental roles. For example, Kanowitz notes that some of the language used by the United States Supreme Court in the famous case of Muller v. Oregon "was unnecessary to the decision."[63] As a result, this case has often been invoked by the courts in upholding a wide variety of sex-discrimination laws. Indeed, when one realizes that the case involved no more than a consideration of the validity of Oregon's law limiting women's hours of work to 10 a day, the language clearly indicates that the Supreme Court had a larger issue in mind—the issue of reaffirming and elaborating on the sexual division of labor implied by parenthood.[64]

> . . . The two sexes differ in structure of body, in the functions to be performed by each, in the amount of physical strength, in the capacity for long-continued labor, particularly when done standing, the influence of vigorous health upon the future well-being of the race, the self-reliance which enables one to assert full rights, and in the capacity to maintain the struggle for subsistence. *This difference justifies a difference in legislation,* and upholds that which is designed to compensate for some of the burdens which rest upon her. . . .

The success of the Supreme Court's effort at legitimation is measured by the fact that this language has affirmed the principle that "sex is a valid basis for classification." This principle, as Kanowitz says, ". . . is often repeated mechanically without regard to the purposes of the statute in question or the reasonableness of the relationship between the purpose and sex-based classification." [65] With forgiveable sociological naiveté, Kanowitz puzzles over and condemns the influence and immortality that this legitimation has achieved.

> . . . The subsequent reliance in judicial decisions upon the *Muller* language is a classic example of the misuse of precedent, of later courts being mesmerized by what an earlier court had *said* rather than what it had *done*. For though *Muller* was concerned only with a protective labor statute which took account of the general physical differences between the sexes, it has been cited, as Murray and Eastwood point out, in cases "upholding the exclusion of women from juries, differential treatment in licensing various occupations and the exclusion of women from state supported colleges."

The language of Mr. Justice Brewer in Muller v. Oregon is so archaic that we may be moved to dismiss its substance as outmoded as well. We may believe that the *operating* norms of modern Americans do not prescribe either men's or women's roles in such polarized terms—protector and economic supporter of the family at one pole, mother and gentle housewife at the other. However, we have seen that potential challenges to the primacy of motherhood for all women have, so far, been neutralized by prescriptive reproductive norms. Even today, Brewer could be cited as an accurate observer of the "real" norms governing the modern woman—more correct than those who believe that higher education, labor force participation, and feminism have effected "basic changes."

The Imprint of Sex Roles on Personality

The magnitude of pronatalist coercions in human societies, ours included, is far from encompassed by the fact that sex roles are so closely identified with the division of labor according to parental functions. As an added precaution, human societies (and American society is no exception) have built the perpetuation of pronatalist sex roles into the structure of personality through socialization "for" personality traits that are congruent with these sex roles, and "against" traits that could produce conflict with them. Such rigid sex-typing of personality traits doubtless explains, in part, why a change in sex role expectations is so difficult to effect. Intra-sex variability is, as we shall see, systematically suppressed by the socialization process which can, in the case of sex-typing, begin to take place from the moment of birth.

Research concerning socially prescribed, preferred, permitted, and proscribed personality traits for the sexes has not been extensive. However, since the explicit research of Komarovsky (on college populations) in the 1940's, it has continued systematically. Hence, we have a long-range body of data concerning the views of college students with regard to the normatively appropriate traits for men and women. Other data on socialization practices generally indicate that the norms expressed among college populations correspond to differential child-rearing practices for the sexes and that, if anything, college students are more permissive concerning a blurring of sex-typed personality traits than are less advantaged groups in the population.

Komarovsky's work on the inconsistent role expectations by parents for their daughters has already been discussed. We saw that the college girls studied by Komarovsky were encouraged to play a "modern" role of achievement in sports and academic life up to the point when this role (if taken seriously by the girl) clearly began to interfere with courtship. At that point, many of the parents (and even male siblings) of the girls began to lecture concerning the advisability of not allowing the modern role to be carried "too far." In effect, the girls were frequently advised to modify their goals and their behavior so as to be in line with anticipated wifehood and motherhood.

The Komarovsky research also showed, as might indeed be expected, that the traditional sex-role expectations were accompanied by expectations that the young women's personality traits would be congruent with the sex role. In Komarovsky's research, the young women perceived young men as the principal enforcers of such traits since, of course, the men were the active agents in initiating dates and marriage. Girls who did not exemplify the appropriate traits risked being sanctioned by unpopularity with the opposite sex and endured the threat of non-marriage. Komarovsky points out that the desired female personality is "often described with reference to the male sex role as 'not dominant, or aggressive as men' or 'more emotional, sympathetic'." [66]

One of the principal findings of the Komarovsky study was the extent to which her subjects felt called upon to dissimulate their real personalities, to "fake" traits that they did not have and did not evaluate highly—traits of helplessness, dependency, lesser intelligence relative to men, etc. Such deprecating presentations of self were seen by these women as catering to their escorts' need to live up to the role expectation of males—higher dominance, security, and intelligence than that of females. Clearly conveyed to these young women was the fact that existing social roles for the sexes presupposed that males would typically have the personality traits that are congruent with occupational achievement and the demonstration of superior physical strength. Since, in actuality, a high proportion of men may not have these traits in as great abundance as a high proportion of women, maintenance of the male image requires collusion by women. These young women, although at the outer reach of "modernity" for American girls, nonetheless were impressed that "success" for a woman, namely the achievement of the wife-mother role, meant subordinating their personality traits to the personality requirements of sex-role differentiation on the basis of parenthood. The following quotations from Komarovsky illustrate the problem as perceived by her subjects: [67]

> When a girl asks me what marks I got last semester I answer, "Not so good—only one 'A'." When a boy asks the same question, I say very brightly with a note of surprise, "Imagine, I got an 'A!' "
>
> On dates I always go through the "I-don't-care-anything-you-want-to-do" routine. It gets monotonous but boys fear girls who make decisions. They think such girls would make nagging wives.
>
> I am a natural leader and, when in the company of girls, usually take the lead. That is why I am so active in college activities. But I know that men fear bossy women, and I always have to watch myself on dates not to assume the "executive" role. Once a boy walking to the theater with me took the wrong street. I knew a short cut but kept quiet.

Later research has served to substantiate and elaborate Komarovsky's roster of personality traits normatively expected of each sex. The work of McKee and Sherriffs in the 1950's clearly documented that women believe men demand traits of them that are exclusively feminine and restrict them from masculine virtues.[68] And, McKee and Sherriffs found that men actually do wish to restrict women from such "male-valued" traits as being "aggressive," "courageous," "daring," "deliberate," "dominant," "forceful," "independent," "rugged," and "sharp-witted." On the other hand, women are found to desire more of a combination of both masculine and feminine traits in men, than men consider ideal for themselves. That is, women would be more tolerant of a less polarized male, than men would be of a less polarized female.[69] This result may well be because in general, the traits chosen as appropriately "feminine" by both sexes are *evaluated* by both sexes less positively than are the masculine traits.[70] Although women select the more highly valued feminine traits as being also desirable for men (gentleness, sympathy, etc.), men apparently wish to avoid the roster of traits listed as feminine since, on the average, these carry relatively low esteem.

More recently, Rosenkrantz, Bee, Vogel, Broverman and Broverman have also studied college students and found that even in the late 1960's there is clearly defined recognition of personality traits expected of men and women, and that agreement on these traits is very great by both sexes.[71] Moreover, men and women agree that a greater number of traits typically associated with masculinity are socially desirable than those associated with femininity. The list runs as follows: [72]

STEREOTYPIC TRAITS

Male-valued traits

Aggressive
Independent
Unemotional
Hides emotions
Objective
Easily influenced
Dominant
Likes math and science
Not excitable in a minor crisis
Active
Competitive
Logical
Worldly
Feelings not easily hurt
Adventurous
Makes decisions easily
Never cries
Acts as a leader
Self-confident
Not uncomfortable about being aggressive
Ambitious
Able to separate feelings from ideas
Not dependent
Not conceited about appearance

Skilled in business	Thinks men are superior to women
Direct	Talks freely about sex with men
Knows the way of the world	

Female-valued traits

Does not use harsh language	Interested in own appearance
Talkative	Neat in habits
Tactful	Quiet
Gentle	Strong need for security
Aware of feelings of others	Appreciates art and literature
Religious	Expresses tender feelings

The authors also examined whether the self-concepts of their subjects correspond to the stereotypes. The self-concepts and the stereotypes were found to be very similar. The authors say: [73]

> . . . The self-concepts of men and women are very similar to the respective stereotypes. In the case of the self-concepts of women this means, presumably, that women also hold negative values of their worth relative to men. This implication is particularly surprising when it is remembered that the data producing the conclusion were gathered from enlightened, highly selected college girls who typically more than hold their own vis-à-vis boys, at least in terms of college grades. The factors producing the incorporation of the female stereotype along with its negative valuation into the self-concept of the female Ss, then, must be enormously powerful.

Although the results of these studies are not placed by the authors in the context of Komarovsky's older work on dissimulation by women, the data suggest that women find themselves in a situation in which personality traits are expected of them that they do not particularly admire, and that they are inhibited from manifesting traits that they do admire. The generally less-admired traits are those that are judged to be congruent with wifehood and motherhood—concern for appearances, concern for the feelings of others, gentleness, quietness, expressivity of succorant and nurturant emotions. The generally more-admired traits are those making for success in the outside world, but incompatible with the wife-mother role as this is defined vis-a-vis the husband-father and the traits his role requires. A more recent study by Broverman, Broverman, Clarkson, Rosenkrantz, and Vogel brings out the double-standard of evaluation for male and female traits even more clearly.[74] The subjects in this study were 79 clinically trained psychologists, psychiatrists and social workers, all involved in clinical practice. They were given the questionnaire concerning bi-polar traits previously used on college students and asked to designate which pole would be closest to a mature, healthy, socially competent adult male, adult female, and adult of sex unspecified. The male, female, and adult instructions were given to separate groups of subjects. The traits these clinicians assigned the adult (sex unspecified) agreed closely with the traits deemed socially desirable by college students, and, as might be expected, male-valued traits were more commonly designated for the healthy male and female-valued traits for the healthy female. However, such designations when examined substantively meant that: [75]

> . . . clinicians are more likely to suggest that healthy women differ from healthy men by being more submissive, less independent, less adventurous, more easily influenced, less aggressive, less competitive, more excitable in minor crises, having their feelings more easily hurt, being more emotional, more conceited about their appearance, less objective, and disliking math and science. This constellation seems a most unusual way of describing any mature, healthy individual.

As a corollary of this finding, the researchers also discovered that the "adult" and "masculine" concepts of health do not differ significantly, but that a significant difference does exist between the concepts of health for "adults" versus "females." In effect, as they say, ". . . the general standard of health is actually applied only to men, while healthy women are perceived as significantly less healthy by adult standards." [76] Why do clinicians hold such double-standards of health for the sexes? Broverman *et al.* suggest that: [77]

> . . . the double standard of health for men and women stems from the clinicians' acceptance of an "adjustment" notion of health, for example, health consists of a good adjustment to one's environment. In our society, men and women are systematically trained, practically from birth on, to fulfill different social roles. An adjustment notion of health, plus the existence of differential norms of male and female behavior in our society, automatically lead to a double standard of health. Thus, for a woman to be healthy, from an adjustment viewpoint, she must adjust to and accept the behavioral norms for her sex, even though these behaviors are generally less socially desirable and considered to be less healthy for the generalized competent, mature adult.

We thus see that although the differentiation of sex roles based on parenthood is sociologically complementary and unstratified, the personality traits expected of the people who fill these roles differ greatly, on the average, in social esteem. The lower evaluation of feminine personality traits relative to "adult" traits generally, constrains men to attempt to achieve "masculine" traits at all costs (or to avoid feminine ones). One might expect women to have the same reaction, and indeed Komarovsky has shown that many really do at some time in their lives, but such a reaction carries severe sanctions because such women run the risk of not being selected for marriage, or being unsuccessful within it. The absence of alternative sex roles for women forces conformity to the personality traits that are congruent with the parenthood roles and no other. As a result, most women are not psychologically equipped to seek out alternative sex roles, or to switch gears from motherhood to success in the outside world. By virtue of a trained incapacity, their personalities are geared to failure, or only very marginal achievement, in the world of business and professional competition. Consequently, most women are more permanently attached to motherhood as their primary status than might be expected given the economic opportunities in American society. It is thus simplistic and unrealistic to expect economic and career incentives to affect women in the same way that they affect men. Women's personalities have been "adjusted" to sex-role expectations that assume a lifetime of home-centered priorities.

By what mechanisms do the adult subjects of the research cited above acquire such sex-typed personality traits and the belief that these traits are appropriate to each sex? Such research as has been done on this subject—whether on parent-child socialization, social pressures by peers in high schools, or public treatment of individuals who do not conform to sex-typing of personality traits and behavior—all have a common theme. This is the theme of social coercion—of punishment, withdrawal of affection, ridicule, unpopularity, ostracism. Moreover, these sanctions are brought into play not only for major deviations from sex-typing (such as, for example, overt homosexuality), but for what might seem to be relatively minor variations such as being a brilliant and achieving female high-school student (in a coeducational school) instead of a cheerleader and fashionable dresser. One has to appreciate the social pressure leading to "adjustment" to reproductively-oriented adult sexual roles in order to understand that fertility behavior in American society is, at present, far from "voluntary."

Let us begin with a brief discussion of sex-typing by parents (and adults with whom a very young child is likely to be in contact). This process is documented widely in books on child development and indeed is tacitly accepted as part of what parents do "for" their children. Mussen, Conger and Kagan say: [78]

> . . . in general, overt physical aggression, dominance, competence at athletics, achievement, competitiveness, and independence are regarded as desirable traits for boys. On the other hand, dependence, passivity, inhibition of physical aggression, competence at language skills, politeness, social poise, and neatness are some of the characteristics deemed more appropriate for girls.
>
> More parents reward behaviors that they view as appropriate to the sex of their child and punish responses that are considered inappropriate. . . . definite patterns of praise and punishment from both parents and playmates during the preschool and school years put pressure on the child to adopt sex-appropriate behaviors.

The authors point out that, in personal interviews, both boys and girls at ages as young as four to nine say that they feel their parents prefer them to adopt sex-typed behaviors.[79] Mussen, Conger, and Kagan go on to state that the learning of "appropriate" sex-role behaviors in early childhood has its results in adulthood. The degree to which the authors accept as "appropriate" that women are socialized into a feeling of inability to cope with life is well-demonstrated by the following paragraph: [80]

> . . . A large group of young adults was presented with a list of adjectives and asked to select those attributes that they felt were most and least characteristic of themselves. In comparison to men, women felt less adequate, more negligent, more fearful, and less mature. These adult attitudes about the self may be traceable, to some degree, to sex-appropriate attitudes and characteristics inculcated in the preschool boy and girl.

More pressure is apparently required to enforce identification by girls with the feminine role than by boys with the masculine one, since studies have shown that children of both sexes regard fathers as more powerful and competent than mothers, are more likely to imitate a man than a woman, and that boys typically identify with the father but that girls identify about equally with the mother and father.[81]

Pressure for sex-typing occurs at a very early age not only through parental channels, but also it is strongly reinforced in childhood as the peer group takes over increasing control in the young person's life. Mussen, Conger, and Kagan point out that the child's "acceptance or rejection by his friends is determined in part by the degree to which he has adopted traits that are appropriate for his sex role." [82] They go on to point out how pervasive and primary in the child's life is the sex-typed assignment by peers to most activities and behaviors.[83]

One of the largest-scale documentations of coercive sex-typing is in Coleman's study of 9 highly diversified high schools in Northern Illinois.[84] Coleman found that, among adolescents of both sexes, the effect of high school as a scholastic system was neutralized, and even nullified, by the counter-effect of adolescent control over the operating daily goals and activities of the students. Since all of the high schools were coeducational, one aspect of adolescent control was extreme differentiation of sex roles in the school along the lines of physical (athletic) prowess for males and beauty coupled with "activity" (party giving) for females. To be a bright, scholarly student was the least desired "image" for both sexes, and indeed students answering to this description were simply ignored. As Coleman points out, the students were actually expressing in the school situation the real values and goals conveyed by most parents, in counterdistinction to the parental lip-service paid to educational achievement and sexually neutral but desirable character traits. For parents (and many teachers) as well as adolescents, the male athlete is the super-hero and the beautiful, popular girl (the athlete's choice) the super-heroine.

Clearly, in paying the enormous bill that it does for high school education, American society is buying, for most students, not intellectual stimulation and the acquisition of valuable cognitive skills, but rather, just the opposite. Being provided are expensive arenas for male athletes and female cheerleaders, together with their hopeful imitators. Compared with the all-important task of competing in the sexual jungle, school work is defined by adolescents as externally imposed and juvenile. Coleman has suggested that scholarly achievement could be stimulated by making inter-scholastic competitions as widespread as inter-athletic ones. Then the creative scholar could win for his school (like the athlete) instead of merely for himself (as is currently the case). However, Coleman's own data indicate that the situation will not yield to such a tactic. This is because, perhaps unwittingly, parents tend to regard the practice adolescents receive, in activities that are intensely differentiated by sex, as "good training" for adult adjustment. These sexual roles, and not the "new math," are typically what parents themselves understand, and it is to these that they can, by and large, relate. After all, it is in these images that they themselves were socialized.

In sum, although we may take it for granted that the process of socialization is a legitimate and necessary constraint on human freedom, research suggests that socialization for sex-typed personalities goes well beyond the constraint on individuals required for social order. It actually represents the enforcement of the society's commitment to a specific goal—reproduction. One may or may not agree with the goal, but it is hard to deny that the process of reaching it constitutes a mammoth feat of social engineering. Individuals, especially women, are channelled in the direction of reproductive activity, and diverted away from other activities, just as inexorably as if they were under orders from a master planning board. Under such circumstances, the notion of reproductive "choice" is an illusion. Indeed, it may always be an illusion, but there is nothing more voluntary about an illusory pronatalist choice than an illusory antinatalist one.

Conclusion

The formulation of explicit antinatalist policies requires an awareness of existing pronatalist ones. Lacking such awareness, action is side-tracked by a spurious controversy as to whether coercion should be instituted or voluntarism maintained. Actually, as this paper has tried to show, our society is already pervaded by time-honored pronatalist constraints. Thus, I have argued, we cannot preserve a choice that does not genuinely exist, and, by the same token, it makes no sense to institute antinatalist coercions while continuing to support pronatalist ones. Insofar as we wish to move in the direction of stabilized zero population growth, the first job for policy would seem to be to eliminate coercive pronatalist influences in a manner that is minimally disruptive of social order.

The scope of this task reminds us that a demographic revolution has more profound implications than might appear from a mere consideration of birth, death, and growth rates. These are only indicators of a society's ability to cope with the survival problem in a particular way. Behind them lie the social organization and control mechanisms that channel resources into the production and rearing of offspring on the one hand, and the effort to avert death, on the other. Population policy, therefore, inevitably goes to the heart of our way of life. To move from one policy (albeit implicit) to another (perhaps explicit) raises issues that threaten many of our established norms and habits. We are bound to experience anxiety in even thinking about the changes that may lie ahead. On the other hand, to allow a diversion of resources from reproduction may help to resolve social problems that are currently engendered by pronatalist constraints. Certainly our increased reproductive efficiency does not, of itself, imply the need for greater regimentation but rather the opposite. It makes possible a fuller expression of human individuality and diversity. After all, each generation provides us with the raw materials for evolutionary adaptation. The problem of adapting to low mortality is, therefore, not one of browbeating biologically specialized individuals out of behavior that is "natural" for all. Rather, it is one of directing cultural and social institutions into the use of human variability for meeting the new functional demands of a modern, low mortality society. In this endeavor, freedom for the development of individual potential may be greatly enhanced. I seriously doubt that it will be curtailed.

3

Pronatalism in Women's Magazine Fiction *

HELEN H. FRANZWA

Department of Communications, Hunter College, New York City

The birth rate in this country has been declining steadily since 1956, but you would never know it if you were a frequent reader of women's magazine fiction. In that never-never land of romanticism and pronatalism, the birth rate has risen steadily since 1955, and motherhood, recently more than ever, is presented as the ideal condition of woman.

It is becoming increasingly apparent that concepts associated with the traditional feminine role are influential determinants of family size. Clarkson et al. (1970) demonstrated that women who perceive themselves as being "rational, competent, active, mature individuals who are capable of functioning effectively in our society" (traditional masculine stereotype) had significantly fewer children than did women who described themselves as "gentle, sensitive expressive individuals" (traditional feminine stereotype). Although unable to draw a causal relationship between self-concept and family size from their study, Clarkson et al. note that these results provide "support for Davis's and Blake's thesis that the stereotypic feminine social role is a critical factor affecting family size in our society."

Both Blake (1969) and Davis (1967) argue that the stereotyped

Unpublished article, 1973

* The material on which this article is based is drawn from research on the image of women portrayed in women's magazine fiction conducted in 1971. This and related images of women are presented in full in "Female Roles in Women's Magazine Fiction, 1940–1970" in Rhoda Unger and Florence Denmark, eds., *Woman: Dependent or Independent Variable,* Chicago: Aldine-Atherton (in press).

female role specifying motherhood and housekeeping as a woman's sole occupation in life motivates women who accept that role to desire at least moderate-sized families—one or two children not being enough to occupy a significant portion of one's life.

Similarly, Hoffman and Wyatt (1960) argue that the mother of two school-aged children is a "woman of leisure" whereas the mother of five is just as hard a worker as is a working mother. If a woman adopts the traditional female stereotypic role of housewife-mother she may elect to have more children in order to assuage any guilt she may have in living a leisureful life.

The fiction of many women's magazines portrays women in the stereotyped female role of housewife and mother. The research reported here explores the way in which the role is presented. Secondly, the potential influence of this fiction on readers is considered.

Method

Short stories appearing in three women's magazines—*Ladies' Home Journal, McCall's* and *Good Housekeeping* were sampled (every story appearing in two randomly selected issues per year at five year intervals) between the years 1940 and 1970. There were 122 stories in the entire sample. The number of children per fictional family and themes associated with motherhood make up the data that is reported here.

Results: I. Fictional Birth Rate

There were more children per fictional family in the 1960s than at any other time in the study and this birth rate remained relatively high into 1970. At the same time, the number of married major female characters with no children decreased substantially and the number of families with three or more children increased somewhat coinciding with the first and only instances of families in the sample with four or five children.

Discussion

Fictional birth rates have not always been so high nor so unreflective of reality. In a study of fertility values in American magazine fiction, Middleton (1963) demonstrated a close parallel between the actual birth rate and the number of children per fictional family. The real birth rate and the magazine fiction birth rate were com-

TABLE 1

Average Number of Children per Fictional Couple *

Year	*Number of Couples*	*Number of Children*	*Mean*
1940	7	11	1.6
1945	10	10	1.0
1950	11	21	1.9
1955 **	5	3	.6
1960	8	19	2.4
1965 **	3	7	2.3
1970	11	21	1.9

* Couples newly married (less than one year) are not included. Pregnancies presented as the focus of a story are counted as one child. (Most couples were portrayed as being young, only five couples had children who were in their teens or older; it is therefore possible to infer that some of these fictional families were not yet fully formed.)

** The number of stories devoted to married women was comparatively small during these sampling periods.

pared during three time periods—1916, 1936, and 1956. Fictional birth rates rose and fell just as they had in "real life." (The mean number of births per fictional family in the stories Middleton sampled was highest in 1916—1.39; lowest in 1936—.74; it rose again to 1.08 in 1956.)

Earlier studies of magazine fiction explored the hypothesis that it reflects popular cultural values and norms. Berelson and Salter (1946), Johns-Heine and Gerth (1949), and Albrecht (1956) all found support for the hypothesis that magazine fiction reflects popular culture. If magazine fiction does reflect popular culture, then the fictional birth rate of the 1960s and 1970 should have decreased. Instead it rose. Why might this have happened?

Perhaps the fictional birth rate jumped in the 1960s as a part of a deliberate effort of women's magazine editors to intensify their pronatalist editorial stance. Ellen Peck (1971, p. 50) in her book *The Baby Trap* quotes an "editorial merchandising specialist" in support of her argument that editors promote motherhood on behalf of their advertisers:

> So, inasmuch as we're selling domesticity, I guess we're selling motherhood. The situation is kind of a paradox since no matter how merchandisers try to show that being a mom and a homemaker is fascinating, it's essentially not. Breeding is not chic, it is not fun, it is not glamorous . . .
>
> But the simplest way out of the problem is through spending. I mean, you know the old saw about the wife feeling depressed, buying a new hat, and feeling better. Well, it's true. Spending money is

therapeutic. If we can keep her spending, she'll be more satisfied with her role. Now, doesn't that make sense?

How does a magazine editor keep her spending? Peck argues that if the housewife is encouraged to have another baby she will continue to play the role of vulnerable consumer. The fiction in these magazines plays no small part in the promotion of the idea that another baby is a solution to the housewife blues. They also encourage their readers to believe that the housewife-mother role is the best career of all and that the childless woman has wasted her life.

Results II: Themes Promoting Motherhood

A major part of this study was the analysis of the plots for themes indicative of the way women should view themselves. These themes, more than the number of children per family, demonstrate the pronatalist nature of these stories. There were basically two kinds of stories about married women—one promoted the idea that she should be a selfless, devoted and loving helpmate to her somewhat helpless husband. Toward this end, she did not work outside the home (of 55 married women, only four worked; of these, only one —a black woman—did not suffer emotionally for it). The other stories were devoted to her role as a mother and it is the themes associated with this type of story that are reported here.

The Housewife-Mother Career Is the Best of All

Mothers in these stories are portrayed as being the heart and soul of the family. The formula typically revolves around the woman's doubt about herself and her role in the family and it ends with confirmation and validation of her role. It should be noted that this particular theme did not appear in the sampled stories prior to 1960. During the 60s, nine stories had this theme. (Not only were there more children in the families in the stories of the 60s and 1970, but more emphasis was placed on the importance of motherhood in them.)

The most obvious defense of the role appeared in a 1960 story in which a mother of five visits a childless friend who is now fabulously wealthy. The visit is a disaster except that it provides her with validation of herself as a mother. Discovering her emptiness as a person, the mother ends her visit abruptly, answering her protesting friend: "There's nothing left of me to see. I don't exist anymore without my family. That's why I've got to go. I'm a wife and mother. For better or for worse. That's all I want to be." The story ends as she returns to the bosom of her family feeling immense pity for her friend's childlessness.

To Solve Your Problems Have Another Baby

There were four stories published in the 1960s whose formula went beyond the simple reiteration of how wonderful it is to be a wife and mother to the children one already has. In these stories the mother's feelings of loneliness, uselessness and boredom were solved by a timely addition to the family. Regardless of the age of the woman (one woman was in her mid 30's; another was 44) or the size of the family she already had (one had three children already, the others had two) this "solution" was presented as being universally applicable.

Typical of these is the 36-year-old housewife-mother of two (17 and 12) who spends a "long, lonely day" daydreaming about how babies had made her marriage "fresh and young." She decides privately to become pregnant again and then announces to her family that she is expecting a baby. She defends her decision by saying that she feels "lonely and unneeded by everyone. . . . Just a piece of furniture." Although her husband and children accept the idea of a new baby readily, they are astounded that she should feel useless. Her husband validates her role:

> Don't you know the home is built around you? Don't you know it's you we come back to always? What would we do if you weren't here when we come back? . . . The house would be empty and cold, just four walls and a roof, all its warmth and spirit gone . . . a house without a soul.

This theme certainly lends support to the Blake, Davis and Hoffman-Wyatt thesis that the mother who commits herself to the home and family on a full-time basis will feel bored and guilty and will solve her problems by adding to her family.

Pregnancy Takes Precedence over Everything Else

Magazine stories are pronatalist in other ways as well. In two of the stories sampled at an earlier time period, 1950, birth control had apparently not yet been invented. The arrival of a baby in each was totally unplanned and disruptive of the couple's life (to the extent that they were both forced to rely on their parents for financial assistance), but the stories suggested that this is the way life is and that everyone should grin and bear it.

The Childless Woman Has Wasted Her Life

Twelve stories explored the feelings of the childless woman.

In some she was featured; in others the heroine derived personal satisfaction from favorable comparison to childless women. They were frequently described as having wasted their lives. They were characterized as being lonely, bored, guilty, unfulfilled, and unhappy. Those few who had careers (college professor, director of a girl's school) did not appear to derive personal satisfaction from their work. Most childless women were portrayed as dependents who had no outlets for self-expression at all save the unfulfilled one of motherhood.

Typical of these women is the wife of a college professor. A school teacher prior to marriage, she resigned in order to become a housewife despite an agreement that she and her husband would remain childless. After three years at home she is bored and says to her husband, "A good marriage has children in it. . . . It didn't seem to matter at first, but I feel useless. As if I'd cheated life." Her husband finally agrees to have children.

Similarly, a spinster, speaking of herself and her two maiden sisters, says, "Alice and Mae had such empty lives. They never married, they've never had children. . . ." In order to avoid wasting her life and being "a drain" on her parents, a woman marries a man she doesn't love: "She wanted a home; she wanted children." Another childless woman is accused of turning "her husband into the baby she can't have." Still another is described by a mother of five as being "a pauper in this highest bracket of wealth."

TABLE 2

Themes from Stories About Married Women and/or Childlessness

Theme	*Number of Stories with the Theme*
1. Married Women Don't Work	14
2. To Keep Your Husband:	
a. Be Less Competent than He	7
b. Be Passive	1
c. Be Virtuous	4
3. Being a Housewife-Mother Is the Best Career of All	9
4. To Solve Your Problems Have Another Baby	4
5. The Childless Woman Has Wasted Her Life	12
6. Pregnancy Takes Precedence Over Everything Else	2
	53 *

* There were 122 stories in the entire sample. See Franzwa (in press) for the themes of the stories devoted to single women and to widows and divorcees.

No childless woman was portrayed in a way that could possibly be construed as positive. Not one was characterized as happy or contented with life; not one believed she was doing anything worthwhile with her life. In their own indirect way these stories are at least as pronatalist as the ones glorifying motherhood directly, for no woman wants to *waste* her life.

Traditional women's magazine fiction is definitely pronatalist. In those stories in which the woman started out single, the ending was either an engagement or a wedding (only 5 of 65 young, single females in the entire sample did not get mated by the end of the story). The stories that featured married women glorified housewifery and motherhood, and the stories which featured "spinsters" bemoaned their empty, childless lives.

Assessment of Influence

Sociologists and other students of the mass media have been concerned with the effects of the mass media on its audience for some time. Specific interest in the potential influence of the media on women to bear and rear children goes back at least to 1901. In his book, *Social Control,* E. A. Ross stated, ". . . The breeding function of the family would be better discharged if public opinion and religion conspired, as they have recently, to crush the aspirations of woman for a life of her own. But the gain would not be worth the price."

Hollingworth (1916) argued that various social institutions including religion, education, medicine, and law as well as various forms of the media including newspapers, magazines, and art all present women with only one viable alternative in life—that of motherhood. She pointed out that women who have had interests and aptitudes other than motherhood have been stigmatized in articles appearing in the popular press as "dangerous" and "abnormal," "indicative of decay" and having "melancholy." She also noted that only positive images of motherhood are portrayed in the media so that "motherhood will appear to consist of compensations only and thus come to be desired by those for whom the illusion is intended." Quoting articles against higher education for women, she found that the major argument opposing it was that education would divert women from maternity: "the population will suffer"; "the birth rate would fall." Hollingworth ended her article on the following optimistic note: "As soon as women become fully conscious of the fact that they have been and are controlled by these devices the latter will become useless. . . ."

To demonstrate the ability of the various forms of the media to control or even to influence the receivers of their messages is a particularly difficult undertaking. Any decision or behavior that an individual makes is the result of any number of inputs—a message from a segment of the media may be but one of those inputs. Assessing the potential influence of that input is not easy, however, there are ways to infer the nature of the influence.

In regard to women's magazine fiction, one way to infer its influence is to analyze the available data on the readership of these magazines. W. R. Simmons and Associates Research, Inc., a magazine readership data firm, has been collecting data on magazine readers' age, sex, occupation, income, marital state, ages of children, social class, education etc. since 1963. A composite picture of the readership of *Ladies' Home Journal, Good Housekeeping,* and *McCall's* (there being no significant differences in the readership among the three) indicates that the typical reader of 1970 was married (72%), had no more than a high school education (70%), belonged to either the lower middle or working class (82%), had a median age of 42 (this figure is accurate for both 1972 and 1973; the median age of readers was unavailable in 1970), was almost as likely as not to have a job outside the home (44%), and was as likely as not to have had at least one child at home under age eighteen (50%). Except for the proportion of married women readers who work, there was relatively little change in these figures since 1963.

TABLE 3

Percentage of Adult Married Female Readers Employed Outside the Home

Year	*Good Housekeeping*	*Ladies' Home Journal*	*McCall's*
1963	32	34	32
1964	36	33	36
1965	38	38	38
1966	41	41	40
1967	43	42	42
1968	47	43	43
1969	39	40	40
1970	44	44	43
1971	45	46	46
1972	44	46	43
1973	44	46	47

SOURCE: W. R. Simmons. *Selective Markets and the Media Reaching Them,* 1963–1973.

If these magazines do have pronatalist influence, we would

have to predict that their readers would have more children than is true for women as a whole. Although a higher number of children for women's magazine readers than for women as a whole would not *prove* influence, failure to find such a relationship would deny support for the hypothesis. Unfortunately, the necessary data to test such an hypothesis is unavailable. Because Simmons' data only details the presence (not the number of) children in the home for a series of age groups under eighteen there is no way to know the actual number of children a reader has.

It should be noted in passing, however, that the proportion of married readers who work outside the home has increased markedly over the past ten years. In contrast, the vast majority of the married women in the fiction do not work. Leavitt (1973) has found that this is still true of the stories published in 1971 and 1972. If the characters in the stories serve as models to emulate, we would not expect to see such a rise in the number of married readers who work outside the home.

A second way to infer the influence of this medium is to assess the extent to which the readers take the fiction seriously. Again, there is no readily accessible data to indicate reader acceptance of magazine fiction. Anecdotal evidence, however, provides support for the hypothesis that readers take confession-type magazine stories (admittedly another genre) seriously. Kosinski (1973, p. 204) reports amazing acceptance of the realness and importance of these stories. On two occasions he appeared on the "Tonight Show" to discuss his research into the nature of confessional stories, arguing that the stories are not true confessions at all but are fictional and follow highly predictable formulas. He was astonished by the audience response to these remarks: "The countless letters sent to both the network and to me revealed that the majority of the readers considered the magazines accurate in their reflection of 'real events' and accepted the stories uncritically, as vivid slices of contemporary life." He argues that it may be easy to ridicule these magazines and to expose them as unrealistic and biased but ". . . it is impossible to ignore their enormous popular support."

During the 1940s a number of studies explored the possible influence on radio listeners of soap operas. Warner and Henry (1948) carried out an elaborate field research study utilizing as subjects women who typified soap opera listeners (the wife of the "Common Man" whose characteristics appear to be identical to those of the readers in the Simmons data with the exception that the soap opera devotees were all full-time housewives). Warner and Henry found that their subjects believed that the stories and characters in the specific soap opera under study, "Big Sister," were believable and real and they readily identified with them. In contrast, a sample of career women, tested to see if such subjects would respond differently, found "Big Sister" to be unrealistic. They could not identify with the characters, they disliked them and in no way wished to emulate them. Warner and Henry concluded that the soap opera is "essentially an emulatory device where the behavior and morals of the heroine are copied by the listeners . . ." (p. 61).

Conclusion

It is obvious that if a magazine has a particular editorial position that its nonfiction articles would explore and develop that position. It makes sense, too, for the advertising to follow the same editorial line. Although fiction can have anything for its subject, the stories in women's magazines appear to follow an overall editorial position projecting an image of the ideal woman as a home-oriented mother. The extent to which this image of woman is accepted and emulated by readers is difficult to assess. Perhaps it has only the effect of reinforcing decisions already made by those who read it. We might conclude as Warner and Henry did twenty-five years ago:

> Our society, by offering a choice to women between being housewives or career women (usually professional), frequently creates a dilemma for them: The career woman's role is attractive because it is usually of higher status than the occupation of the Common Man level and offers more moral and emotional freedom. On the other hand, such a role is frightening, demands hard work, ability to buck the system, and the capacity for self-initiated action. Most of the life of such women is outside the family. The Big Sister program plays up the importance of the role of the wife and therefore obliquely depreciates the role (career woman) the ordinary listener has avoided, or not been able to take. It helps resolve any conflict she may have within her for not choosing the other role (that once might have been open to her) and reinforces her present position.

4
Television's Romance with Reproduction

ELLEN PECK

Note: "Television's Romance with Reproduction" was prepared for the National Academy of Television Arts and Sciences under the auspices of the Population Institute as part of a preliminary investigation by PI into maternal themes and media images: therefore the project was approached with an alertness to population-ecology implications of these themes and images.

Part I: Programming

Susan, in "As the World Turns," is pregnant.

She is not the only one.

Turning the daytime dial, we see that Susan in "Days of Our Lives" is also pregnant, as are Kate in "Love of Life," Mrs. Donovan in "Love of Life," Ann Jones in "Bright Promise," Kathy in "The Doctors," Alice in "Another World," Chris Cameron in "Where the Heart Is," and Iris in "Love Is a Many-Splendored Thing."

Further, Janet in "Search for Tomorrow" has just had a baby, as have Meredith in "One Life to Live," Edie in "All My Children," Angel in "Love Is a Many-Splendored Thing," Diana in "General Hospital," Linda in "Days of Our Lives," Iris in "Love Is a Many-Splendored Thing," Mary in "Where the Heart Is," Sally in "Love of Life," two women (other than Janet) in "Search for Tomorrow," Carolee in "The Doctors . . ."; and "Another World" 's Pat Randolph has twins.

Prepared for National Academy of Television Arts and Sciences, under the auspices of the Population Institute, 1972

Actually, the birth rate on daytime TV seems to rival that of Latin America!

If the pregnancies *per se* are demographically questionable, the way in which they are presented is often psychologically alarming. All too frequently, pregnancy is shown as woman's way to become the center of attention, retreat from unresolved conflicts, or compete for men.

In "Days of Our Lives," for example, both Laura and Linda are romantically linked to Mickey—Laura as his wife, Linda as his mistress. When Linda's baby was born, Linda said to Laura (rather smugly), "Now we both have a child by Mickey" (the implication being, you no longer have that advantage over me). Laura accepted this natalist competition: when Linda challenged her by saying, "I have never seen a man so thrilled and happy over a baby," Laura counters by replying, "I have—when my son was born."

Another natalist competition is going on in "As the World Turns." Susan is married to Dan, who is in love with Liz (and is, in fact, the father of Liz's child.) Sensing her husband's attraction to Liz, Susan decided to become pregnant, in the hope that this would counteract Dan's attachment to Liz.

Actually, that pregnancy was planned—at least by Susan—which seems to be a rarity on the daytime dramas. Most pregnancies are accidental—for example, Carolee's pregnancy by Steve was "accidental," the result of one weekend spent together. (It might be worth noting that Carolee is a supervisor of nurses and Steve a doctor. Neither, apparently, is aware that the Pill is available, on prescription, at most drugstores.)

Similarly, Kathy now finds herself unexpectedly pregnant by *Dr.* Nick Bellini; Ann Jones, Dean of Women at a college, is pregnant by *Dr.* Brian Walsh; and Chris Cameron, in the midst of a love affair with *Dr.* Hugh Jessop, was very surprised to find that pregnancy can result from intimacy.

(Dr. Jessop happens to be the focal point of yet another "competition by conception." Since Hugh Jessop's affair with Chris began, Hugh's estranged wife, Allison, has tried desperately to seduce her husband and become pregnant as a result, with no success. In a recent episode, Dr. Jessop rejected his wife's advances, then left to spend the remainder of that segment cuddling Chris, who is now very visibly pregnant with his child. The message to viewers is clear: whoever conceives, wins.)

In still another show, no one challenges a new bride's decision to have a child "right away." (Perhaps someone in "Another

World" *could* point out to Alice that the presence of a child during the first two years of marriage *doubles* a couple's chances of eventual divorce.)

In other daytime situations, a mother of two teen-agers has just given birth to her third child; Liz has told her husband, "I want your children—a dozen of them"; and Carolee isn't through yet! Even though her baby is only a few months old, and even though she and Steve are not yet married, she is already searching for an apartment large enough for "half a dozen little Steves."

There is more.

Althea, who is childless, has told Carolee, "I'm so envious of you, you and your beautiful baby." ("Love of Life"), Kate who was not sure she wanted to have a child, was advised, "Don't let any feelings of uncertainty keep you from having a baby. Every new life is a new chance." And Diana, when unhappily pregnant on "General Hospital," was told, "Motherhood is the most wonderful experience a woman can have. Think of the first time the baby splashes you in the bathtub, the first time he sleeps through the night without crying . . ."

Actually, were all pronatalist, glory-of-motherhood-and-reproductive-function comments to be combined and presented to the FCC Fairness Doctrine Committee, daytime TV would owe Zero Population Growth, National Organization for Non-Parents and other similar organizations approximately 18,200 minutes of "equal time" *for the past year's shows alone.**

If the totality of life's joys is to be found in parenthood, then loss of reproductive function is the specter which must haunt every daytime TV character. Sandy reacted to her hysterectomy with nothing short of blind hysteria: "Empty, empty, empty—I'll never feel life inside me again." Women who miscarry are usually institutionalized (Liz seeks psychiatric help in England, Laura at Verde Valley) . . . and men are no less threatened.

In "All My Children," Nick's sterility is causing him such mental duress that his marriage to Anne is troubled; in "Days of Our Lives," Mickey is carefully shielded from knowledge of his sterility because of the traumatic effect this would surely have on his sense of manhood (yes, *Mickey is sterile:* Linda's child was in truth fathered by another man, and Mickey's wife's son resulted from a chance encounter between Laura and Mickey's brother, Bill); and in "General Hospital," Philip, who is impo-

* Figured on an absurdly modest basis of 5 minutes pro-natalist dialog or plot content per show, per day.

tent(!) due to a recent accident, seems more upset by loss of *procreative* ability than sexual ability: remembering a time when he had observed Diana with their baby, he says "Diana—feeding *my son.* I'll never forget it. It was beautiful, just beautiful. That must be what it's all about. My God! How I've been robbed!"

He feels cheated, not of the joy of sex itself, but the chance to procreate more babies to watch Diana feed.

Strong impressions are conveyed here: pregnancy will save your marriage . . . pregnancy will bring you attention . . . motherhood will fulfill you . . . bearing a man's child will make you supremely important to that man.

Any population "positives" on the daytime shows (employment of women, predominance of one-child families) are weak and easily overshadowed by the following factors:

1. Low dramatic value given to women's careers
2. Predominance of pronatalist dialog and plot lines
3. Antinatalist dialog generally reserved for unsympathetic characters (e.g., cold and selfish Erica in "All My Children")
4. The fact that it is pregnancy which unfailingly propels a woman to center stage of dramatic action

Presently, eleven of the fourteen daytime dramas carry strong reproductive themes. Sometimes, several interweave—e.g., in "All My Children," Edie's "earth mother" contentment, the selfish and cold behavior of childless Erica, Nick's temporary sterility. Similarly in "Days of Our Lives," the Laura-Linda natalist competition, Susan Martin's dramatic pregnancy by rape, Mickey's sterility.

We should perhaps say a word about daytime quiz and talk shows. Recently, on "The Dating Game," a contest question was "How many children do you want?" The responses were three, three, and five.

That same week Garry Moore asked a "To Tell the Truth" contestant, "And what do you do?" When she replied, "I'm a housewife and mother of seven children," the audience applauded mightily.

Also that week on the "Mike Douglas Show," someone chatted with an actress about her many hobbies, tennis, art, etc., *then asked: "But when are you going to be a mother?"*

The actress conceded that many friends asked her this, too, often taking her on shrewdly routed shopping trips through baby departments; she felt forced to speak further, explaining rather uncomfortably that she had had a miscarriage or two . . . and in short had to try to answer a question that was *none of anybody's business* but which well illustrates how a woman without children is put on the defensive by society's (and television's) assumption that the duty, glory, and destiny of every woman lies in motherhood.

A chat with talk show interviewers about the impropriety of "maternal chauvinism" on the air might change such unfortunate patterns of questioning. Breaking the conditioned responses of studio audiences to multiparous women is a more challenging matter: one useful approach might be to forego marriage-and-maternity centered "getting to know you" questions for game show guests, and ask contestants instead what they think about the China trip or spring hemlines.

Eventually, as the world turns, day turns into prime evening time, and television sets in 40 million homes continue to glow with projected messages, direct and implied, about the desirability of family life and children.

We are familiar with the happy but fatherless "Partridge Family" (are all fatherless families so happy?), the wholesome, six-kid "Brady Bunch" (can all families that large expect easy affluence and a live-in maid?), the rare mutual devotion of all "Smith Family" members, one to another (all seeming, at times, to be nothing less than commercials for the more-than-two-child family).

Then, recently, "Colombo" explained to a jilted girl, "Don't worry, same thing happened to my niece. But now she's married to a nice guy and got six kids." (Could eventual happiness have been equated to something other than "six kids?") In a "Walt Disney World," a girl who runs a riding academy explains why she didn't marry a wealthy equestrian and travel the world: "I didn't want the patter of little hooves. I want a two-legged family."

In February, "Marcus Welby" action centered around a pregnant woman in an episode that was excellent dramatically but heavy with pro-pregnancy propaganda. Sample dialog. Mr. Carpenter to his wife: "Pregnancy agrees with you. You get more beautiful every month." Dr. Welby to Mrs. Carpenter: "You've got a pretty good track record—secretary to bookkeeper to wife . . . and now motherhood." Later, referring to pregnancy, Dr. Welby says, "It's a pretty good prescription." (A good prescription, Dr. Welby, for the estimated 250,000 women who physically abuse their children every year? A good prescription for those 30,000 women who will, in 1972, abandon their homes and children? The prescription of pregnancy, Dr. Welby, has a side-effect: parenthood. While pregnancy can seem pure romance, parenthood involves responsibilities: responsibilities which not every woman is equipped to face.)

And . . .

The writers of the "Dick Van Dyke Show" have taken Dick's beautiful and talented middle-aged wife (who has already raised two children) and sent her back to the diapers!

A few episodes from last season's Dick Van Dyke series deserve examination. (They call this one "Off and Running," I call it "I Didn't Mean Us.")

> *Situation.* Dick hosts his own talk show. After interviewing author and commending the book *Overpopulation Begins at Home,* Dick returns to his own home to learn that another child is on the way. He and Jenny already have a 16-year-old son and a 9-year-old daughter.
>
> *Sample Dialog.*
>
> JENNY: You've always been so outspoken about the dangers of overpopulation and how responsible couples should replace only their own number . . .
>
> DICK: Honey . . .
>
> JENNY: Didn't you mean what you were saying?
>
> DICK: Yes, but . . . I didn't mean us.
>
> (*I didn't mean us . . . Not Forest Hills . . . not in my neighborhood . . . I didn't mean us . . .*)
>
> *Later.*
>
> JENNY: What are you going to say to our son, the ecologist?
>
> DICK: I'm going to tell him that Mommy and Daddy are good and concerned citizens . . . but that we love babies a lot . . . and to have only two kids when he gets married.
>
> *Denouement:* The profound discussion on which the final decision is ultimately based:
>
> DICK: Do you want three?
>
> JENNY: Yes.
>
> DICK: So do I. So let's.

There is a new message here—not "with blithe disregard for the population crisis, have as many children as you want," but "be aware of the population crisis; *then* have as many children as you want."

Frankly, that is small improvement.

Add to Jenny's pregnancy this one . . .

In an episode they call "The Birth" (I call it "The Birth," too) Jenny picks up a hitchhiker and brings her home to stay overnight. The girl is unwed and in her ninth month of pregnancy. A heartwarming story unfolds . . . in contrast to the real fates of many unhappy, abandoned pregnant girls, the boy who had left Debbie returns to her; the parents who had rejected her find and forgive her; and all ends happily in the hospital (where she and Jenny deliver babies at the same time).

In still another episode, Carol leaves Bernie because of his resistance to having a family: he's not ready, he says. Dick invites Bernie to move in. Carol is lonely, so Jenny invites her to stay in their home as well. After much maneuvering by Dick and Jenny, there is a happy ending. Bernie finally says he's willing to start having a family. . . . (Now, it is common in sociology to regard as "unwanted" a child who is unwanted *by either partner*. And it is common in marital counseling to find trouble resulting from this. Surely, children should result from neither carelessness, nor coercion.)

The Barbara Eden-Larry Hagman network movie "Howling in the Woods" carried a similar theme, however, featuring this closing dialog between the estranged husband and wife:

> HE: Why did you leave me?
> SHE: You didn't want to have children.
> HE: Yes, I always said I wasn't ready for children. But when I read your note and realized you'd left me . . . suddenly I was ready for children.

I'd like to suggest a variation that might have worked just as well:

> HE: Why did you come back?
> SHE: A better question might be, why did I leave?
> HE: I know why . . . you were bothered that I didn't want to have children.
> SHE: Yes, but after being away from you for a while, I realized that it's not children that matter—it's you . . . it's us.

Notable in "The Jimmy Stewart Show" was an echo of the "never too late" theme: an older man proving his virility by having a child late in life. (Might he not just as easily have proved his altruism by *adopting* a child late in life?)

There seemed something dangerously Panglossian about Jimmy Stewart's town, Easy Valley, as reflected in such speeches as, "We need a college of our own, here in Easy Valley, so that we can keep our young 'un's here . . . so they won't have to go dashin' off to the big cities and the big colleges . . . so that they can stay right here in Easy Valley and have young 'un's of their own to raise . . . 'cause it's towns like this that give our country its real strength" (and social myopia? and population problems?).

Television has done a good job with some old messages: "We've got a big country here," say the Westerns; "Motherhood is destiny," say the soaps; "Kids are fun for everyone" imply the evening story lines; "Life's real and high adventure is wiping up spills," say the advertisers. (Any problems? Drop two Crayolas in water. . . .)

The measure of the extent to which these messages have been absorbed into the public consciousness may lie in the following story:

Last year Senate-House Joint Resolution 108 was introduced, cosponsored by 35 senators. Recognizing the dangers posed by this country's continued population growth, S.J. 108 would have called for "a United States policy on achieving population stabilization *by voluntary means consistent with human rights and individual conscience.*"

S.J. 108 was endorsed by a commission created by Congress last year to study population issues. During hearings on the resolution, various experts testified that, with continued population growth, we will have more pollution . . . more congestion . . . more social disorganization . . . more destruction of wilderness and wildlife . . . more government controls and restrictions . . . and higher and higher taxes. Stewart Udall warned that we are "at the edge of" rationing of our national parks and wilderness areas *and will see such rationing within the decade;* it was Assemblywoman March K. Fong's regretful opinion that "our children's children are likely to wake up one morning to find that space and materials are too scarce to sustain them."

What happened to this resolution? Despite widespread support on Capitol Hill, significant negative public reaction and much misunderstanding resulted. One senator reported receiving several hundred negative letters within a few days, some blindly objecting to "total government control and restriction of American families."

S.J. 108 was a gentle and democratic resolution that would have been important symbolically for all our citizens. It was dropped by the Senate Labor and Public Welfare Committee, Senator Alan Cranston reluctantly announced in late November.

And it will not be reconsidered this year.

Meanwhile, Janet in "Search for Tomorrow" had her third child . . . a program on vanishing wilderness was being prepared which would not mention population . . . Dick Van Dyke laughingly gave only lip service to population problems . . . a contemplated abortion did not occur in "Bright Promise" . . . eighteen product commercials featuring four or more children appeared on network TV within one week . . . and, sometime late in 1971, even as newscasters brought us reassuring reports that our birthrate was dropping, the population of the United States rose from the 207 millions into the 208 millions.

It is not all television's fault.

Yet—if we are concerned for the survival of a planet already overburdened and exhausted by excess of human life, we must also be concerned about the power of television to affect natalistic attitudes. For television certainly has this power.

Surely, we all have seen how the media *can* reach out, re-shape attitudes. In just four years, for example, public attitudes regarding the Vietnam war changed dramatically—due in no small part, it is agreed, to exposure and examination by the media.

If the media could raise to consciousness our motives for an unjust war, the media might, likewise, bring to light motives for reproduction other than "convenience" or romance.

Television, as a particularly powerful medium of communication and entertainment, has a clear responsibility to create new, non-natalist programming approaches. Such new approaches will better serve a society in which children have too often been the victims of our casual attitudes towards reproduction—and a society which is just beginning to learn that it exists within the context of a finite world.

Part II: Commercials

No overview of television's influences would be complete without a look at those persons and industries who pay for air time: the advertisers. Thus, for one week in February 1972, a staff of volunteers conducted an unusual (and somewhat nerve-shattering) survey, observing and monitoring all network commercials aired during that period.

The intent of this report is to provide a sampling of *typical* pronatalist influences in commercials; and, by these examples to alert the television viewer to the existence of pronatalism in other commercial and media messages.

Since the nature of the pronatalist influences within commercials varied discernibly, categories of commercial pronatalism have been defined. Sample commercials cited within each category are representative but do not in all cases constitute a complete list: in some instances, only one example was chosen to illustrate a category, with this one example being more fully described and commented on.

Throughout, researchers' parenthetical remarks will be found.

No excuse is offered for the frankly subjective nature of these remarks: viewing thousands of commercials (which were overwhelmingly trivial in content when not clearly pronatalist in bias!) during the same time period when the M.I.T. population-ecology study *Limits to Growth* reached public attention was sufficient to provoke occasional indignation and even sarcasm.

The ratings and categories were arrived at by the Special Projects staff of the National Organization for Non-Parents, with advice and comments from insurance company executive Kenneth P. Veit and psychiatrist E. James Lieberman, M.D.

After examining a sample of two thousand commercial exposures (some repeats), researchers found that 33 percent of daytime commercials and 14 percent of those seen after 6 P.M. were objectionable for one or more of the reasons stated herein.

Examples of Objectionable "Pronatalist" Commercials, Grouped According to Reason for Objectionability

I. Large Families Used as Product Sales Tool

Notable among the many such commercials viewed were St. Joseph's Aspirin ("I'm Alice Cook. I have six children, and they come in all shapes and sizes. So do their colds"); Cold Power ("Mrs. Ray Dennison has four kids, and endless laundry"); Rain Barrel ("Anita Scheem has a growing family. She does fourteen loads of laundry per week"); Ruffles Potato Chips ("I have a large family and nine grandchildren"); and Hour After Hour Deodorant ("I have four kids and I really need it").

Large family scenes were also presented by Q-Tips, Carnation, Fleischmann's Margarine, and Florida Orange Juice Association, among others.

The cumulative effect of such presentations works at counter purpose to population awareness, by creating the feeling that having many children is still to be regarded casually; it may mean you need a little extra laundry power or more deodorant, but there is no suggestion that such a reproductive decision carries any implication for the larger society.

Particularly worrisome in this regard was the Swanson TV Dinner commercial which showed five children at the family dinner table. The announcer began, "Man has been eating meat for a long time . . . ," and went on to extol the virtues of the product in question. Actually, though man has been eating meat for a lengthy period of time indeed, the stark rules of overpopulation are beginning to nudge people of many nations down the food chain toward vegetarianism. The size of our future population here in the U.S. will be a factor in how often meat can appear on our tables. If many couples choose five-child families, that won't be often!

II. Idealized Family Situations

These were considered objectionable, even if only one or two children were presented. An example we will cite is an Oldsmobile Cutlass commercial. Here, the car is a gift to Mom from Dad and the (two) kids. The picture given is one of easy prosperity: a nice home, a spacious lawn, well-dressed family members—and a new car as well.

The fact that the average family of four experiences some financial strain seems virtually uncontestable; thus our concern in this category and several others is that "idealized" really amounts to "falsified." In this Oldsmobile commercial, information about the economics of a two-child family is being transmitted along with the product information. Two messages are being telecast: (1) Oldsmobile Cutlass is a nice car; (2) the two-child family is a nice family unit. Though the first message is direct, and the second subliminal, in effect both Oldsmobile Cutlass and the two-child family are being "sold."

III. Idealized Father-Son, Mother-Daughter Relationships

Part of the myth of motherhood and apple pie is a close, sisterly relationshp between a teen-aged girl and her mom; and accompanying the "mom-and-apple-pie myth" is a "fatherhood-and-outdoor-activity-with-son myth."

These strict sex-role segregated images of parenthood are among the greatest sales tools going; and we see them in such commercials as Con-tac (Dad "takes the boys up to the cabin"), Wheaties (Dad shoots rapids with son), and Geritol (teen-aged daughter says, "Mom, you're incredible. . . . I hope I look as good as you when I grow up").

Now, in these commercials the *direct messages,* or product claims, are possibly to be believed: Con-tac cures colds, Wheaties taste good, Geritol builds blood. But the *indirect messages* which say that parenthood brings loving respect from children and a wonderful companionability are to some extent unreliable (given the evidence of generation gap and alienated youth which surrounds us). We have a sneaking suspicion that "Mom, you're incredible . . ." is not always said in a loving tone of vóice.

Mother-daughter closeness *happens,* certainly, as do father-son camping trips; but that isn't all there is to parenthood. Sibling rivalry, illness, school problems, minor accidents, and trips to the dentist are realities of family life too—as is occasional overt hostility between the generations.

False claims about products are regulated by the FTC; false "claims" about parenthood are not: therefore advertisers should assume a certain responsibility for *fair* representation of parental relationships and family life when they use these as sales tools.

It might seem to be asking a lot to suggest that advertisers abandon idealized situations as backgrounds which frame their products in an alluring way. But the time may come when viewers are so sensitized to the unreality of such settings that this commercial technique will no longer work. Direct information about products, given *with* supportive evidence and *without* emotional gimmicks, might be an alternative worth considering.

IV. Problems of Parenthood Solved by Product

Franco-American Spaghetti (child decides not to run away from home when Mom fixes it), Del Monte Dessert (child decides not to run away from home when Mom fixes it), Pine-Sol ("cleans up any dirty thing that happens"), Johnson's Floor Wax (deals with Jimmie the Scuffer), and Scott Towels (which easily wipe up the "45th spill of the day") are examples here.

Here, problems of parenthood are at least presented—but with a total lack of gravity. These power-of-the-product commercials should certainly be used with less extravagance.

No doubt Johnson's Wax can erase scuff marks, and Scott Towels absorb the forty-fifth spill of the day; but these cleaning products can*not* be expected to be of emotional aid to the distraught mother who faces these minor but cumulatively annoying cleanup tasks. Scott Towels may *help*—we doubt that they will turn a frantic mother into a serene one, as in the commercial!

V. Sentimentalized Image of Children as Sales Tool

In a Pampers commercial, several children stand over a baby's crib and discuss Pampers. One child then says, "I'm going to tell *my* mommy that *I* want a new baby brother, too." Frankly, one wonders what is being sold: Pampers? Or babies?

A Hershey Chocolate commercial tells us, "There is nothin' like the face of a kid eatin' a Hershey bar." There is also nothin' like the face of a kid havin' a tantrum! Here more camera time and more song copy are devoted to children than are given to the product. Again, what is being sold? Hershey bars or children's faces?

This category also includes commercials which simply use children gratuitously; in instances where children are irrelevant to the product message, their use seems nothing less than exploitation of the sentiment associated with children. Such exploitation represents questionable advertising ethics. A few such examples include Ivory Snow (men compare diapers washed with different products and cuddle the "Ivory Snow baby" at the end of the commercial); Maxwell House Coffee ("It was our first house in the suburbs, our first baby. Fran dropped over for coffee and I fixed Maxwell House"), FDS Feminine Deodorant Spray (mother and child run through meadow as announcer discusses product), and Sterling Salt (a baby in a highchair is asked if he does not prefer Sterling brand salt!).

VI. "Madonna Image" as Sales Tool

Though closely related to the preceding category, it is felt that this particular and distinctive image needs special attention. Enshrined in art and poetry as it has been through the centuries, the devotion of a mother to a new infant has probably become the most potent of all pronatalist media devices.

We will cite a Gerber commercial which features a beautiful mother and baby, with the following gentle song as background: "Jenny Rebecca, four weeks old, how do you like the world so far? There'll be slides to be sliding on, toys you can wind up. . . ." After other childhood delights are alluded to in the song's lyrics, an announcer's authoritative voice concludes, "Gerber makes strained foods for the most important person in the world: your baby."

The response of Dr. E. James Lieberman, former Chief of Child and Family Studies, National Institute of Mental Health, to this commercial was strongly negative. In Dr. Lieberman's opinion, the suggestion that one's baby is the most important person in the world is "indefensible . . . an effort to promote a product by exploiting parental sentiment, at the expense of children and the larger society in general."

We are reminded of a story once told by author Martha Wienman Lear, a story about "a courageous loner who quit the PTA because others refused to broaden their horizons. 'I told them we couldn't help ourselves unless we helped others,' she said. 'I told them, We need a new school. Ten blocks away they need a new school too. Now why don't we think about this and examine our needs and theirs and see where it is really needed more?' And they jumped on me and yelled, *'What do you mean, needed more? Our children come first!'* "

("Our children come first" . . . "The most important person in the world: your baby.")

We are reminded also of family counselors Rustum and Della Roy, who have written of "the gross selfishness in our culture that encourages noble phrases such as 'It's your duty to your children' and 'The family comes first.' The family ends up as a veritable sponge, sopping up any loving concern which might reach the world outside. . . ."

The world outside? Does that matter—compared to "the most important person in the world: your baby"?

It seems to us that it is dishonest to lull viewers into thinking that the future of today's children will be filled with naught but beautiful things, when, given ecological realities, the future world may be filled with difficulties beyond description. Just as regrettable is the microcosmic view of this commercial, which suggests that "your" baby is better somehow than other babies (or children, or adults). Such a point of view abets an unconscionable egoism.

VII. Pregnancy Used as Product Sales Tool

This technique should be placed high on a list of advertising practices to be abandoned! When pregnancy is used to push a product, pregnancy is often pushed, *along with* the product. Consider the following examples:

Rolaids. "When I was pregnant, I took Rolaids . . ."

Cheer. Husband says, "Thought I'd help out around the house before Joan gets home with the baby." (Suggestion: could a husband be helpful in a non-natal situation?)

A-1 Sauce. Her husband says, "Now that you're expecting, I don't want you to lift a finger . . ." (Here, too, the message is pregnancy-brings-solicitousness: thus the pregnancy becomes more than just a background situation for a product sell but a condition that is in itself enticing.)

Playtex Nurser. A pregnant woman tells viewers that she used Playtex Nurser for her *last* baby, thus projecting a "baby machine" image. (Could a woman instead possibly say, "Having a baby is serious business these days. You're not sure what the future will be like, or what kind of parent you'll be. But one thing I am sure of is Playtex Nurser . . ."?)

Pregnancy is also suggested to viewers by the "Have a baby"

themes of Johnson's Baby Shampoo and Johnson's Baby Lotion commercials. The latter, for example, begins: "Having a baby can do great things for your hands." Is this *really* what is meant? If it's the *lotion* that helps hands, why not simply suggest that viewers try it? Similarly objectionable is "There is nothing like having a baby to help you discover the best shampoo for your own hair."

VIII. "Generation After Generation"

A Nationwide Insurance commercial shows a closeup of a baby in a crib. An off-camera voice announces, "Some day, little fellow, years from now, believe it or not, you're going to retire. But meanwhile Nationwide will give you insurance protection *for the years when you're raising your own family. . . .*"

This type of commercial assumes that the pattern of the past will be the pattern of the future—that parenthood for all will continue to be the expected norm. Other examples include:

Bumblebee Tuna. ("Do you remember when you were little, your mother served you Bumblebee tuna. Now that you're a mother, you'll serve Bumblebee tuna to your own child") and a Gold Medal Flour spot in which Mom remembers baking her first cake with *her* mom, and is now baking that same cake for her child. Jell-O, Polaroid, and Campbell's Soup were among other advertisers who presented commercials with this theme.

Our objection here is to the suggested inevitability of parenthood ("for the years when you're raising *your own family*"), to say nothing of the incredible implication that the future will be cozy and untroubled.

IX. Supermom

This particular variety of pronatalist commercial message presents motherhood as synonymous with superior wisdom or abilities. The image of the overly devoted mother is a common one in this category. Examples include:

Safeguard. Wife tells husband of its advantages.

HE: What are you, a soap expert?
SHE: I'm a *mother*.

(Preferable responses: "No, I'm just clever." "Not really, but I'm learning." *"Yes."*)

Nyquil. "To husband, kids, and dog, she's the Rock of Gibraltar." (Could we request some variations on this theme? Perhaps, "To her husband, office staff, and Sierra Club chapter, she's the Rock of Gibraltar"?)

Correctol. "You the mother, you the wife, you the woman . . ." (Note order of importance!)

Hunt's Snack Pack. "Tastes like somebody's *mom* just made 'em." (A radical thought: is it possible that people who aren't mothers might be good cooks?)

Geritol. Man to wife: "Gee, honey, you're incredible. You take care of the house and kids all day, you meet me at the train . . ." To Geritol goes the dubious distinction of being cited in two of our categories.

During daytime hours, of the 1000 commercials sampled, a total of 326 (approx. 33 percent) were found objectionable. The food and beverage product category contained the highest percentage of objectionable commercial exposures (39 percent objectionable) followed by household products (35 percent objectionable) and health, personal hygiene and other personal use categories (31 percent objectionable). All other product categories considered together were found to have only 14 percent objectionable commercial exposures.

Specifically, the daytime figures reached are:

Of a total of 308 personal products commericals sampled
97 (31%) objectionable
204 (66%) unobjectionable
7 (2%) commendable

Of a total of 340 food and beverage commercials sampled
133 (39%) objectionable
205 (60%) unobjectionable
2 (⅔%) commendable

Of a total of 223 household product commercials sampled
78 (35%) objectionable
143 (64%) unobjectionable
2 (less than 1%) commendable

Of a total of 129 sample commercials from other product categories
18 (14%) objectionable
111 (86%) unobjectionable
0 commendable

We note that (1) category most in need of improvement is the food and beverage category, with 2 out of 5 offensive; further, a very high percentage (33 of 133 or about one fourth) of objectionable commercials within this category use two-or-more-child families as sales vehicle; and (2) "commendable" positive, nonparental daytime images were practically nonexistent, outweighed 30 to 1 by pronatalist commercials. (The evening ratio here was somewhat better: 12 to 1. Still hardly "equal time.")

Of the one thousand after 6 P.M. commercials sampled, a total of 139 (14 percent) were found objectionable. In contrast to daytime hours, here 19 percent of personal product commercials were objectionable; 15 percent of food and beverage commercials were objectionable; 15 percent of household product commercials were objectionable. All other product categories considered together were found to have 6 percent of commercial exposures objectionable.

In the after 6 P.M. hours,

Of the total of 304 personal product commercials sampled,
57 (19%) objectionable
237 (78%) unobjectionable
10 (3%) commendable
Of the total of 272 food and beverage commercials sampled,
41 (15%) objectionable
231 (85%) unobjectionable
0 commendable
Of the total of 170 household cleaning products sampled,
26 (15%) objectionable
142 (84%) unobjectionable
2 (less than 1%) commendable
Of the total of 254 sample commercials from other categories,
15 (6%) objectionable
239 (94%) unobjectionable
0 commendable

We note (1) the sharp drop in objectionable food and beverage commercials, from 39 percent objectionable in daytime hours to 15 percent objectionable after 6 P.M. and corresponding sharp drops in other categories, which suggest strongly that advertisers need not be tied to pronatalist approaches; but that (2) while there was a definite *decrease* in objectionable commercials and a definite *increase* in unobjectionable commercials, the overall rate of commendable commercials did not improve—but remained constant, at just about, or just under, 1 percent. We had expected better.

Though the purpose of this study of commercials was to evaluate pronatalist and pro-parental influences, we must add a word about certain commercials which are objectionable from a somewhat different frame of reference. We call these "Growth is Good" commercials. An example is the series of Eaton commercials, one of which proclaims, "EATON MOVES IT. EATON HARVESTS FORESTS. EATON SHOVELS THE EARTH. EATON MOVES ALL KINDS OF MATERIALS . . ." We are left with the uncomfortable feeling that Eaton will bury us.

The underlying "Man vs. Nature" theme is unjustifiable. Given a finite world and limited resources, Eaton's continuing projection of a growth mentality makes little sense. Eaton might well investigate the recent, major study conducted at M.I.T. and published under the title *The Limits to Growth.* We suggest that Eaton associate itself with a new word: *equilibrium.*

Much as we regret this Eaton commercial series and other "Growth is Good" commercials, we again note that they do not fall within the framework of this particular study, and were therefore not rated as "objectionable" within our percentage figures.

Similarly, though the intent of this project was to investigate pronatalism rather than sexism, we could not help but note a dominant theme of the subjugation of women in commercial messages: when a woman was not serving children's needs, she was usually serving *someone;* often, a fully capable adult woman was shown docilely taking orders from a male announcer about how to cook or clean her floors. Again, for purposes of this particular study, sexist commercials were rated "objectionable" only if they contained pronatalist elements as well.

Unobjectionable Commercials

The majority of commercials in our sample were "unobjectionable" (64 percent in daytime hours, 86 percent after 6 P.M.). These were not pronatalist, did not exploit parenthood, children, or family life. Generally these were product descriptions, demonstrations, or animations; or, if situational or emotional, they employed situations or pulled on emotions other than parental ones (e.g., many personal products used romantic themes).

Commendable Commercials

We found some small number of commercials (less than 1 percent) to be commendable. These did not exploit maternity, extol family life, or glorify parenthood or children. Further, they illustrated positive (sometimes imaginative) alternatives to such advertising practices—by showing modern images of women in non-maternal roles and even non-domestic situations. Examples:

Bayer Aspirin. Features fashion designer Betsey Johnson, who exemplifies career woman, new lifestyle

Olivetti. A secretary finds *her career* aided by an Olivetti typewriter! (The woman is finally out of the kitchen—but only a secretary; not yet the boss.)

Handi-Wipes. "Have 1,001 uses and can be used over and over," says a woman who is polishing furniture in an antique shop. (We applaud the "re-use" emphasis as well as the imaginative departure from the domestic setting in which most commercials for such products occur)

Drive Detergent. Again, we are out of the house. Women test the detergent in a laboratory setting and prefer it without enzymes

Vicks Formula 44. "Karen Jackson, teacher, has withstood all kinds of attacks. But when she gets a cough . . ."

We would like to see more commercials such as these, which show women in new roles. No product or service need rely on glorified family images in their advertising. This becomes obvious when the following contrasting examples of products and services within the same general category are considered:

Examples:

Objectionable	*Unobjectionable*
Rain Barrel. Mother plus many children. "Anita Scheem has a growing family. She does 14 loads of laundry a week. She uses Rain Barrel . . ."	*Nu-Soft.* product closeup. "Nu-Soft smoothes out wrinkles you used to have to iron out. Nu-Soft is recommended by the following famous manufacturers: Martex, Lady Pepperell . . . (others)"
Mutual of Omaha. girl to boy: "What if I marry you and you get sick and we have babies to take care of? I can't marry you until you call Mutual of Omaha . . ." *Nationwide.* (baby in crib) "Some day, little fellow . . . you're going to retire. Meanwhile, Nationwide has insurance for the years when you'll be raising your own family . . ." *Lincoln National Life Insurance.* Children, children, children, and more children at a birthday party scene. "Love plus children equals life insurance."	*Metropolitan Life Insurance.* "Florida's everglades are dangerous. Here's a man who volunteers for civil air patrol to rescue those lost here. He's a Metropolitan agent. Helping others is what Metropolitan people do on their job—and on their own time, too. At Metropolitan, we sell life insurance, but our business is life."
Fleischmann's Margarine. One commercial has four children and	*Blue Bonnet Margarine.* "At Pavillon d'Elysee in Paris, we asked

husband in background, another has four children, parents and grandparents . . .

some of the most famous food authorities in France to taste gourmet dishes cooked in butter —and those cooked in Blue Bonnet margarine." In French accents, the experts conclude that "There is no *difference!*"

We are not against commercial advertising. We commend, in fact, commercials which are straightforward (Nu-Soft), socially aware of the larger world of the community (Metropolitan Life Insurance) and those which explore non-domestic sales situations with imagination (Blue Bonnet Margarine). We suspect that such approaches would meet with more positive consumer response than the tired, domestic, fix-your-child-this-and-he'll-smile dramas, anyway.

We *are* against commercial advertising which ties itself to mother's apron strings. We are against natalistic commercial advertising.

It is 1972. Demographer Nathan Keyfitz foresees chronic levels of semi-starvation for all nations within the lifetime of today's children. Other demographers, such as Dr. Lincoln Day, advise us that we need, not zero population growth, but *negative* population growth (*fewer* than two children per family) if we are to survive. Dr. Aurelio Peccei, director of Fiat, Olivetti, Italconsult, and other corporations, has created the Club of Rome to warn all nations of crucially destructive economic and ecological effects of continued population growth. Jacques Piccard, reporting in Geneva in late 1971, warned that we have already destroyed 30 to 50 percent of all ocean life, and our rate of destruction is accelerating. Others in Geneva spoke of changes occurring in the oxygen balance of our planet, while the impartial computer banks at M.I.T. were preparing for us a solemn message: all population growth projections end in collapse.

Bringing all this to our doorstep, demographer Judith Blake has warned us that this nation must immediately substitute antinatalist policies for pronatalist ones. Advertising, as a source of wealth and influence, should lead towards this goal.

In view, in fact, of the demographic, nutritional, economic, and environmental projections, any continuing pronatalism on the part of advertisers can only be judged as grossly irresponsible and grossly anti-social. We hope such policies will not continue.

"Some day, little fellow, believe it or not, you're going to retire . . ." *Maybe.*

5

Pronatal Influences in Home Economics Texts in a Junior High School

NANCY COX

State of Maryland Commission on the Status of Women

Sexism in textbooks is under attack. From pre-school picture books, to post graduate texts, traditional attitudes about women's (and men's) abilities, assertiveness, and emotional "nature" are being challenged. Those sweet, passive little girls who were in the shadow of adventuresome, slightly troublesome little boys are beginning to be replaced with more realistic models. Pressure is mounting on schools to buy course materials that show examples of women in non-traditional vocations. These are the success stories.

There are stories less successful. In home economics and family life texts, assumptions about the inherent natures of men and women are obviously and blatantly misguided; nonetheless, they have been virtually ignored in the critiques of textbooks. Feminist criticism has invaded nearly every academic discipline, but perhaps because the role structuring in the home economics field has been so readily apparent, there was not enough challenge in listing what was objectionable about this education of young women.

Elements of Pronatalism

What is objectionable (but often overlooked) are the persistent assumptions that women will become wives and mothers—that motherhood is automatic in marriage, and that all future life choices will be in addition to this fate. In general, women have

Unpublished, 1974

been the targets and victims of these pronatal ideas. Women are being programmed to want children and to feel primary responsibility for children. So far, women's liberation has only focused on "liberating" women from being or feeling primarily responsible for the care of children and the home. But until women are really free from the social precepts proclaiming that every woman's duty and destiny is motherhood, we will have to acknowledge that freedom from 50% of baby and home care is just another form of tokenism.

The following criteria are helpful in identifying pronatalism in textbooks:

1. Inevitability of parenthood assumed
2. Childfree lifestyles and/or marriages not acknowledged
3. Childfree marriages treated as problematic or undesirable
4. Adherence to theories of maternal instinct or maternity as central to women's life
5. Bias against abortion, adoption, or the only child
6. Failure, when appropriate, to discuss methods of contraception

The fight to eliminate pronatalism is the last battle against sexist thought. Legally and socially, women are being recognized as athletes, students, professionals, and laborers. Discriminatory laws are being attacked with vigor by civil libertarians who recognize that the time for sexual equality is at hand. Men and women are filing complaints of sex discrimination in record numbers. (In Maryland, slightly over one-third of all complaints of job discrimination filed with the Equal Employment Opportunity Commission for the first nine months of 1973 were based on sex discrimination. The pattern is nationwide.)

In addition to equal educational and employment opportunities, sexual equality has been translated into demands for:

1. pregnancy leave compensation, defining pregnancy as an illness
2. programs for universal day-care
3. men and women sharing, 50–50, the task of raising children.

But these demands do not remove the heavy chains of "biological destiny." There is not enough emphasis placed on equal opportunity to bear or not bear children, and the battle for universal contraceptive and abortion services is merely a skirmish. In *Everyone Was Brave: The Rise and Fall of Feminism in America* (1968) by W. L. O'Neill makes this comment: "The original feminists had demanded freedom in the name of humanity; the second generation asked for it in the name of maternity." It's not my point to question the demands for day-care, pregnancy compensation, or male/female sharing of childcare. It is my point to question these demands as the rallying cry of "every woman's rights."

There are deeper, more vital needs that are central to establishing women's total sense of freedom from all cultural and biological constraints, and these needs must be voiced. It's not enough that women can "have their cake and eat it too" (i.e., have children and day-care), if they are still denied "the staff of life," the right to make their own decisions about rearing children.

This background about what are the present concerns of the women's movement is important for an investigation of texts that deal with young women's futures. For no matter how many photographs are used depicting men performing household chores and taking care of children (not just "helping" women do these tasks), these books will remain objectionable if they perpetuate the attitudes that the route to happiness is through parenthood, that mature people will find the greatest joys in their lives in being parents, or that the greatest gift a woman can present her husband is a baby. As often as these statements are true, they are unconscionable as statements of *universal* truth.

One other point should be raised. Great strides have been made in the legal fight against "channeling" girls into home economics without giving them any chance to take an industrial arts course. At this early stage of the struggle for non-sexist education this fight has been crucial. That may be one of the reasons why a frontal attack hasn't been waged against the home economics textbooks. The reasoning might be that it's more important to remove the barriers preventing girls from taking printing or metal working or drafting, than to challenge the home economics curriculum.

Even if girls in home and family courses are there by choice, they should not be misled by a glorified picture of motherhood. We cannot ignore the real need to examine home economics textbooks to see what attitudes and pressures prevail.

Textbook Selection

In an effort to arrive at an objective and representative sampling of actual books in use, this paper will survey all the textbooks being used in the 1973–4 school year by one junior high home economics department in the Baltimore County school system. Of the eighteen books in use, nine could be considered as strongly pronatal. Some claimed to be written for the students' future needs as wives and mothers; others imagined the reader as the bride (for "your" wedding) or mother (when "your" child); all nine presented an unbalanced, strongly idealized view of the nature of children.

Six of the texts were mildly objectionable. If they made assumptions about parenthood, they were not continually reinforced; they were, in general, concerned with the present needs of the students in the course.

Three were frankly excellent books, free of any overt pronatal bias. They were designed for the students' present and future needs and directed the students toward professions where they might practice the home economics skills they were learning. These texts were remarkable in that they were attempting to provide the female student with skills that would help her become self sufficient.

Specific comments on texts follow:

Child Growth and Development
Elizabeth B. Hurlock, Ph.D.
Webster Division, McGraw-Hill (4th Edition, 1970)

Dr. Hurlock debunks the myth of parental instinct yet assumes the inevitability of parenthood. Note the beginning and conclusion of the following paragraph from the preface:

> Gone are the days when it was believed that bringing up children was guided by a 'parental instinct.' Today it is recognized that men and women must learn to play the role of parents just as they must learn to play any other role in life. . . . It is hoped that the material in this book will help the students of today, who will be tomorrow's parents.

If Dr. Hurlock had written ". . . this book will help the students of today, *some* of whom will be tomorrow's parents," her book would have acknowledged the idea of free choice as regards parenthood.

Preparation for parenthood is mentioned, but what is suggested is too little, too late.

> Ideally, all preparation for the new baby—physical, material, and psychological—should begin as soon as the doctor informs the woman that she is pregnant.

Where does the notion come from that the preparation for a baby is something that begins *when a woman is already pregnant?* Is this an "ideal" situation?

A caption under a picture of a baby reads: "But whether it is a boy or a girl, most families soon accept the child to be exactly what they need to make a happy family." No evidence is offered to support this idea. Dr. Hurlock did write "*most* families," so perhaps she is aware of exceptions. Then the question is: why has she failed to discuss why *some* families do *not* find a child "exactly what they need to make a happy family." Certainly, such sentimental over-simplification as this photo caption offers seems unsatisfactory.

In studying a book on child growth and development, certain questions arise: Why study this material? Is this topic relevant to students' needs? Should this material be studied at this time? (The book does not provide satisfactory answers.)

Should we be teaching child care in junior and senior high school with no prior mention of birth control and family planning? (This book does.)

Should we assume that all girl students who take this course will be mothers? (This book makes that assumption.)

Should a book on child care be directed only to females? (This book is.)

Should we assume a desire for motherhood, apart from marriage? (This book emphasizes a woman's relationship with a child and does not develop satisfactorily the idea that the decision to have a child should be *mutual* and based on a good *marital* relationship.)

Or could this book be set up to give its readers a course of instruction which equips them to care for children, without making the assumption that child care means a mother-child relationship? (Hopefully so. Love between adults and children need not be based on biological ties.)

The Developing Child
Holly E. Brisbane with Dr. Audrey Palm Riker
Charles A. Bennett Co., Inc., 1965

Photographs and text frequently conspire to idealize parenthood. For instance, opposite the title page is a full page picture of a beautiful couple; the husband's hand rests on his wife's back while they lean over to watch their baby smiling up at them from a crib. The caption reads: "Caring for and guiding the development of your own children is one of the greatest experiences —and rewards—in life." The preface continues this theme: "Another intent of this book is to help adolescents in their preparation for parenthood." Lest there be any doubt that this book is pronatal, the first unit is titled: "Looking Toward Parenthood."

The authors dabble in what could be an invigorating discussion of how girls and boys assimilate their "sex-roles." That the discussion never materializes is a definite shortcoming of the text.

If you are a girl you are engrossed in accepting and clarifying a

> mature feminine role, pointing toward the kind of woman you want to be. . . . Without conscious awareness you absorbed an entire set of cultural expectations: girls become wives and mothers; girls wear skirts; girls don't have fist fights . . .
>
> If you are a boy you must learn to become a man with all the attendant responsibilities imposed by Western culture: men become husbands, fathers, heads of families, breadwinners.

While the text does suggest that much of these roles is imposed by the outside society, it does not encourage the student to question if he fits (or wants to fit) the type casting.

The following is a somewhat balanced view of what motherhood entails. Unfortunately, the authors do not consider that with the possibility for "disillusionment and unhappiness," motherhood may not be best for all, that some women may not "accept and welcome" this role.

> On the mother, more than anyone else, rests the responsibility for a healthy family relationship. Her adjustment is perhaps the most difficult to make, especially if the coming baby will be her first child. Though she accepts and welcomes her new and deeply satisfying role as a mother—at the expense of her former freedom—there are adjustments that she may find at times emotionally trying.

To mc, the most disturbing point in the book is its myopic disregard for the condition of children of the rest of the world. The authors totally disregard that the U.S. might have its own population and poverty problem. They make an irresponsible statement about the future of the American baby, without any thought that this might not be so. There is no sense of connection between the U.S. and India; instead, the contrast between the U.S. and India seems purposefully drawn to show how the situation in one country has no bearing on the other.

> The average American baby today will grow taller, heavier and suffer fewer illnesses than any one of his ancestors. He will live seventy or more years. This is because he will eat better food and enjoy more material comforts—television, automobiles, prepared foods—than most other people in the world.
>
> If this same American baby were born in the streets of Calcutta, India, his daily diet would consist of a little rice and whatever else he could scavenge. He might never know a roof over his head. He would live half as long and his growth would be stunted.

There is no discussion of the need for family planning in either India or the U.S. On the following page the text reads: "Children come with marriage. Well adjusted parents, even if the baby is not planned for, will accept and welcome him with love and affection." This is a totally indefensible statement. Instead of being fed this kind of pablum, students need information about family planning and the responsibilities of parenthood.

Homemaking for Teenagers
Book II (3rd Edition)
Irene E. McDermott, Jeanne L. Norris, Florence W. Nicholas
Charles A. Bennett Co., Inc., 1972

Some simple arithmetic might sum up this book's viewpoint.
"Marriage and a Home of Your Own" gets 11 pages.
"The Single Woman" gets ⅔ of a page.
"Child Development" gets 43 pages.
The Childfree Adult gets 0.

"Why study child development?" the text asks rhetorically, and then proceeds to list a number of reasons ending with:

> Are you really so much younger than your friends who are marrying and starting a family?

This kind of question not only acknowledges the fact of early marriage, but has the appearance of approving of teen-age parenthood.

Because this text was designed for high school use, it was used only as a resource book in the junior high. The high school student would benefit greatly if the section on "The Single Woman" were augmented to give practical advice to help a young woman feel that she could be self-sufficient if she did not marry.

Learning About Children
Rebekah M. Shuey, Elizabeth L. Woods, Esther Mason Young
J. B. Lippincott Co., 1969

To their question, why is it important to learn about children, the authors respond:

> An understanding of children is necessary for future parents. The . . . reason for learning more about children is that most of you will be parents yourselves in the not too distant future . . . Good parenthood depends on an understanding of children . . . If you have a chance to watch and think about them now, your role as a parent will be more satisfying both to yourself and to your offspring.

The authors assume an eventual parental role. Their advice would be better if it encouraged students to observe children with an open mind and an attitude of questioning *whether* they would actually find the role of parent "satisfying."

The blanket assumption that "*Most* of you will be parents in the *not too distant future* . . ." (emphasis mine) is unfair. It is particularly irresponsible in a textbook written for junior high school students. For these students, whose average age is fourteen in the ninth grade, the "not too distant future" may often mean months and not years. This book gives no suggestion of an optimum age for parenthood and no suggestion of other priorities that a student might have before embarking on parenthood.

The authors develop a checklist quiz asking "What are the characteristics of a good baby sitter?" Sample considerations include, among others:

1. Do I really like children?
2. Am I dependable and responsible?
3. Do I think of children's interests before my own?
4. Am I calm in emergencies and can I be firm when necessary?

A similar checklist should cover "What are the characteristics of a good parent?" but unfortunately this does not appear.

A chapter entitled "Looking Ahead to Marriage and Children" begins:

> Many of you are looking ahead to the time when you will be independent and *will marry and have children* . . . Young people planning to *marry and have children* carry a responsibility for having good physical and mental health. (emphasis mine)

There is no discussion of marriage without children. It is misleading to presume that these two institutions (marriage and parenthood) are unfailingly "wedded" and irresponsible to imply that everyone who marries will, or should, decide to have children.

Continuing, we find a value judgment applied to the decision to have children:

> Most new babies are looked forward to with eager anticipation. However, parents-to-be have to be ready to give up some of their former *more self-centered life* together. They must be ready to care for the baby they have created and to *share their own love in a more mature way*. (emphasis mine)

That first word, "*most*," raises an unanswered question about some of the other new babies whose parents are *not* looking forward to their arrival "with eager anticipation." What are the contraindications for deciding to have children?

Another question needs asking: is it fair to program a student to believe that a childfree marriage is more "self-centered" than is having a baby for the sake of whom a couple will "share their love in a more mature way"? Or, does such an attitude reflect a discriminatory bias in attitudes of the authors?

Later, the authors say

> After experiencing the birth of their first baby, parents are more at ease when additional babies come.

Is this patently true? What are parents more relaxed about? The amount of time they have to spend with each other? Or perhaps their eased financial situation with the added children? These are considerations the authors failed to take into account.

Visual elements of this book must also be mentioned: captions under photographs of babies and children served no useful purpose of instruction. Rather than pointing out a child's needs or requirements based on the photos, the authors felt it would be more entertaining to offer cute comments such as "I love my big hat and I am not going to take it off." This may be an endearing gimmick to use in a family album—it seems entirely out of place in a junior high school text which purports to be an objective and meaningful guide to *Learning About Children.*

Personal Adjustment, Marriage and Family Living
Judson T. Landis and Mary G. Landis
Prentice-Hall, 4th Edition, 1966

This book is suggested as a resource book. Let us proceed immediately to what is objectionable:

1. *Pro-Nuptial Bias.* "Most marriages are happy," say the authors, offering as evidence only one questionnaire study in which 80% of 792 married people indicated that, if they had it to do over, they would again marry the same person. For the statements, "75% of the married people *in your town* (emphasis mine) are happy or very happy in their marriages," and "Even in Hollywood, the majority of marriages are happy," the authors offer no evidence at all.

2. *Pronatal Bias.* "Evidence in our society indicates that many couples are not prepared to be good parents," the authors say. "Homes fall down on the job in many ways," they admit. However, they then proceed to urge "preparation" and "education" for child-bearing in order to fit all adults into the Procrustean bed of parenthood. The premise that all adults should be parents has been criticized by diverse authorities, none of whose views surfaces here.

3. *Bias Against the Only Child.* The one-child family is not viewed as acceptable by the authors. Couples unable to have more

than one biological child are urged to consider adoption.

4. *Bias Against Adoption.* The authors then proceed to warn: "Couples need to examine their own motives as honestly as they can before adopting a child. If they want him because they believe having a child will help hold together a shaky marriage, they are expecting the impossible . . . If they wish to adopt in order to have a child to carry on the family's business or continue the family's achievement socially or in a profession, they are likely to try to fit the child into a mold that may not be right for him . . ."

These reasonable considerations are viewed as a bias against adoption principally because the authors do not suggest that it might be in order to examine one's motives before having bio-children.

Teen Guide to Homemaking
Marion S. Barclay, Frances Champion, Jeanne Hayden Brinkley, Kathleen W. Funderburk
Webster Division, McGraw-Hill Book Company, 1972

Assumption number one is made in the first chapter: "As boys and girls mature, they find joy in fulfilling their roles as males or females . . . many women find fulfillment in working roles *as well* as in their roles as wives and mothers." (my emphasis) Whether a woman works or not, she is expected to become a mother.

The photographs in the text are advertisements provided by various manufacturers. The view of "family life centered around growing children" provided by these professional models posing before carefully planned backgrounds is idealistic, unrepresentative, misleading, and in questionable taste.

The following are quotations taken from the text ("Being a Parent"):

> The job of parenthood is, in a sense, the most responsible job a person ever accepts. With parenthood comes the responsibility for the growth and well-being of a child, whether natural or adopted.
>
> The father's role includes financial, child care and family leadership responsibilities. Even when the mother works, if there is a father in the home, he is usually the major wage earner . . . He is a family leader and projects this image to the children . . . It is not at all unusual to see a father and his children buying the week's groceries. Nor is it strange to see him doing the laundry.
>
> The mother's role usually includes the major responsibility for the smooth running of the household, whether or not she works outside the home.

This idealized concept of "father" and "mother" playing their respective roles is often unrealistic. The discussion would be of greater benefit if it asked what factors are considered most important by researchers, psychologists, doctors, and parents for success in being parents.

A chief criticism is the over-emphasis on the study of the child's development without more directly relating this study to the life of the child who is reading this textbook. Or is the relationship merely the assumed one that every girl in the junior high who studies this book is eventually to become a mother? The emphasis of the book is misplaced because the parent-child theme is dominant (not the baby-sitter-child theme) and the effect is to assume a life pattern that teens will be "homemakers."

The discussion about children begins with visits to obstetricians. Where is there mention about visits to Planned Parenthood or discussion of birth control, which many couples choose to practice before embarking on their first child? The omission is glaring.

Teen Horizons at Home and School
Dora S. Lewis, Anna K. Banks and Marie Banks
Macmillan Company, 1970

On the cover of *Teen Horizons at Home and School* is a photograph of a wooden doll house. Its four compartments are filled with what represents, in all probability a teen-aged girl's horizons. The first room contains a large baby bottle, teddy bear and rocking horse; the second contains buttons, thread, scissors and thimble. In the third are lipstick, nail polish, mirror, comb and a porcelain doll's head. The fourth is filled with antique furniture in an elegant living room. From first glance, it is apparent that these teen horizons are somewhat limited.

The opening definition of "family" is good:

> What does the word "family" bring to your mind? Probably a picture of a group of people who provide for one another's basic needs and who perform special functions for one another . . . the purposes of *most* (emphasis mine) families are to bear children and raise them . . . We *often* (again, emphasis mine) think of a family as a father, mother, and their children . . .

From this point, however, the book fails to live up to its promise of providing an enlightened, modern view of family lifestyles. Quickly, the words "husband" and "wife" interchange with "mother" and "father." The text does *not* discuss childless families or families with adopted children. It does acknowledge that "sometimes cousins live as 'children' in a family" . . . Family ties are thus regarded as biological.

Here is how the family life cycle is described:

> A wedding ceremony brings a young couple into the *newlywed* stage . . . After the first baby comes they enter the *expanding family stage* . . . As more children come into the family, the family reaches the *crowded years* . . .

and finally, the text discusses the *empty nest* and *retirement* stages. Families are thus assumed to have quite a few children—and when they're gone, the home is an "empty nest." (Implication: something's missing?)

While there is a discussion of the advantages and disadvantages of siblings (and even the advantages of being an only child!) the emphasis is on the normality of sibling groups. A caption under a photo of four children says, "In a large family, children have a chance to adjust to many different personality types and . . . different ages." Are the authors saying that children in small families cannot have similar opportunities to adjust to others?

The book was published in 1970 and has made certain accommodations to the women's movement. However, despite a discussion of how sex roles are developed, the authors don't encourage the student to question the assumptions of sex role stereotyping:

> Sex was the first factor to influence your role in life. You know that people treat boys and girls differently almost from birth . . . Such differences in treatment continue throughout life, and they explain why men and women form strong ideas concerning what is "right" for each of them to do.

It is interesting to note the caption under a picture of a little girl playing with her doll: "Children's games are a preparation for life's roles. Playing with dolls strengthens a little girl's idea of the roles of *wife and mother*." (emphasis mine) The authors present this early stereotyping as an automatic way of life.

The section entitled "Manners and Morals for Moderns" is totally inadequate, especially since the entire discussion of sexual development is viewed as a matter of morals. Whereas great care is taken to tell teens how to make proper introductions ("It is good form to say 'Jane, may I present Bill?' ") no such specifics are offered regarding matters of sex. Further, note the pronatal progression from developing sexual interests to an interest in parenthood:

> Sexual maturity moves from shared interests and relations with members of the opposite sex, to the development of real love, and to the foundation of new families.

The authors neatly sidestep any frank talk about sex development, totally ignore contraception, and face the consequences of sexual activity with a short burst of morality: "When young people misunderstand the nature and purpose of sexual feelings, they may act in ways they later regret."

Might there not be far less "later regret" if writers of books such as this abandoned their marriage-push and baby-sell and answered relevant questions that junior high school students have about their own sexuality?

Better Homes and Gardens Baby Book
The Editors of Better Homes and Gardens
Meredith Corporation, 1969

This book is highly sentimental, conveying a sense of almost reverential excitement about the satisfactions of having a baby. Such a perspective may not be inappropriate for adult, expectant parents for whom the book is intended; it *is* out of place for junior high school students.

Any teacher wishing to use this book as a resource should take great care to develop a balanced view about childbearing, since the book itself will do nothing to build students' concepts of reproduction as a great responsibility.

The New Seventeen Book of Etiquette and Young Living
Enid A. Haupt
David McKay Co., Inc., 1971

The book jacket reveals a pronatal bias when it assumes that "girls will be accepted as workers and thinkers, as well as being potential wives, mothers and hostesses." Again the old pitch is made that it's fine for a female to think and work—as long as she doesn't lose sight of her future role as wife, mother and hostess. In support of this conjecture: five chapters are directed to the reader's own engagement and marriage. From the chapter, "You're Engaged," through to the actual ceremony, the subject of the wedding is "you."

Discussion of wedding etiquette generally is not appropriate for this age student. Often getting involved in the pomp and circumstance of weddings can influence a young girl into believing that what she wants is to be married, when all she really wants is to be the bride in a big show.

The six following books were rated mildly objectionable.

Experiences in Homemaking
L. Belle Pollard, Helen H. Laitem, and Frances S. Miller
Ginn and Company, 1968

This book concentrates on the student's present needs. For instance, the section on childcare is geared to what the babysitter must know.

However, the authors do promote parenthood when they say, "One of the most rewarding experiences of life is to have your own home and *your own* children." (my emphasis) They also add that, "Most children compensate for any trouble they cause by bringing their parents much joy and pleasure." This kind of unsupported statement is not in the best interests of the students. Nor is it socially responsible to over emphasize the biological relationship between parent and child ("your own children") when the emotional and intellectual relationships are so much more affecting.

Foods in Homemaking
Marion L. Cronan & June C. Atwood
Charles A. Bennett Co., Inc., 1965

The authors discuss the matter of teen-age marriage and motherhood as an outgrowth of the nutrition section. They point out the importance for girls to have mature bodies with established habits of good nutrition before embarking on motherhood. In its favor, the tone of the discussion is matter of fact. On the other hand, the text could have developed more discussion on teen-age marriage and childbearing practices, instead of simply accepting the trend toward teen-age pregnancies.

Guide for Today's Home Living
Hazel M. Hatcher and Mildred E. Andrews
D. C. Heath and Co., Inc., 1966

This is a fine book for teen-agers. It treats students in the context of being a member of their family and does not try to motivate the student for some future time as parent. At one point in the text, the authors do state that what students will learn about child development can help in earning money as well as in marriage and parenthood. The chief objection to an otherwise well-balanced text is that once marriage is mentioned, parenthood seems to be close behind.

Practical Nutrition
Alice B. Peyton
J. B. Lippincott Co., 1962

This is a resource book on nutrition. Intended for the practical nursing student, the author notes she hopes it "will serve as an authoritative source of information for the homemaker and individual." Note the use of the term "individual" outside of any role. This is an example of role-free writing.

However, the author falls into the stereotyping trap in discussing the goals of adolescents. She assumes that "since girls of this age are looking forward to marriage, they should have some understanding of the importance of good nutrition in preparation for pregnancy." This is an example of pronatal, sexist writing. However, the remainder of the book is excellent in its objectivity.

How You Plan and Prepare Meals
Byrta Carson and MaRue Carson Ramee
Webster Division, McGraw-Hill Book Company, 1962

There is no discussion of the single woman, although a distinction is made between "wife and mother" so that the two are not always synonymous. In other parts of the text, however, the "host" is also called "father" and the "hostess" is interchangeable with "mother." To the extent that this exists, the book would be considered pronatal; and to the extent that virtually only men are shown in professional roles related to food handling and women as homemakers and consumers, the text is sexist.

In its favor, the book presents a Child Care section in which the student is considered the babysitter, not the future mother.

Understanding and Guiding Young Children
Katherine Read Baker and Xenia F. Fane
Prentice-Hall, Inc., 1971

This book was anomalous: it clearly states that some couples will find personal fulfillment without having children; however, occasional generalizations to the effect that most readers are awaiting the time of marriage and parenthood weaken this insightful statement.

And, in future editions, could the topics "The Only Child," "The Adopted Child" and "Children Whose Mothers Work Outside the Home" be placed in a section other than "Handicaps and Crises"?

The following three texts were considered free of pronatal bias:

Becoming Myself
Walter J. Limbacher, Ph.D.
Pflaum Standard, 1972

Teachers wishing to discuss how children learn the sex roles that society casts them in will find Chapter 14, "My Growth Into Adolescence," an excellent resource. This is an innovative book which presents young people's real experiences and emotions with which students can identify and gain in self-understanding.

First Foods
Marion L. Cronan and June C. Atwood
Charles A. Bennett Co., Inc., 1971

The text does not assume that cooking is done for a family or by a woman. Consequently the book is relevant to male and female students and encourages learning about foods as an essential part of becoming self-sufficient. Especially significant is the last chapter, "Jobs Ahead," which focuses on careers in food and gives tips on how to succeed in interviews.

Lessons in Living
Martha J. Davis and M. Yvonne Peeler
Ginn and Company, 1970

The subject of child development is introduced in the following way:

> Someday you may be working with children. You may be a baby sitter or work in a nursery school. You may have children of your own . . . You will enjoy children more when you understand them.

In the section "Love and Understanding," emphasis is not on parent-child relationships but rather on how everyone, including the reader, can show affection for a child.

Conclusion

Textbooks will not change overnight and old editions will remain on bookshelves. But if teachers and students are aware of a pronatal bias in some of their texts, they can begin openly to question biased statements or underlying attitudes.

Simply recognizing pronatalism can help to counteract its effects.

6

Is There a Relationship Between Childlessness and Marriage Breakdown?

ROBERT CHESTER

Department of Social Administration, University of Hull, England

Summary

The common belief that childlessness is positively associated with instability of marriage derives from official statistics which appear to show higher divorce rates for childless than for fertile couples. The official findings are a procedural artifact, however, and the relationship shown is certainly exaggerated and possibly spurious.

The appropriate strategy in determining whether divorcees are relatively infertile is to find a population with disrupted marriages and measure its fertility experience. In doing so it is necessary to take note of the definition of fertility, the remarriage factor, and (most importantly) the duration of marriage. The official statistics use the conception of legal duration of marriage. Since this ignores separation before divorce, its use exaggerates the infertility of divorcees, as does failure to exclude remarriages. *De facto* duration of marriage (wedding to separation) is a superior statement of opportunity to conceive, and calculations on this basis eliminate or even reverse the fertility differential between divorcing and stable couples. Local figures are used to illustrate this effect, and the finding is supported by evidence from a sample of marriages ending in legal proceedings lesser than divorce. It is concluded that the alleged relationship between childlessness and instability of marriage is probably either non-existent or the reverse of that normally assumed, and that in any case measure-

From *The Journal of Biological Science,* 1972

ment of the net overall effect of childlessness does not provide a helpful datum. An alternative strategy of research is suggested, which would seek patterns of effect rather than net overall effect, taking heed of relevant variables, and also considering all forms of marital breakdown including marriages in which cohabitation continues only with disharmony.

Introduction

There is a common and persistent belief that childlessness is positively associated with instability of marriage. Popular credence is documented by Slater & Woodside (1951) and Klein (1968), but the notion that childless marriages are more prone to disruption is also widely manifest in professional literature on the family in this country. The alleged relationship is variously interpreted, but its existence is for the most part somewhat casually assumed, and is deduced from official statistics showing that childless couples figure more prominently among those divorcing than among those remaining married. Only Dominian (1968) among recent writers seems to question the proposition, despite the fact that American research findings cast doubt on the existence of the relationship in the USA, and despite also the general failure of research to find a uniform relationship between children and marital satisfaction (Hicks & Platt, 1970). The question at issue is whether couples who divorce are more often childless (or have fewer children) than comparable couples who remain married. This paper seeks to show the need for a more refined approach to the analysis of the relationship between childlessness and marital stability, and will suggest that (a) the association found in our official statistics between childlessness and divorce is at least in part a procedural artifact; and that (b) the deduced association between childlessness and marriage breakdown is in consequence certainly exaggerated and possibly spurious.

Terminology

At the outset it is necessary to be clear on meanings, since there are differences between disciplines in terminological usage which sometimes create confusion. Bio-medical (and French demographic) convention uses "fertility" to refer to reproductive potential, whereas English-speaking demographers use this term to denote reproductive performance, and reserve the word "fecundity" to describe potential. Because of the nature of the data to be used it is intended here to follow English demographic usage, so that an infertile woman is one who has not yet produced a live-born child, irrespective of her potential capacity to do so. The terms "childless" and "infertile" are therefore used interchangeably in what follows, and this should be kept in mind. In some discussions it seems likely that the author has slipped from one meaning of infertile to the other, with consequent loss of clarity in argument. For the present purpose, all marriages and functionally equivalent sexual unions are initially infertile, and cease to be so when the woman has produced a live-born child. Matters relating to infecundity and its possible effects on stability of marriage are not an issue here, although, of course, they are proper topics for other investigations.

The Alleged Relationship and Its Interpretation

A relationship between childlessness and divorce is commonly asserted or assumed rather than examined. Walker & Whitney (1965, p. 161), for instance, claim that "Divorce rates are highest for childless couples, and progressively decline with size of family." Similar statements can be found in Johns (1965, p. 49), Fletcher (1966, p. 141), Turner (1969, p. 62) and Farmer (1970, p. 133) who states, "Divorce rates are comparatively high between childless and one-child couples who have been married for some years." Humphrey (1969, p. 6), in a study of involuntary infertility, claims that one in five of childless couples divorce, against only one in twenty of fertile pairs. This fallacious conclusion is reached because, having defined infertility as being without issue after 15 years of marriage, he attributes all childless divorces to the small group of ultimately infertile couples, not noticing that at any time the proportion of the married population not yet fertile is higher than the percentage who never have children. Misunderstanding of statistical data is found also in McGregor, Blom-Cooper & Gibson (1970, p. 76) with regard to matrimonial proceedings lesser than divorce. Taking for granted a relationship between childlessness and divorce, these authors comment apropos of one table that, ". . . childlessness is as much a factor in the breakdown of marriages which come to the magistrates' court as it is in those which result in divorce." But the same page reports that the infertile proportion of the sample was 18%, which in fact is less than the figure (20%) reported for married women in the 1961 Census.

Those cited above share an unsatisfactory strategy in that they treat childless marriage as a category of inquiry, and comment on the marriage breakdown experience of the infertile married population. This approach is unfruitful, because the likelihood of fertility has a temporal dimension, and the currently infertile population ranges from those just married to those with more than 50 years of marriage duration. The more appropriate procedure is to seek a population of disrupted marriages in order to measure its comparative fertility, holding relevant variables (and particularly duration) constant. This approach is used by the Registrar General (1964) in arriving at the conclusion that those divorcing are relatively infertile, but, as will be shown, some inappropriate units of comparison are employed in this calculation.

Interpretations of what is taken to be a fact vary. Sometimes there seems to be an assumption that the presence of children stabilizes the marital relationship, while sometimes the emphasis is less on the positive effect of children and more on the negative effect of childlessness. Alternatively, and more subtly, it is suggested that childlessness may be an index of unsatisfactory marital adjustment rather than a causal factor in marriage breakdown. Here it is supposed that there may be abstention from parenthood by couples who are uncertain of the viability of their marriages, or that childlessness is manifest among those reluctant to forego personal freedom and therefore resistant also to full marital commitment. Other contributory possibilities suggested are latent homosexuality, repugnance to childbearing, "selfishness," and accommodation problems. Popular opinion finds support in the commonsense notion of couples remaining together "for the sake of the children," ignoring the fact that divorce may thereby be postponed rather than averted, and that sometimes the presence of children may itself be productive of marital disharmony. What these diverse ideas have in common is that they may be seeking to explain a relationship which does not in fact exist.

Official figures published in 1964 appeared to show both that family size is smaller for those divorcing and that the rate of infertility is higher. The proportion infertile was given as 30% for the divorcing couples, against 18% for those remaining married, with mean family sizes of 1.44 and 1.80 children respectively. However, although the correct logic of analysis is followed in this calculation, the data to which it is applied are unsatisfactory in various ways. Several American writers, and most notably Monahan (1955), have examined the apparent parallel association between childlessness and divorce in the USA, and have been sceptical of its validity. Some evidence now available prompts similar scepticism of the alleged relationship in Britain, and in considering this issue three matters in particular require scrutiny. These are (a) the definition of "children"; (b) the remarriage factor; and (c) the duration of marriage. The distinction must also be kept in mind between divorce and the more embracing concept of marriage breakdown. Childlessness need not necessarily bear the same relationship to both categories, since extrapolation from divorce to the wider concept is a hazardous exercise (Chester, 1972b).

The Definition of Children

The official comparison of fertility experience is based on divorce court returns on one side and census figures on the other, and "children" are differently defined in the two cases. The Census enumerates all legitimate live births, irrespective of survival. The divorce courts, however, are concerned with surviving "children of the family." This is a legal concept, and includes issues of the marriage, children born to one party and "accepted" by the other, and adopted children. The court returns thus include some children not born to the couple and omit any of their children who have died before proceedings are commenced. The figures do not therefore constitute an accurate fertility record, and it is perhaps dubiously legitimate to refer to the "fertility" of divorcing couples. For convenience the term will be retained, but the distinction should be noted.

The net effect of these different definitions is uncertain. Divorcing couples are credited with some children not born to the marriage, but debited by the number of their own children who have died. More than merely infant and child mortality is relevant here, since many couples divorce after lengthy legal durations of marriage. Again, the Registrar General comments (1961, p. ix) that contrary to intention the Census returns may include some children born illegitimately, and this must be seen against the fact that approaching one-third of illegitimate children are born to married women, or those who would describe themselves as such on the Census return. In the case of both divorcing and stable unions some children may have been adopted out. Such children would count in the fertility of those remaining married but not for those divorcing, since they would no longer be children of the family. We cannot currently know whether the fertility of divorced women is understated or exaggerated in divorce court returns, but certainly the issue is problematic, and our knowledge of the total fertility experience of divorcing women is unsatisfactory.

Remarriage

American writers (e.g. Kephart, 1954; Monahan, 1955) have proposed that in the analysis of divorce patterns there is good reason to differentiate primary marriages (bachelor-spinster marriages) from remarriage situations. To begin with, there is reason to suppose that remarriages are more unstable than primary marriages (Monahan, 1952, 1958). Additionally, the age-at-marriage distribution for remarriages is different and, at least partly in consequence, the fertility pattern is also different. Furthermore, it is probable that when remarriage leads to divorce it does so at characteristically briefer durations, and that the antecedent separations also occur earlier within marriage (Registrar General, 1966; Chester, 1971a). The concept of children of the family is also relevant here. Widows who remarry at mature ages may have had children, but these may not have become children of the family because they were themselves married or otherwise independent. Since such a remarriage is unlikely to produce further children the woman would be regarded as infertile at subsequent divorce, and this would create a marginal element of spuriousness in the figures. The recognition of complications such as these led Rowntree & Carrier (1958) to base fertility comparisons on primary marriages only, but other writers on divorce have ignored the remarriage factor.

In making fertility comparisons it would be possible in principle to eliminate the remarriage factor on the remaining-married side of the calculation by the use of appropriate census tables (such as "women married once only and enumerated with their husbands"). In fact, the comparison group used in the official statistics is all married women, and this is presumably because remarriages cannot currently be discriminated on the divorce side of the comparison. Since remarriages probably contribute more than their share of divorces and less than their share of fertility, an unknown biasing effect is built into the computation, and it would therefore be desirable to separate primary marriages in the analysis. An indication that this would make a difference is given by figures from the local sample which is to be further discussed. Of primary marriages in this sample 23% were infertile, against 40% of the remarriages. Consequently, whereas 75% of the total 1000 marriages had children, this figure became 77% when remarriage was excluded. These figures are given as exemplary only, but they support the general point made here.

The Duration of Marriage

Independently of the foregoing points, and more important than either, there is a further difficulty in seeking to discover whether divorcing marriages show more childlessness than stable unions. This relates to marriage duration, since in measuring the comparative fertility experience of different social categories a vital variable is opportunity to conceive. For divorcees, the official statistics measure this by the legal definition of marriage duration, which is from wedding day to date of decree absolute. As Kephart (1954) and Monahan (1955) insist, however, the *de jure* duration of marriage is a poor statement of opportunity to conceive, since it ignores the length of time spouses may have been separated before divorce. Clearly it is imperative that comparative fertility should be measured at comparable durations, and much hinges on the extent to which sexual cohabitation is overstated by legal durations. This pitfall has long been recognized by American writers, although it has been overlooked by British commentators on divorce except for Rowntree & Carrier, who point specifically to the desirability of data on effective duration even though unable to obtain it for their own work.

Precise calculation of opportunity to conceive is probably not possible, because other factors than duration of marriage are involved (coital rates, for instance). However, a better index than legal duration is offered by *de facto* duration, defined as the period from date of marriage to the date of separation or break-up. It is probable that sexual activity will have typically declined or ceased before this latter date, although the force of this point is diminished by our ignorance of patterns of sexual activity among the stable married population. Nevertheless, whenever *de facto* durations have been substituted for *de jure* the apparent differential in fertility between divorcing and remaining-married couples has been reduced or eliminated. Jacobson (1950) presents evidence that this was the case for Sweden in 1938, and recognizes that the use of separation dates for his own analysis would have altered his conclusions. His methods in arriving at the claim that nevertheless there was a fertility differential in America were severely criticized by Monahan (1955), whose own analysis casts doubts on the existence of such a differential. Day (1964), in examining Australian divorce, also recognized that use of *de facto* data would diminish the differential he found. He regarded a 5-year interval from break-up to divorce as an "extreme assumption," but even on this assumption found a residual differential. However, as will be shown, a 5-year interval is by no means extreme, and Day does not examine the remarriage factor or the definition of children.

In a study described elsewhere (Chester, 1971a) it was possible to collect material relating to both the date of separation and the date of divorce, and the results indicate that in Britain as in America the *de facto* and *de jure* durations of marriage differ considerably. Separation dates were available for 805 (91%) of the 881 primary-marriage divorces studied. For these there was a 4.6-year difference in means between the legal and effective durations of marriage, and a 4.3-year difference in the medians. The median interval from separation to divorce was 2.9 years, and in one-third of the cases the interval was greater than 4 years. Such figures show that *de jure* duration does seriously overstate opportunity to conceive, and that in the official comparison those remaining married have in fact enjoyed significantly longer periods in which to have children.

Furthermore, the calculation showed not only mean differences in the two kinds of duration, but also that the differences in the duration-distribution of cases are greatest in the immediate post-marriage period. To illustrate, 38% of the cases broke up within the first quinquennium of marriage, during which period only 16% of divorces occurred. During the first decade of marriage 62% of separations occurred, against 45% of the divorces, and during the first 20 years the figures were 90% of the separations and 78% of the divorces. This temporal skew of *de facto* durations is crucial when fertility comparisons are made, because first births are overwhelmingly concentrated in the first quinquennium of marriage. Standardization of duration is therefore imperative, and while the official compiler rightly follows this procedure his results are nullified by the inadequacy of the duration data available to him. Indeed, given the magnitude of the discrepancies between the two kinds of duration it is not clear that the official comparison serves a helpful purpose, since the casual use made of it by secondary commentators issues in misleading interpretations.

There are further complications in computing the comparative fertility of divorcees even when analysis is restricted to primary marriages and based on *de facto* durations. Youthful marriage, for instance, is associated both with higher divorce propensity and with higher fertility. The implications of age-at-marriage were recognized by Rowntree & Carrier, who noted that allowance for this factor would have somewhat increased the fertility differential they found (based on legal durations). On the other hand, it is probable

(Chester, 1972a) that youthful marriage is also associated with brief duration of marriage to break-up and with above average intervals from separating to divorcing, so that for young marriages the legal duration of marriage may exaggerate duration even more than it does for others. (This analysis is further complicated by differential proneness to premarital pregnancy, to which attention must return in due course.) It is true that the official calculation offers figures for different age-at-marriage groups, but these still have the defect of deriving from data on *de jure* duration.

The figures for *de facto* duration given above derive, of course, from a local sample, but there seems no reason to suppose that they represent a local peculiarity since they are supported by some recent evidence reported by McGregor *et al.* (1970). Looking at magistrates' court applicants who went on to divorce, these authors found a mean interval of 5 years between the lower court action and divorce, and it is reasonable to assume that this is approximate to the difference between *de facto* and *de jure* duration. Such evidence creates confidence in the local duration data, and the conclusion seems inescapable that the Registrar General's finding of differential fertility between divorcing and stable marriages is to an unknown extent an artifact of reporting procedure and statistical method.

The Fertility of the Local Sample

It would not be appropriate here to provide an extended analysis of the fertility experience of the local sample, but information relating to this group can be presented in a way that makes clear the difference which can be made to fertility comparisons when *de facto* duration is substituted for *de jure*. In this exercise the local nature of the sample is relatively unimportant, since the purpose is to illustrate an effect rather than to offer an alternative and definitive measurement of the comparative fertility of divorcees.

As noted above, 77% of the primary-marriage divorces involved children, and the durations of the marriages concerned ranged from the briefest periods up to more than 40 years. In order to calculate the effect of substituting effective for legal duration it is necessary to impose an upper time-limit on the durations considered, since otherwise the handful of divorces at the very advanced durations create distortions. Analysis is therefore concentrated on the 833 cases (94%) where legal durations were up to 30 years. For this group the proportion infertile was 23.7%, and in 800 cases the *de facto* duration was known. When the 1961 Census figures for the fertility of women married once only and enumerated with their husbands are standardized for the two kinds of duration a significant effect occurs. Standardizing the census women on the *de jure* durations of the divorcees provides a figure of 18% infertile. Since the proportion for the divorcees was 23.7%, this figure appears to confirm the official finding of a fertility deficit. When, however, the census women are standardized for *de facto* duration, their proportion infertile appears as 27.9%. The divorcees, that is to say, were more fertile than those remaining married.

It must be remembered that these figures do not allow for age at marriage, and also that *de facto* durations were not available for all cases. Nevertheless, the results show strikingly the difference which can be made to fertility comparisons when a more realistic notion of marriage duration is employed, and it is unlikely that they are seriously misleading. Although, however, the divorcees now appear to have a surplus rather than a deficit in fertility, no explanation of this will be pursued because the results may themselves be affected by a further (and final) complication in the data which must be noted. So far it has been assumed that the problematic aspect of measuring opportunity to conceive is to establish a terminal date. The frequency of premarital conception, however, indicates that the commencing date is also problematic, and that it often antedates the wedding day. Since premarital pregnancy is itself divorce-disposing, and is associated with other divorce-disposing variables such as age at marriage, then to measure opportunity to conceive from the date of marriage will artificially exaggerate the fertility of divorcing couples (particularly those with brief duration) in the same way that to measure such opportunity to the date of divorce understates their fertility. If it may be assumed that differential premarital pregnancy reflects differential intercourse behaviour rather than different contraceptive practice, then divorcees must be credited with additional periods of opportunity to conceive by comparison with their non-divorcing marriage peers. There is no currently available way in which this corrective factor may be calculated or even estimated, although it might be noted that on the evidence of Kinsey *et al.* (1953) and Schofield (1965) intercourse between future marriage partners tends to be concentrated in the year or so before marriage and has a relatively low frequency-rate. Intercourse rates are likely to be much higher in the year following marriage than in the year preceding it, and again, in partial 'compensation' for their premarital abstention, it is likely that intercourse-frequency is greater for the remaining-married group at the latter end of any given duration than for a couple approaching the break-up date that will determine their *de facto* duration.

The effect of these different factors is uncertain, but it is clear that the question of differential fertility is complicated, and that the official comparison based on legal duration provides no warrant for believing that divorcees are less fertile than those in comparable stable unions. *De facto* duration, as defined here, is not totally satisfactory as a measure of opportunity to conceive, but it is superior to legal duration, and calculations based on it provide a different picture of the relationship between childlessness and divorce from that which is normally assumed.

Fertility and Other Forms of Marriage Break-Up

Not all marriages which break up terminate in divorce. Many result in proceedings before magistrates, and these form a significant fraction of disrupted marriages (see Chester, 1971b). If attention focuses on the relationship between childlessness and marriage breakdown (rather than simply divorce) it is appropriate to notice these cases, and the available evidence suggests that this group of marriages is not characterized by excess infertility. Women in the national sample of matrimonial cases studied by McGregor *et al.* (1970) were slightly less inclined to infertility than married women in the 1961 Census, and markedly so at the briefer durations. The data reported do not permit full comparison, but for women in the matrimonial sample with durations up to 7 years the proportion infertile can be calculated as 20%, against 38% infertile for comparable census women, with mean family sizes of 1.26 and 0.95 children respectively. In this analysis of a different aspect of marriage breakdown the authors were in effect measuring *de facto* duration, and once again it can be seen that when such duration is used the alleged deficiency in fertility is much affected. Certainly these couples were at least as fertile as those remaining married, and probably rather more so.

These findings still leave unaccounted for those marriages which break up unremarked by the legal system. Informal separations undoubtedly occur, although the numbers and trends are unknown and probably unknowable (Chester, 1972b). It might be argued that informal separations may more commonly involve childless couples, since no question of child maintenance arises and there might be less incentive therefore to take court action.

Again, an informally separated mother who applies for income assistance may be encouraged by the social security authorities to apply for a maintenance order (Marsden, 1969), and clearly mothers would be more likely to require public support than an unencumbered wife who could more readily support herself. There may, therefore, be selective processes operating such that fertile women are transferred from the informally separated group to the category known to the statistics via divorce or magistrates' court proceedings. However, the absence of dependent children does not necessarily imply infertility, since there may be mature children for whom no question of maintenance arises. Furthermore, although there may be over-selection of the fertile for court action, leaving the informally separated group relatively infertile, the relationship may equally go the other way at least so far as divorce is concerned. If separated wives without children are more likely to marry again, there would be over-selection by the infertile of the divorce option to make this possible, thus leaving the informally separated group over-representative of mothers. In fact we do not know about the relationship of fertility and remarriage, or anything of significance about the informally separated, and there is no particular case for believing that informally separated wives are more infertile than those whose breakdown is signified by divorce or maintenance orders. They may be relatively infertile, but any such conclusion is purely speculative, and it is unlikely that any fertility deficit here would outweigh the findings above and thus indicate an overall relationship between childlessness and marriage breakdown.

Conclusion

An adequate answer to the question of the relationship between childlessness and divorce or marriage breakdown must await a more refined analysis than is possible with currently available data. From the considerations above it cannot be definitively concluded that there is no relationship between these variables, but it is clear that previous deductions from official statistics have been incautious, and that by the use of legal durations these statistics create a spurious fertility differential. It remains, perhaps, somewhat odd that commentators have almost unanimously accepted (and tried to explain) the existence of the relationship without subjecting it to serious question, and we may wonder whether the reason for this lies in the normative orientations and cultural assumptions of those concerned. Certainly, by linking marital pathology with abstention from parenthood, belief in the relationship is supportive of traditional family values and the ideological assumption that children are the natural fulfilment of marriage.

Parenthood doubtless influences patterns of marital adjustment, but its effects are probably not in a uniform direction, and the way in which such effects are mediated is not well understood. The historical dimension is also important, because parenthood has different meanings in different temporal contexts, and the recent increase in the proportion of divorcees with children may reflect this. It may be, however, that in any case the style of analysis commented on above, which seeks to discover the net effect of childlessness on the stability of marriage, is not the most fruitful for either pragmatic or theoretical purposes. More meaningful knowledge would derive from an alternative approach which looked for syndromes or patterns of effect rather than net overall effect, seeking to discover in what ways childlessness was important for which groups of marriages. Such an approach would examine the feelings of the spouses about the desirability of children and whether these were mutual, whether the childlessness was voluntary or involuntary, whether childlessness has different meanings at different stages of married life, and similar questions. It would pay attention also to such matters as marriage type, marriage duration, definition of fertility, etc., and any variations in these by occupation, social class, religion or region. Consideration would be given to forms of marriage break-up other than divorce, and also to marriages which remain unbroken but continue only in the deepest disharmony or disengagement. This alternative approach would seek, that is, a rounded picture of the kinds of relationship which exist between fertility, inter-spousal adjustment, marital satisfactions, and the stability of the marriage. Even valid knowledge of the net overall relationship between childlessness and marital stability would not greatly aid our understanding of marriage behaviour, and whether this relationship ultimately proved to be positive or negative it could conceal patterns of effect which indicate diverse consequences of infertility in differently situated contexts. It is the understanding of such diversity which research could most profitably seek.

Acknowledgments

The work for this article springs from current research which has been financed by the Eugenics Society, the Social Science Research Council, and the Department of Health and Social Security, to all of whom my thanks are due.

7

Burgess and Cottrell Data on "Desire for Children": An Example of Distortion in Marriage and Family Textbooks?*

EDWARD POHLMAN

Director of the Birth Planning Research Program, University of the Pacific, Stockton, California

Burgess and Cottrell reported on "desire for children" and "marital adjustment." Marriage and family textbooks have typically misrepresented the data in citing it. As one example of six criticisms, Burgess and Cottrell warn that the data refer to couples married only a few years; failure to mention this leads to gross misinterpretations. Textbook reporting of these data raise questions about the adequacy of marriage and family textbooks and, indeed, textbooks in the social sciences generally. Possibly a tightly organized, collaboratively prepared text would permit more depth in scholarship behind each chapter than is possible when one author must cover a huge range of material.

Burgess and Cottrell[1] reported some data which have been typically distorted in those marriage and family textbooks which we have found citing the data.[2] This seems of interest, not only in itself as a flaw which should be corrected, but as a possible example of distortion that may be fairly widespread in secondary sources—in the marriage and family field and out of it.

The data in question are typically presented by adapting or copying a bar graph presented by Burgess and Cottrell which bears the following labels on the left side:

Journal of Marriage and the Family, August 1968

* Supported by grants from Syntex Laboratories, Inc., and from the Social Science Committee of Planned Parenthood-World Population.

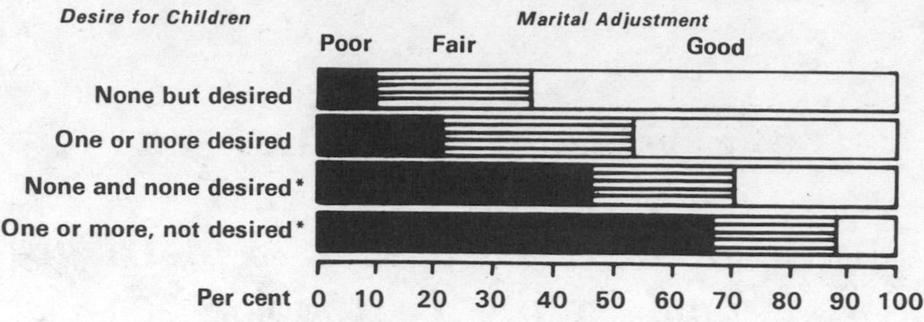

Adapted from E. W. Burgess and L. S. Cottrell, Jr., *Predicting Success or Failure in Marriage,* Englewood Cliffs, New Jersey: Prentice-Hall, Inc., 1939, p. 260.

The bar graph then shows a progressive decrease in the proportion with "good" marital adjustment, as one goes from the top to the bottom category.

Six Criticisms

1. Sample Atypical as to Marriage Duration

The first fault to be noted is particularly glaring, because the original authors explicitly warn against it:

> Because of the small number of years married that is characteristic of the cases in the study, it would be unwise to draw hasty conclusions from the data presented.[3]

This warning is ignored; as a result, although couples in this sample had been married only one to six years, the bar graph is given a sort of timeless and absolute validity. For example, it is made to seem that parents in the "none but desired" category are permanently childless but wish they had children. However, since many couples had been married only a year or two and since fecundity problems are not typically known this soon, the "none but desired" category might be better interpreted as involving primarily a group who wanted children but had not had them yet.

Burgess and Cottrell support the latter type of interpretation by citing the study of Lang[4] and quoting him. Lang concluded that, in the first two years of marriage, childless marriages were happier but that, for couples married five years or more, the opposite held true on the average. (Incidentally, neither Lang nor Burgess and Cottrell noticed a crucial weakness: all Lang's differences in happiness ratings for the first few years might readily be explained as the result of Lang's failure to control for premarital conception and presumably associated unhappiness.) The intent of Burgess and Cottrell, in interpreting their own data, was clearly to warn that the picture might be different with longer marriage durations. The warning has typically been ignored. Judson and Mary Landis [5] do mention it in a somewhat ambiguous way but fail to relate it specifically to the Burgess and Cottrell graph which they reproduce.

2. Depression-Era Data

Although students reading the footnotes and references for the graph can see that this study was published in 1939, textbooks need to emphasize that the data are over a quarter of a century old and came from the depression period. Especially in view of financial pressures then, relationships might have been true that would not hold true today. Possibly, economic hardships meant that children served as more of a problem in the first six years of marriage than is true today.

3. Cause-Effect Relationship Not Shown

The data are typically handled in a manner that would imply that, if couples decide they do not want children, this decision will produce marital maladjustment. The slogan is just between the lines: "Procreate for a happy marriage." Students should be specifically cautioned against such conclusions, since there are two other major possible lines of explanation: (1) People who are unhappy in general tend to have less happy marriages and are also more likely to want to remain childless; and (2), when marriage turns out to be somewhat unhappy, couples may wish to avoid children. Marriage and family textbook writers may have biases toward seeing parenthood as happy and holy, and childlessness as a strange deviation which makes people less interested in family life education. Bernard [6] suggests that the marriage and family people may have encouraged parenthood and even big-family-mindedness in ways that are quite oblivious to population problems. Probably many couples who are parents under our present norms and expectations would be better off childless (to say nothing of their offspring) and might even wish for this possibility. Pressures toward parenthood are already strong in our culture;[7] this particular misinterpretation (by implication) of the Burgess and Cottrell data does not help matters.

4. No Controls for Premarital Conception

Premarital conception might be expected to lead to problems in marital adjustment. Hence controls for the premarital versus postmarital status of conception are extremely important. Lacking such controls in the Burgess and Cottrell data, one may speculate that the relatively miserable couples who had "one or more, not desired" may have contained an unduly high proportion of premarital conceptions. Incidentally, the N for this group was only 36 couples, with a large standard error implied, although the secondary sources do not list the N's.

5. No Controls for Marriage Duration

The fifth criticism is like the fourth: there was a failure to control for length of marriage in this particular analysis of data. Elsewhere, Burgess and Cottrell[8] show that, in general, marriage adjustment ratings are less good as marriage goes on for a longer time. Among those married between one and six years, those who want children but have none were probably married for a shorter time than those who had children and wanted them. Although inspection of the two graphs[9] suggests that duration of marriage is not enough of a factor to account for all the correlation noted, it may be a contributing factor.

6. Poor Labels

This writer's sixth criticism has to do primarily with the extremely cryptic nature of the labels on the bar graph. Burgess and Cottrell had reason for such abbreviations, since in their presentation the abbreviated sentences referred to fuller statements they had made about the four classifications. But the secondary sources never give these fuller statements. What happened to the families who wanted some children but had had more than they wanted? Were they in the "one or more, not desired" or "one or more desired" categories? Or what happened when the wife wanted all the children but the husband did not want them all? More recent research suggests that, at least in 1960, such problems were very frequent.[10] The column heading for the labels of the bars is not adequately descriptive: the variable involved is not simply "Desire for Children," even though this is the heading Burgess and Cottrell used. Some idea of the number of cases in each of the four bars (160, 186, 111, 36) might also be helpful.

General Comments

Several of the above criticisms implicate the original source; this is true of the fourth and fifth criticisms and of some parts of the sixth. But a secondary source is not free from responsibility to smell out problems in the presentation just because the primary source fails to do so.

One might argue that it would be impossible, in a secondary source geared to undergraduate college students, to make the changes implied by the writer's six criticisms and still present the data within a reasonable amount of space. But the secondary-source author must decide whether he is justified in bringing in a given fragment of data at all. If he must choose between reprinting material which will inevitably be seriously misunderstood and omitting it, the latter may be more desirable. The writer is not assuming that this is the case with the data in question, however. . . .

8
Pronatalism in the Army

CAPT. H. P.
Arizona

Discrimination against childfree Army couples seems to fall into two categories: institutionalized and non-institutionalized. By "institutionalized" we are referring to discriminatory practices carried out by the Army as a matter of policy, whereas subtle or non-institutionalized discriminations are largely matters of how Army people with children behave toward those without children. Examples of both will follow.

The most highly visible form of institutionalized discrimination involves housing. The Army provides larger housing for larger families at exactly the same rate as it provides small houses for small families, according to rank. The amount of money received each month for housing depends on an officer's rank—the amount of housing space provided for that amount of money depends on family size! It's as simple as that. For instance: one officer receives $195 a month for housing; but under Army regulations he does not qualify for an on-post house any larger than a 2-bedroom house because he and his wife have no children.

Another officer of the same rank also receives $195 a month and therefore qualifies for a 4-bedroom house for the same amount of rent. Why? The second officer has two children. This is the sole determinant.

There are instances where *only* large-unit housing is available on post, yet the empty 3- or 4-bedroom units are "unavailable" to a single Army man or Army couple without children, who must then find housing off the base.

Children are a definite requirement to qualify for even substandard housing on one Army base we know of.

Although the housing situation is probably the primary case in institutionalized discrimination, another instance that might be mentioned is travel allowance for Army personnel, which also varies according to family size. As the number of his family members goes up, so does his mileage allowance when an Army man is transferred.

The Army policy on childbirth can be viewed as discriminatory. Childbirth is free in the Army, but abortions are not even allowed: thus the Army acts as guardian of pronatalist policies of the past, denying to Army wives freedom of reproduction control which the Supreme Court has granted to other women in the country.

When an Army wife has a baby, hospitalization and delivery are absolutely without cost. (Actually, it does cost something like $7.25 to have a child on most bases. That small amount covers the cost of food for the mother during her stay in the hospital.) It is so inexpensive to have children in the Army that many Army officers and non-commissioned men do so for just this reason.

In one Army class of 73 captains, 56 are married. Eleven of their wives either gave birth or became pregnant during one recent six-month period. Since the class members average only 28 years of age and had, collectively, a previous total of 91 children, there would be some case for correlating Army life with childbirth and for viewing these Army policies as *actively* pronatalist (that is, encouraging of childbirth) as well as discriminatory against those who do not have children.

An Army doctor at first tried to leave the service and take a job on the staff of a civilian hospital. When he discovered his wife was pregnant again he commented, "I guess I won't leave the Army until I'm sure Grace has had all the children she wants."

One gets used to following orders in the Army, and it is easy to interpret these institutionalized discriminations as an implicit "order" for an Army man to marry and have children.

Subtle, non-institutionalized forms of discrimination are harder to pin down—but they do exist and can be painful at times for childfree couples.

Commissaries carry items packaged in huge sizes, with the obvious intention of allowing large families to save pennies. This can also, however, train couples to "think big."

Another example comes from an extremely important Army manual, *The Officer's Guide*. On page 75 of the 1970–71 edition is a chapter entitled "Customs of the Service." The following statement appears:

> When a child is born to the family of an officer the unit commander sends a personal letter of congratulations to the new parents on behalf of the organization.

Note the authority of the word "sends": this is not regarded by officers as an optional courtesy. (Why not a yearly letter of congratulations to all officers whose wives have not had a child that year?)

The *Guide* then goes on to discuss the tradition of the silver baby cup given to the new parents with an appropriate engraving. This is another example of a tradition that perpetuates the idea that having a child is automatically deserving of a personal gift or reward.

Probably the saddest, most insidious discrimination occurs on the social level, where officers' wives are thrown together in an inevitably close society by being confined to a relatively small area. If you have no children, you can expect to be excluded—from conversations, and from decision-making involving group plans, and from that subtle sense of belonging and sisterhood that can give your temporary environment a much-needed network of friendships.

PART II

Parenthood: Motivation, Myth, and Consequence

It is probably safe to say that marketing experts have given more attention to motives for soap-buying than social scientists have given to motives for reproduction.

Much of the force behind pronatalism results from the strong feeling that desire for children is natural, and conversely, that those who don't want children are somehow "unnatural." Thus pronatalist forces throughout society are considered an accurate reflection of this desire, and are uncritically accepted and then in turn reinforce the childbearing norm. Investigation of the complexity of motivations for parenthood has been hampered by this assumption that the overriding motive is built-in. Thus, some even argue that consideration of "motive" for reproduction is pointless because reproductive impulses result from deep, mystic, immutable (and of course "natural") yearnings for immortality through one's descendants. This point of view is well expressed in a contemporary college text (*Marriage for Moderns,* Harold Bowman, McGraw-Hill, 1970) which quotes from a 1966 article in *Bride's* magazine entitled "Why Men Marry":

> A man without children is not complete. . . . Children establish my place in the long chain of generations who have carried my blood from the dark caves of the past and who will carry it endlessly forward into time. Children are my continuity. Through children I fling my seed into the future. Reproduction is the act of life, is life itself. In reproducing, I affirm my place in the system of life inhabiting the earth. The man without children has lost his place in history.

Similarly, Margaret Reynolds, fecund heroine of Anne Roiphe's novel *Up the Sandbox,* muses on contemplating her fourth pregnancy:

> . . . We are part of history. . . . We are doing what the Neanderthals, the Indians, the Babylonians and the Assyrians, the Egyptians and the Hittites, the Tartars and the Mongolians, the Indo-Europeans, and the Twelve Tribes of Israel have all done. We will not be spun off the planet's surface, unlinked to our kind. . . .

Is such rhetoric an explication of a fact or a convenient emotional argument? There is good reason to believe it's the latter. But it is not our intention here to lay down all the arguments for and against the existence of a "maternal instinct" or attempt to sort out the influence of cultural versus biological factors. Such an approach would be futile primarily because few scientists agree on how to define an instinct. Each scientific discipline has developed its own set of criteria: ethologists, for example, no longer use the term "instinct" alone, but see instinctive behavior as a select class or grouping of specific motor acts that are invariant in their development and expression. Thus the pouncing movement of the domestic cat is considered instinctive as it is unlearned, remains the same throughout the life of the animal, and is displayed by all members of the species. By comparison maternal behavior seems to be at least largely learned (for example, people have to learn how to handle and care for their babies), can vary according to the individuals' circumstances (a woman may want a child at one time of her life but not at another) and can vary from person to person and culture to culture. Therefore most psychologists and social scientists avoid describing a desire for childbearing as an instinct.

The notion persists, however, in the popular mind where the need for proof and consistency is obviously less relevant. Here the term instinct is used loosely and as a catchall for any kind of behavior that seem to be prevalent and long-standing, motherhood naturally included. A major exception among professions is some psychoanalysts, largely influenced by Freudian ideas about sexuality. Dominant among these is the theory of "penis envy" which suggests that a child is desired to make up for the missing organ in the female. This line of thought resulted not from scientific proof so much as from Freud's imaginative interpretations of the human body, neatly depicted to fit observed psychological conditions. But, along with other of Freud's theories, such as the "death wish," the penis-envy concept has fallen out of favor in most contemporary psychoanalytical thought.

Today most scholarly analyses of childbearing behavior, while not flatly denying that a desire for children might be in part at least innate, turn rather to social and cultural forces that bear on the issue. Margaret Mead, for example, in her classic study *Male and Female,* discusses innate tendencies, but emphasizes the learning process as the critical factor. Women, she notes, have to learn to want children only under socially prescribed conditions and, in the same way, can learn not to want children. Those who choose the latter life-style, and suffer for it, do not suffer because they are denying something so biologically basic that it results in a trauma, but rather because women *learn* they must bear children to be socially respectable. Childbearing practices, and individual attitudes toward them, she concludes, depend upon how each culture values parenthood and what it teaches the young as correct behavior in this respect.

There are differences not only among cultures, but within them as well. It is apparent from data on individual couples and aggregate birth trends that far from being the same among all members of a society, there is great variation in childbearing behavior, particularly at times of social change. Thus in the United States during the depression years of the 1930s, 20% of ever-married women had no children. By contrast, in 1960, the authors of the important Growth of American Families Study found that childlessness had dropped to 7–8%. They further concluded from the incidence of voluntary childlessness in this group (1%) that this phenomenon "is nearly extinct."

More recently we see indications of a change back to a greater incidence of childlessness. Census Bureau figures, reported in 1972, indicate that 4% of young wives expect to have no children. In more select studies, a survey of university students indicates that, in 1970, an average of 12% desired no children (see Pohlman, "Changes in Views Toward Childlessness," Part IV); and a survey of high school students in a California community (1972) shows that 17.2% of those responding intend to be non-parents (Larry Barnett, Ph.D. and Shirley Radl, "Childbearing Predictions of Students in a Cupertino, California High School," 1972, unpublished).

Were reproductive behavior truly instinctive, it would not be expected to be subject to such variability—to changes of style, as it were—nor would it seem logical to label the fluctuating numbers of those who reject reproduction completely "instinctively deficient."

Many long-standing notions of instinct, along with Freud's continuing impact, die hard in popular literature and thought. After all, it is tempting to call an action or desire "instinctive" when it seems to reflect commonly felt and deep emotions such as those associated with reproduction. The fact, however, that such emotions are now *less* commonly held than before may force an eventual widespread change of concept.

The readings that follow begin with a selection from popular literature that denies the maternal myth (or the myth of the existence of a maternal instinct). Betty Rollin touches off her rebuttal by citing an array of authoritative opinions from different disciplines. The role of instinct is here rejected on the basis that these theories are fundamentally arguments of perceived *need:* society, because of overpopulation, no longer needs every woman to bear children and women do not need motherhood to be complete, though they still think they do. She speaks to many of the long-standing arguments favoring motherhood and explains how, out of "need, inevitability and pragmatic fantasy" the myth took hold.

In line with current realities, Rollin suggests a shift away from the "biology is destiny" frame of reference. A few militant voices would even replace Freud's "biology is destiny" with "biology is dead"; certainly it can at least now be said that biology is *choice*—or presents the opportunity for it.

In "Motivations in Wanting Conceptions," psychologist Edward Pohlman presents an important review of the literature. He dismisses the term *instinct* because of its ambiguity; and after giving a list of possible innate (unlearned) factors that make child-bearing desired or rewarding, he concludes that "much of what is attributed to innate factors may be explained readily as a matter of social learning."

Although he finds no systematic evidence to support Freudian theories, he outlines numerous psychoanalytical hypotheses that may relate to childbearing decisions. The male, for example, could find parenthood—particularly when a large family is involved—a reassurance of his virility, potency, and sexual prowess. Competition with one's parents or siblings and a sense that parenthood represents extension of one's ego, or self, are cited as other possible factors that may influence one's attitudes toward having children.

Social pressures, Pohlman feels, play a major role in child-bearing behavior, with observable fad or fashion aspects within given cultures. A fashionable motive expressed by many is a "liking for children"—a catchall sentiment which includes desires for human interaction and also reflects dependency needs of the parents. Providing a role for the woman, in motherhood, is a powerful motivation, for as he suggests, it "may be the chief means of establishing her identity."

Pohlman's work is of great value to the serious student of reproductive dynamics. His book, *Psychology of Birth Planning* (1969), (a term Pohlman prefers to *birth control*) is highly recommended, as are the various studies to which he makes reference.

The next two selections clearly do make value judgments, both delineating "wrong reasons" for having children. Neither presentation, Planned Parenthood's sixty-second television message or Robert Gould's popular article "The Wrong Reasons to Have Children," pretends to be scientific or objective. The advertisement, part of a large multimedia campaign begun in 1971, introduced millions of Americans to a roster of motivations which had previously received little public articulation. But while the delineation of "wrong reasons" for a mass media audience cannot practically be expected to be an incisive analysis of an issue, this series contains a serious verbal evasion and visual bias that could have been at least partially avoided.

Note that after exposition of several "wrong" reasons, the spot cites *wanting a child* as a "right" reason.

However, *want* is obviously a complex term. Most parents, for whatever reasons known or unknown to them, claim they "want" their children. Having a child to avoid the draft, to stay busy or to feel important, to keep up with the Joneses—all can be construed as wanting a child. The ad essentially ends up where it begins: people want children for many reasons and depending on the perspective or interpretation, they may be right or wrong. And obviously the mere feeling of wanting something, like wanting the fastest car on the block, does not make it personally beneficial, socially rewarding—or right.

Visually, note that the mother who wants her child for the "right" reason in this ad is more beautiful in traditional terms than the individuals who have the "wrong" motives for having children. We should recall once more, perhaps, Leta Hollingworth's comment about "the ideal (maternal) type" which is publicized as a means of social control, of encouraging childbirth. By such an interpretation, this Planned Parenthood commercial might be considered pronatalist.

While Planned Parenthood's "wrong reasons" present mainly external, surface social pressure, Gould, a professor of psychiatry at New York University Medical Center, presents a list more balanced between outer, and inner, pressures. Examples of inner pressures include the motives: "I want to be somebody, . . ." "I need to be needed, . . ." "I want my child to get the things I never had, . . ." and the sexist-pronatalist "A baby will keep a woman in her place."

Even though many people would consider such a feeling as legitimate or "right," the motive of childbearing as an avenue to immortality ("I fling my seed into the future") is seen by Gould as a wrong reason. He comments that a productive life will also leave its mark on the world. And actually, are not the men and women noted by history remembered for their achievements rather than for how many (if any) children they had?

Gould in his article was able to explain and analyze undesirable reproductive dynamics in a way which Planned Parenthood's ad could not; he thus provides a more ambitious confrontation with ego-extension motives for reproduction. Gould's list of "wrong reasons" for having children is more challenging. For some, it is sure to be less comfortable.

A great deal of literature has dealt with the effects parents and various types of parental behavior have on children. The corresponding concern—how the presence of children to be raised affects the adults who must raise them—has received relatively little thoughtful attention.

In our culture, as in almost all cultures, it is commonly presumed that parenthood enriches one's personality, stabilizes one's position within the community, and solidifies the marital bond. There is a widespread idea as well that becoming a parent increases one's maturity.

These attitudes serve as subtle encouragements of parenthood and are part of the general pronatalist bias of our society.

If our selections here emphasize the negative aspects of parenthood (and we freely admit this to be the case) there is no intention to replace *Parenthood Enriches!* with *Parenthood Destroys!* as a predominant attitude: but merely an attempt to counterbalance a heretofore prejudiced perspective, and to present some new considerations.

A basic concern must obviously be the nature of parenthood and the realities of childrearing. It is our observation that too many new parents face too many surprises. This situation stems in large part from a general lack of questioning about the changes that will take place in the new situation, but also results from the persisting taboos about discussion of the less pleasant aspects of childrearing. As one of LeMasters's interviewees comments, "We knew where babies came from, but we didn't know what they were like."

Because the realities of having children come as a surprise, this section is a direct attempt to tell "what they are like." Without questioning the basic value of parenthood, and without denying the satisfactions it can hold for some, we simply mean to demonstrate what has been too little pointed out before: that parenthood involves work, sacrifice, and most of all *change:* there is not only change in the relationship between husband and wife and others but change in each parent's own self-concept. The nature of that change is not always positive.

Indeed, the nature of the change is perceived by 83% of couples interviewed by University of Wisconsin sociologist E. E. LeMasters as a "crisis" of adjustment. In his paper, "Parenthood as Crisis" (which was awarded the Ernest Burgess Prize by the National Council on Family Relations in 1957), LeMasters begins by hypothesizing that the adding of a child to a marital union necessitates reorganization of established patterns. Particularly because of the small size of the modern nuclear family, he asks, would not the addition of a member be as drastic as the removal of one? The 83% "crisis" figure seems to confirm his conjecture. An important interpretation of these findings involves the specific nature of introducing a first child into a two-person family situation: the family unit immediately changes from a dyad to a triad. LeMasters cites two studies indicating that a pair grouping is one of the most satisfactory forms of human relationships, whereas the triad is one of the most volatile.

The LeMasters study again confronts us with a troublesome ambiguity in the term *wanted* as applied to childbearing. Most couples in the crisis group have planned and "wanted" their child. But, due to a romanticized perception of parenthood to which LeMasters several times refers, these couples may not have correctly comprehended the nature of either the institution (parenthood) or the object (child) they "wanted."

It is well worth noting, by the way, that the crisis sample is not viewed as neurotic exceptions to a general pattern of easy adjustment; indeed, LeMasters comments that the crisis group seemed generally average or above average in preparental personality adjustment.

Though LeMasters cautiously notes that most of the crisis couples eventually made what "seems to be" a satisfactory adjustment to their new roles as parents, it is worth wondering how many of them might have weighed costs against benefits as regards parenthood—and perhaps made different reproductive decisions as a result—had they but known the costs.

It is probably no news that children are expensive. According to the Commission on Population Growth and the American Future, the cost of raising a child can easily approach $100,000.

There is, however, a less-well-examined theme: that is, that the true "costs" of raising children cannot be measured in economic terms alone, and that emotional costs of tasks involved are no less real than economic ones.

Is not the anxiety over doing the "right" thing when raising children a common plight? And what of the resultant guilt over a child's perceived defects or misbehaviors? From the fatigue almost universally experienced by new parents to the painful sense of loss when children leave home, diverse conflicts and strains, lack of serenity and spontaneity, feelings of isolation and confinement, hours of energy and simple hard work add up to significant emotional "expenditures" indeed.

The old idea had it that couples who could "afford" children in monetary terms shouldn't hesitate to have them. (Part of this attitude may have had a certain elitist base: there are certainly those who view income as a rough indicator of intelligence and feel it is the duty of the intelligent to reproduce. . . .)

Increased attention to "emotional" costs and requirements of parenthood might bring us to a more valid point of view—one which sees suitability for parenthood as a matter of psychological aptitude, not a matter of income or IQ. As yet, there are no credible guidelines for potential ability to cope with the stresses and demands involved, no *Would You Be a Good Parent?* profiles. But it would certainly be helpful for those contemplating parenthood to make themselves aware of "job descriptions" and ask themselves if indeed they do have the probable aptitude and desire for what is involved.

A previously mentioned researcher, Pohlman, has noted that the very fact of pregnancy can bring emotional costs as well: in contrast to the idea that pregnancy is a time of blooming health and radiant happiness, a survey comparing the emotional state of pregnant and nonpregnant women found that crying spells, "the blues," and extreme irritability were far more common among the former group. Pregnant women were also concerned about their appearance and loss of sexual attractiveness.

Appearance presents a major focus of conflict for the mother-housewife as well. The idealized woman in American society is glamorous, sexy, charming, and gracious—and especially *youthful.* Can a woman beset by the responsibilities and chores of parenthood easily maintain those qualities of surface attractiveness? Though television and the media tell her yes, her own experience often does not confirm this.

In "Changes in Marriage and Parenthood: A Methodological Design," sociologist Harold Feldman of Cornell University concentrates his study on how parenthood affects marital satisfaction. His survey results indicate that husbands and wives *with* children had a significantly *lower* level of marital contentment than did those without children; and that when a couple has a child, their level of marital satisfaction decreases from that of their former, childfree state.

He, like LeMasters, suggests that the triad is perhaps a more unstable form of relationship, but the nature of the dyad that was being disrupted was here significant: in the companionate (or closely knit) relationship, the level of marital satisfaction decreased, whereas it was more apt to increase given a "differentiated" relationship. In the latter case, a previously nonexistent closeness between the parents was hoped for and sometimes achieved with the new, shared interest in the child.

When turning to changes in marriage other than marital satisfaction, Feldman found that the first child had a unique effect on the attitudes of the parents. Some of the consequences he found include a feeling of being more overwhelmed, an increase in sex problems, and a rise in negative attitudes about the self. He found that the wife/mother gained in one area at least—(she felt more needed)—but to some extent at the expense of her marriage.

A second child brought to the marriage "an even greater negative effect" it was found, apparently intensifying such perceived changes as: less satisfaction with home; more instrumental conversation; and a lowering of sexual satisfaction after childbirth.

Feldman found that consensus between spouses on matters of childbearing bore an important relationship to marital satisfaction —more important than agreement over issues regarding a wife's career. Thus, the author stresses the need for couples to evaluate their marriage and assess their individual attitudes on childrearing: in short, to prepare for parenthood if they intend to undertake it.

More and more couples, however, seem *not* to choose to undertake parenthood. One of the justifications, or rationalizations, recently used by some childfree women to defend their choice of life-style is the contention that, unburdened by demands of their own biological children, they are freer to participate in affairs of the larger "family" of the community—for example, becoming more active and effective politically.

In fact, *are* nonmothers more politically inclined than mothers?

Professors Naomi B. Lynn and Cornelia B. Flora, both of Kansas State University, have approached this question by conducting an interview survey among 343 women, with and without children.

In their report, "Child-Bearing and Political Participation: The Changing Sense of Self, the researchers found that women without children were more likely to feel a sense of political involvement than were mothers. With a higher educational attainment the difference became more striking. Interestingly, there seemed to be no statistical shift indicated by an increased number of children or by the age of the children—factors obviously directly related to the amount of discretionary time available to the mother. And there was no change in political efficacy between mothers and nonmothers in the lower socio-economic group.

These data suggest that it is the *role of mother* itself which seems to make the important difference in a woman's political participation and political self-concept. Once the status of mother was a reality, the sense of self altered; with the lower socio-economic group wives, however, this status had always been assumed to be their inevitable role and thus made no change in their political self-image.

It is perhaps relevant to note that the role of mother requires particular qualities (such as being adept at promoting harmony within a small group) that are at variance with those of an active political role (propensity for competition within a much larger frame of reference).

The quotations from mothers interviewed will be of interest, and several of the Flora-Lynn observations are challenging indeed for those concerned with the possibility that motherhood may retard expression of political interest by women: for example, the researchers note the likelihood that *mothers* who *do* approach a "political" issue may be prompted to do so only if that issue *directly involves* their own children.

Thus, many issues of general welfare which affect groups other than the children of a certain community may well suffer from "neglect"—from lack of energy and concern on the part of a significant proportion of our population.

There are other possible effects of parenthood on one's politics which might be hypothesized—for example, the question of whether a man might compromise his integrity on an issue in order to safeguard his family's financial security. This theme was strikingly treated by Ibsen in *The Enemy of the People*. The protagonist, Dr. Stockmann, discovers the town baths to be polluted and thus unsafe for the tourists who are to bring prosperity to the town. Dr. Stockmann is warned against publicizing the pollution of the baths by his brother, who admonishes, "A man with a family has no right to behave as you do; you have no right to do it, Thomas. . . ."

The implication here is that, if the town must abandon the

baths, Stockmann's own family will suffer resentment. (In fact, the plot also involves the disinheritment of Stockmann's wife if the lack of safety of the baths is exposed.)

The idea that there may be subtle shifts in one's politics if "duty to family" is in conflict might bear investigation. One recalls the old shibboleth that "a conservative is a liberal with two children."

One might also wonder how parenthood might affect one's career integrity, one's avocations, or philanthropy. . . . Regrettably, this particular paper now stands alone as a statistical report of one specific way in which motherhood affects mothers in the political arena.

9

Motherhood: Need or Myth?

BETTY ROLLIN

Correspondent with N.B.C. Nightly News

Motherhood is in trouble, and it ought to be. A rude question is long overdue: Who needs it? The answer used to be 1) society and 2) women. But now, with the impending horrors of overpopulation, society desperately *doesn't* need it. And women don't need it either. Thanks to The Motherhood Myth—the idea that having babies is something that all normal women instinctively want and need and will enjoy doing—they just *think* they do.

The notion that the maternal wish and the activity of mothering are instinctive or biologically predestined is baloney. Try asking most sociologists, psychologists, psychoanalysts, biologists—many of whom are mothers—about motherhood being instinctive; it's like asking department-store presidents if their Santa Clauses are real. "Motherhood—instinctive?" shouts distinguished sociologist/author Dr. Jessie Bernard. "Biological destiny? Forget biology! If it were biology, people would die from not doing it."

"Women don't need to be mothers any more than they need spaghetti," says Dr. Richard Rabkin, a New York psychiatrist. "But if you're in a world where everyone is eating spaghetti, thinking they need it and want it, you will think so too. Romance has really contaminated science. So-called instincts have to do with stimulation. They are not things that well up inside of you."

"When a woman says with feeling that she craved her baby from within, she is putting into biological language what is psychological," says University of Michigan psychoanalyst and mother-

From *Look,* September 22, 1970

hood-researcher Dr. Frederick Wyatt. "There are no instincts," says Dr. William Goode, president-elect of the American Sociological Association. There are reflexes, like eye-blinking, and drives, like sex. There is no innate drive for children. Otherwise, the enormous cultural pressures that there are to reproduce wouldn't exist. There are no cultural pressures to sell you on getting your hand out of the fire."

There are, to be sure, biologists and others who go on about biological destiny, that is, the innate or instinctive goal of motherhood. (At the turn of the century, even good old capitalism was explained by a theorist as "the *instinct* of acquisitiveness.") And many psychoanalysts still hold the Freudian view that women feel so rotten about not having a penis that they are necessarily propelled into the child-wish to replace the missing organ. Psychoanalysts also make much of the psychological need to repeat what one's parent of the same sex has done. Since every woman has a mother, it is considered normal to wish to imitate one's mother by being a mother.

There is, surely, a wish to pass on love if one has received it, but to insist women must pass it on in the same way is like insisting that every man whose father is a gardener has to be a gardener. One dissenting psychoanalyst says, simply, "There is a wish to comply with one's biology, yes, but we needn't and sometimes we shouldn't." (Interestingly, the woman who has been the greatest contributor to child therapy and who has probably given more to children than anyone alive is Dr. Anna Freud, Freud's magnificent daughter, who is not a mother.)

Anyway, what an expert cast of hundreds is telling us is, simply, that biological *possibility* and desire are not the same as biological *need*. Women have childbearing equipment. To choose not to use the equipment is no more blocking what is instinctive than it is for a man who, muscles or no, chooses not to be a weight lifter.

So much for the wish. What about the "instinctive" *activity* of mothering. One animal study shows that when a young member of a species is put in a cage, say, with an older member of the same species, the latter will act in a protective, "maternal" way. But that goes for both males and females who have been "mothered" themselves. And studies indicate that a human baby will also respond to whoever is around playing mother—even if it's father. Margaret Mead and many others frequently point out that mothering can be a fine occupation, if you want it, for either sex. Another experiment with monkeys who were brought up without mothers found them lacking in maternal behavior toward their own offspring. A similar study showed that monkeys brought up without other monkeys of the opposite sex had no interest in mating—all of which suggests that both mothering and mating behavior are learned, not instinctual. And, to turn the cart (or the baby carriage) around, baby ducks who lovingly follow their mothers seemed, in the mother's absence, to just as lovingly follow wooden ducks or even vacuum cleaners.

If motherhood isn't instinctive, when and why, then, was The Motherhood Myth born? Until recently, the entire question of maternal motivation was academic. Sex, like it or not, meant babies. Not that there haven't always been a lot of interesting contraceptive tries. But until the creation of the diaphragm in the 1880's, the birth of babies was largely unavoidable. And, generally speaking, nobody really seemed to mind. For one thing, people tend to be sort of good sports about what seems to be inevitable. For another, in the past, the population needed beefing up. Mortality rates were high, and agricultural cultures, particularly, have always needed children to help out. So because it "just happened" and because it was needed, motherhood was assumed to be innate.

Originally, it was the word of God that got the ball rolling with "Be fruitful and multiply," a practical suggestion, since the only people around then were Adam and Eve. But in no time, super-moralists like St. Augustine changed the tone of the message: "Intercourse, even with one's legitimate wife is unlawful and wicked where the conception of the offspring is prevented," he, we assume, thundered. And the Roman Catholic position was thus cemented. So then and now, procreation took on a curious value among people who viewed (and view) the pleasures of sex as sinful. One could partake in the sinful pleasure, but feel vindicated by the ensuing birth. Motherhood cleaned up sex. Also, it cleaned up women, who have always been considered somewhat evil, because of Eve's transgression (". . . but the woman was deceived and became a transgressor. Yet woman will be saved through bearing children . . . ," 1 Timothy, 2:14–15) and somewhat dirty because of menstruation.

And so, based on need, inevitability and pragmatic fantasy—the Myth *worked,* from society's point of view—the Myth grew like corn in Kansas. And society reinforced it with both laws and propaganda—laws that made woman a chattel, denied her education and personal mobility, and madonna propaganda that said she was beautiful and wonderful doing it and it was all beautiful and wonderful to do. (One rarely sees a madonna washing dishes.)

In fact, the Myth persisted—breaking some kind of record for long-lasting fallacies—until something like yesterday. For as the truth about the Myth trickled in—as women's rights increased, as women gradually got the message that it was certainly possible for them to do most things that men did, that they live longer, that their brains were not tinier—then, finally, when the really big news rolled in, that they could *choose* whether or not to be mothers—what happened? The Motherhood Myth soared higher than ever. As Betty Friedan made oh-so-clear in *The Feminine Mystique,* the '40's and '50's produced a group of ladies who not only had babies as if they were going out of style (maybe they were) but, as never before, they turned motherhood into a cult. First, they wallowed in the aesthetics of it all—natural childbirth and nursing became maternal musts. Like heavy-bellied ostriches they grounded their heads in the sands of motherhood, only coming up for air to say how utterly happy and fulfilled they were. But, as Mrs. Friedan says only too plainly, they weren't. The Myth galloped on, moreover, long after making babies had turned from practical asset to liability for both individual parents *and* society. With the average cost of a middle-class child figured conservatively at $30,000 (not including college), any parent knows that the only people who benefit economically from children are manufacturers of consumer goods. Hence all those gooey motherhood commercials. And the Myth gathered momentum long after sheer numbers, while not yet extinguishing us, have made us intensely uncomfortable. Almost all of our societal problems, from minor discomforts like traffic to major ones like hunger, the population people keep reminding us, have to do with there being too many people. And who suffers most? The kids who have been so mindlessly brought into the world, that's who. They are the ones who have to cope with all of the difficult and dehumanizing conditions brought on by overpopulation. They are the ones who have to cope with the psychological nausea of feeling unneeded by society. That's not the only reason for drugs, but, surely, it's a leading contender.

Unfortunately, the population curbers are tripped up by a romantic, stubborn, ideological hurdle. How can birth-control programs really be effective as long as the concept of glorious motherhood remains unchanged? (Even poor old Planned Parenthood had to euphemize—why not Planned Unparenthood?) Particularly among the poor, motherhood is one of the few inherently positive institutions that are accessible. As Berkeley demographer Judith Blake points out, "Poverty-oriented birth control programs do not make sense as a welfare measure . . . as long as existing pronatalist policies . . . encourage mating, pregnancy and the care, support and rearing of children." Or, she might have added, as long as the less-than-idyllic childrearing part of motherhood remains "in small print."

Sure, motherhood gets dumped on sometimes: Philip Wylie's Momism got going in the '40's and Philip Roth's *Portnoy's Complaint* did its best to turn rancid the chicken-soup concept of Jewish motherhood. But these are viewed as the sour cries of a black humorist here, a malcontent there. Everyone shudders, laughs, but it's like the mouse and the elephant joke. Still, the Myth persists. Last April, a Brooklyn woman was indicted on charges of manslaughter and negligent homicide—11 children died in a fire in a building she owned and criminally neglected—"But," sputtered her lawyer, "my client, Mrs. Breslow, is a mother, a grandmother and a great-grandmother!"

Most remarkably, The Motherhood Myth persists in the face of the most overwhelming maternal unhappiness and incompetence. If reproduction were merely superfluous and expensive, if the experience were as rich and rewarding as the cliché would have us believe, if it were a predominantly joyous trip for everyone riding—mother, father, child—then the going everybody-should-have-two-children plan would suffice. Certainly, there are a lot of joyous mothers, and their children and (sometimes, not necessarily) their husbands reflect their joy. But a lot of evidence suggests that for more women than anyone wants to admit, motherhood can be miserable. ("If it weren't," says one psychiatrist wryly, "the world wouldn't be in the mess it's in.")

There is a remarkable statistical finding from a recent study of Dr. Bernard's, comparing the mental illness and unhappiness of married mothers and single women. The latter group, it turned out, was both markedly less sick and overtly more happy. Of course, it's not easy to measure slippery attitudes like happiness. "Many women have achieved a kind of reconciliation—a conformity," says Dr. Bernard, "that they interpret as happiness. Since feminine happiness is supposed to lie in devoting one's life to one's husband and children, they do that; so *ipso facto,* they assume they are happy. And for many women, untrained for independence and 'processed' for motherhood, they find their state far preferable to the alternatives, which don't really exist." Also, unhappy mothers are often loath to admit it. For one thing, if in society's view not to be a mother is to be a freak, not to be a *blissful* mother is to be a witch. Besides, unlike a disappointing marriage, disappointing motherhood cannot be terminated by divorce. Of course, none of that stops such a woman from expressing her dissatisfaction in a variety of ways. Again, it is not only she who suffers but her husband and children as well. Enter the harridan housewife, the carping shrew. The realities of motherhood can turn women into terrible people. And, judging from the 50,000 cases of child abuse in the U.S. each year, some are worse than terrible.

In some cases, the unpleasing realities of motherhood begin even before the beginning. In *Her Infinite Variety,* Morton Hunt describes young married women pregnant for the first time as "very likely to be frightened and depressed, masking these feelings in order not to be considered contemptible. The arrival of pregnancy interrupts a pleasant dream of motherhood and awakens them to the realization that they have too little money, or not enough space, or unresolved marital problems. . . ."

The following are random quotes from interviews with some mothers in Ann Arbor, Mich., who described themselves as reasonably happy. They all had positive things to say about their children, although when asked about the best moment of their day, they *all* confessed it was when the children were in bed. Here is the rest:

"Suddenly I had to devote myself to the child totally. I was under the illusion that the baby was going to fit into my life, and I found that I had to switch my life and my schedule to fit *him*. You think, 'I'm in love, I'll get married, and we'll have a baby.' First there's two, then three, it's simple and romantic. You don't even think about the work." . . . "You never get away from the responsibility. Even when you leave the children with a sitter, you are not out from under the pressure of the responsibility." . . . "I hate ironing their pants and doing their underwear, and they never put their clothes in the laundry basket. . . . As they get older, they make less demands on your time because they're in school, but the demands are greater in forming their values. . . . Best moment of the day is when all the children are in bed. . . . The worst time of day is 4 p.m., when you have to get dinner started, the kids are tired, hungry and crabby—everybody wants to talk to you about *their* day . . . your day is only half over."

"Once a mother, the responsibility and concern for my children became so encompassing. . . . It took a great deal of will to keep up other parts of my personality. . . . To me, motherhood gets harder as they get older because you have less control. . . . In an abstract sense, I'd have several. . . . In the non-abstract, I would not have any." . . . "I had anticipated that the baby would sleep and eat, sleep and eat. Instead, the experience was overwhelming. I really had not thought particularly about what motherhood would mean in a realistic sense. I want to do *other* things, like to become involved in things that are worthwhile—I don't mean women's clubs—but I don't have the physical energy to go out in the evenings. I feel like I'm missing something . . . the experience of being somewhere with people and having them talking about something—something that's going on in the world."

Every grown-up person expects to pay a price for his pleasures, but seldom is the price as vast as the one endured "however happily" by most mothers. We have mentioned the literal cost factor. But what does that mean? For middle-class American women, it means a life-style with severe and usually unimagined limitations; i.e., life in the suburbs, because who can afford three bedrooms in the city? And what do suburbs mean? For women, suburbs mean other women and children and leftover peanut-butter sandwiches and car pools and seldom-seen husbands. Even the Feminine Mystiqueniks—the housewives who finally admitted that their lives behind brooms (OK, electric brooms) were driving them crazy—were loath to trace their predicament to their children. But it is simply a fact that a childless married woman has no child-work and little housework. She can live in a city, or, if she still chooses the suburbs or the country, she can leave on the commuter train with her husband if she wants to. Even the most ardent job-seeking mother will find little in the way of great opportunities in Scarsdale. Besides, by the time she wakes up, she usually lacks both the preparation for the outside world and the self-confidence to get it. You will say there are plenty of city-dwelling working mothers. But most of those women do additional-funds-for-the-family kind of work, not the interesting career kind that takes plugging during "childbearing years."

Nor is it a bed of petunias for the mother who does make it professionally. Says writer/critic Marya Mannes: "If the creative woman has children, she must pay for this indulgence with a long burden of guilt, for her life will be split three ways between them and her husband and her work. . . . No woman with any heart can compose a paragraph when her child is in trouble. . . . The creative woman has no wife to protect her from intrusion. A man at his desk in a room with closed door is a man at work. A woman at a desk in any room is available."

Speaking of jobs, do remember that mothering, salary or not, is a job. Even those who can afford nursies to handle the nitty-gritty still need to put out emotionally. "Well-cared-for" neurotic rich kids are not exactly unknown in our society. One of the more absurd aspects of the Myth is the underlying assumption that, since most women are biologically equipped to bear children, they are psychologically, mentally, emotionally and technically equipped (or interested) to rear them. Never mind happiness. To assume that such an exacting, consuming and important task is something almost all women are equipped to do is far more dangerous and ridiculous than assuming that everyone with vocal chords should seek a career in the opera.

A major expectation of the Myth is that children make a not-so-hot marriage hotter, or a hot marriage, hotter still. Yet almost every available study indicates that childless marriages are far happier. One of the biggest, of 850 couples, was conducted by Dr. Harold Feldman of Cornell University, who states his finding in no uncertain terms: "Those couples with children had a significantly lower level of marital satisfaction than did those without children." Some of the reasons are obvious. Even the most adorable children make for additional demands, complications and hardships in the lives of even the most loving parents. If a woman feels disappointed and trapped in her mother role, it is bound to affect her marriage in any number of ways: she may take out her frustrations directly on her husband, or she may count on him too heavily for what she feels she is missing in her daily life.

". . . You begin to grow away from your husband," says one of the Michigan ladies. "He's working on his career and you're working on your family. But you both must gear your lives to the children. You do things the children enjoy, more than things you might enjoy." More subtle and possibly more serious is what motherhood may do to a woman's sexuality. Often when the stork flies in, sexuality flies out. Both in the emotional minds of some women *and* in the minds of their husbands, when a woman becomes a mother, she stops being a woman. It's not only that motherhood may destroy her physical attractiveness, but its madonna concept may destroy her *feelings* of sexuality.

And what of the payoff? Usually, even the most self-sacrificing maternal self-sacrificers expect a little something back. Gratified parents are not unknown to the Western world, but there are probably at least just as many who feel, to put it crudely, shortchanged. The experiment mentioned earlier—where the baby ducks followed vacuum cleaners instead of their mothers—indicates that what passes for love from baby to mother is merely a rudimentary kind of object attachment. Without necessarily feeling like a Hoover, a lot of women become disheartened because babies and children are not only not interesting to talk to (not everyone thrills at the wonders of da-da-ma-ma talk) but they are generally not empathetic, considerate people. Even the nicest children are not capable of empathy, surely a major ingredient of love, until they are much older. Sometimes they're never capable of it. Dr. Wyatt says that often, in later years particularly, when most of the "returns" are in, it is the "good mother" who suffers most of all. It is then she must face a reality: The child—the appendage with her genes—is not an appendage, but a separate person who doesn't even like her—or whom she doesn't really like.

So if the music is lousy, how come everyone's dancing? Because the motherhood minuet is taught free from birth, and whether or not she has rhythm or likes the music, every woman is expected to do it. Indeed, she *wants* to do it. Little girls start learning what to want—and what to be—when they are still in their cribs. Dr. Miriam Keiffer, a young social psychologist at Bensalem, The Experimental College of Fordham University, points to studies showing that "at six months of age, mothers are already treating their baby girls and boys quite differently. For instance, mothers have been found to touch, comfort, and talk to their females more. If these differences can be found at such an early stage, it's not surprising that the end product is as different as it is. What is surprising is that men and women are, in so many ways, similar." Some people point to the way little girls play with dolls as proof of their "innate motherliness." But remember, little girls are *given* dolls. When Margaret Mead presented some dolls to New Guinea children, it was the boys, not the girls, who wanted to play with them, which they did by crooning lullabies and rocking them in the most maternal fashion.

By the time they reach adolescence, most girls, unconsciously or not, have learned enough about role definition to qualify for a master's degree. In general, the lesson has been that no matter what kind of career thoughts one may entertain, one must, first and foremost, be a wife and mother. A girl's mother is usually her first teacher. As Dr. Goode says, "A woman is not only taught by society to have a child; she is taught to have a child who will have a child." A woman who has hung her life on The Motherhood

Myth will almost always reinforce her young married daughter's early training by pushing for grandchildren. Prospective grandmothers are not the only ones. Husbands, too, can be effective sellers. After all, they have The Fatherhood Myth to cope with. A married man is *supposed to* have children. Often, particularly among Latins, children are a sign of potency. They help him assure the world—and himself—that he is the big man he is supposed to be. Plus, children give him both immortality (whatever that means) and possibly the chance to become "more" in his lifetime through the accomplishments of his children, particularly his son. (Sometimes it's important, however, for the son to do better, but not *too* much better.)

Friends, too, can be counted on as myth-pushers. Naturally one wants to do what one's friends do. One study, by the way, found an absolute correlation between a woman's fertility and that of her three closest friends. The negative sell comes into play here, too. We have seen what the concept of non-mother means (cold, selfish, unwomanly, abnormal). In practice, particularly in the suburbs, it can mean, simply, exclusion—both from child-centered activities (that is, most activities) and child-centered conversations (that is, most conversations). It can also mean being the butt of a lot of unfunny jokes. ("Whaddya waiting for? An immaculate conception? Ha ha.") Worst of all, it can mean being an object of pity.

In case she's escaped all of those pressures (that is, if she was brought up in a cave), a young married woman often wants a baby just so that she'll 1) have something to do (motherhood is better than clerk/typist, which is often the only kind of job she can get, since little more has been expected of her and, besides, her boss also expects her to leave and be a mother); 2) have something to hug and possess, to be needed by and have power over; and 3) have something to *be*—e.g., a baby's mother. Motherhood affords an instant identity. First, through wifehood, you are somebody's wife; then you are somebody's mother. Both give not only identity and activity, but status and stardom of a kind. During pregnancy, a woman can look forward to the kind of attention and pampering she may not ever have gotten or may never otherwise get. Some women consider birth the biggest accomplishment of their lives, which may be interpreted as saying not much for the rest of their lives. As Dr. Goode says, "It's like the gambler who may know the roulette wheel is crooked, but it's the only game in town." Also, with motherhood, the feeling of accomplishment is immediate. It is really much faster and easier to make a baby than paint a painting, or write a book, or get to the point of accomplishment in a job. It is also easier in a way to shift focus from self-development to child development—particularly since, for women, self-development is considered selfish. Even unwed mothers may achieve a feeling of this kind. (As we have seen, little thought is given to the aftermath.) And, again, since so many women are underdeveloped as people, they feel that, besides children, they have little else to give—to themselves, their husbands, to their world.

You may ask why then, when the realities do start pouring in, does a woman want to have a second, third, even fourth child? OK, 1) Just because reality is pouring in doesn't mean she wants to *face* it. A new baby can help bring back some of the old illusions. Says psychoanalyst Dr. Natalie Shainess, "She may view each successive child as a knight in armor that will rescue her from being a 'bad/unhappy mother.' " 2) Next on the horror list of having no children, is having one. It suffices to say that only children are not only OK, they even have a high rate of exceptionality. 3) Both parents usually want at least one child of each sex. The husband, for reasons discussed earlier, probably wants a son. 4) The more children one has, the more of an excuse one has not to develop in any other way.

What's the point? A world without children? Of course not. Nothing could be worse or more unlikely. No matter what anyone says in Look or anywhere else, motherhood isn't about to go out like a blown bulb, and who says it should? Only the Myth must go out, and now it seems to be dimming.

The younger-generation females who have been reared on the Myth have not rejected it totally, but at least they recognize it can be more loving to children not to have them. And at least they speak of adopting children instead of bearing them. Moreover, since the new non-breeders are "less hung-up" on ownership, they seem to recognize that if you dig loving children, you don't necessarily have to own one. The end of The Motherhood Myth might make available more loving women (and men!) for those children who already exist.

When motherhood is no longer culturally compulsory, there will, certainly, be less of it. Women are now beginning to think and do more about development of self, of their individual resources. Far from being selfish, such development is probably our only hope. That means more alternatives for women. And more alternatives mean more selective, better, happier motherhood—

and childhood and husbandhood (or manhood) and peoplehood. It is not a question of whether or not children are sweet and marvelous to have and rear; the question is, even if that's so, whether or not one wants to pay the price for it. It doesn't make sense any more to pretend that women need babies, when what they really need is themselves. If God were still speaking to us in a voice we could hear, even He would probably say, "Be fruitful. Don't multiply."

10

Motivations in Wanting Conceptions

EDWARD POHLMAN

Director of the Birth Planning Research Program, University of the Pacific, Stockton, California

Before reading "Motivations in Wanting Conceptions," it is well to have a basic orientation to several important studies that are referred to:

Lee Rainwater's 1965 study *Family Design: Marital Sexuality, Family Size, and Family Planning* (Chicago: Aldine) was a study relating conjugal role relationships to family size desires in 409 individuals.

Lois Hoffman and Frederick Wyatt, *Social Change and Motivations for Having Larger Families: Some Theoretical Considerations* (Merrill-Palmer Quarterly, Vol. 6). An interesting observation of this 1960 study is that some parents are motivated to have *additional* children to assuage guilt over perceived shortcomings in rearing of initial child or children.

Family Growth in Metropolitan America (FGMA) involved a longitudinal study of couples at three times. The first time couples were interviewed, each had just had a second child (in 1957). Follow-up interviews in 1960 and 1963 involved many couples in the original sample.

Indianapolis Study (reported variously between 1946 and 1958) examined the attitudes toward fertility, conception, and family planning among 1000 couples drawn from a white, Protestant population of at least eighth grade education.

Growth of American Families Study (GAF). In-depth interviews conducted in 1955 and 1960 (each sample including about 2400 wives) regarding past childbearing and expected childbearing patterns.

Chapter 4 of *Psychology of Birth Planning* (Schenkman, 1969)

Most parents in most cultures probably want some children. A logical next question is why. In asking this question, we do not consider broad social or economic perspectives, but operate only from the delimited viewpoint sketched previously. The present chapter provides a catalog of possible motives for wanting children, which may serve as a source of hypotheses. The catalog has an American bias, but many of the factors suggested are applicable across a wide range of cultures. The organization below discusses one motive at a time; Rainwater (1965) presents cases that illustrate the integration of many factors.

Important American sources on the question of why people want children are Rainwater (1965), the FGMA reports (1961; 1963), and Hoffman and Wyatt (1960). Probably one should not become entangled in the Indianapolis Study (1946–1958) material on this topic unless one has first studied the FGMA reports. The GAF studies bear on the topic of this chapter only indirectly, with brief exceptions (GAF, 1959; 1966).

Neither the Indianapolis nor the FGMA studies claimed much success in correlating the personal independent variables they studied—such as personality factors or family relations—with desired family size or related variables. In contrast, they found appreciable correlations for the independent variables of socio-economic status (in the Indianapolis Study) and religion (in the FGMA studies, as was true also in the GAF studies). Probably the latter variables tended to be catch-alls that summarized numbers of moderately correlated independent variables. But neither socio-economic status nor church membership per se can explain why people want or do not want a conception (Rainwater, 1965; FGMA, 1961), from the perspective of this chapter. To say that a man wants a larger or smaller family "because" he is lower class or belongs to a certain church is not a satisfactory psychological explanation; we must ask what factors associated with class or church influence his desires for children. Also, if we are interested in changing birth planning behavior (rather than merely chronicling or predicting it), we cannot usually do this by changing either socio-economic status or religion.

Rainwater (1965) criticizes the Indianapolis and FGMA reports for using "overly ambitious" quantitative criteria for judging the value of relationships found, criteria appropriate to the precision of demography but somewhat out of line with standards of social psychological research. In view of the scarcity of empirical evidence, however, most ideas to be presented below must be viewed either as assumptions or as hypotheses for further testing.

Nevertheless the failure of the Indianapolis or FGMA studies to find evidence to support a given hypothesis should make us question that hypothesis but not throw it out, for four reasons. The first two are underlined again and again by the FGMA (1961; 1963) writers: (1) possible insensitivity in measuring the independent variable in question, and (2) highly specific populations. Possibly some hypotheses inappropriate for these populations are more appropriate in other populations in America or elsewhere. Also, a hypothesis might not be supported in *any* one culture at a given time, yet might find support in comparisons across a range of cultures or times, with the wider variations implied.

(3) Reasons for wanting or not wanting *some* children and *more* children may be rather different. Since almost everyone wants some children, in the cultures that have been studied extensively, and since people who want no children tend to be somewhat atypical in many other ways, it is difficult to research the reasons that people may have in common for wanting children. Hence the dependent variables of the major studies have emphasized variations in family-size factors among those who wanted some children. But the independent variables that relate to such criteria may be somewhat different from those leading parents to want some children in the first place. For example, if there should be any innate factors that prompt people toward wanting children, these would presumably be common to almost all people in a given study. The present chapter combines possible reasons for wanting some, and for wanting more, children.

(4) Factors that strongly influence some individuals or small subgroups may not show up in the over-all picture for large groups, even when those groups are controlled for socio-economic status or religion. For example, if it is true that marital *discord* sometimes leads a parent to want a child as a means of saving the faltering marriage, and also that marital *happiness* sometimes leads a parent toward wanting a child, these opposing tendencies might cancel one another out in the group picture. The independent variable may show no correlation with family size and the demographer will probably conclude that the variable is of no value for predicting the fertility of groups. But such a correlation would not rule out possible relationships interesting to those who seek a finer-grained analysis of motives for wanting conceptions. Similarly, a factor might be lost or minimized in a large group if it is very important but to only a relatively few people. Raising such speculations is no substitute for providing evidence that a hypothesized relationship does indeed exist, and many of

the hypotheses mentioned in this chapter have only case study evidence to support them. For example, this is the only kind of evidence for the contention that couples sometimes have a child to save a faltering marriage (e.g., Sloman, 1948). But the negative findings of demographic studies of groups do not prove that a given hypothesis has no merit in understanding individual cases.

People's answers to questions about why they want children, or larger or smaller families (GAF, 1959; 1966; Rainwater, 1965; Clare & Kiser, 1951) are interesting and important but cannot be relied on too heavily to tell us their real reasons. As the authors just cited suggest, rationalizing by providing socially desirable answers is probably rampant.

A. Innate Factors

Many medical and other writers speak of a maternal "instinct" (e.g., Deutsch, 1945; Soddy, 1964; Wengraf, 1953). Some authors use the term only in quotes or to criticize the concept (e.g., Reed, 1923; Seitz, 1958). "Instinct" will be avoided because of its ambiguity. Instead we shall speak of possibly innate (unlearned) factors that make it intrinsically rewarding to reproduce and rear children. It is possible to distinguish, logically, a series of somewhat distinct possible factors, such as those making it innately rewarding or satisfying to (1) have sex relations, (2) have a fetus in the uterus, (3) go through delivery and childbirth, (4) breastfeed a baby, (5) cuddle a baby next to one's skin, and (6) take care of an infant or older child. The first set of factors, involving sex relations, is usually not included in the term "parental instincts," and probably should not be included in our discussion—especially since contraceptive practice makes it possible to have sex relations without children. The remaining factors involve women primarily, although men might be motivated by the last two. We do not usually hear of a "paternal" but only of a "maternal instinct," although Benedek (1959) speculates that there is a drive toward fatherliness. Mead (1949) seems to be saying that women, but not men, have innate needs to have children.

Much of what is attributed to innate factors may be explained rather readily as a matter of social learning, if one cares to use such an explanation (Sears et al., 1957). Little girls learn that they should want and have children. Probably most psychologists, and certainly this writer, would lay primary stress on explanations involving learning. However, there is no decisive evidence that separates possible innate from learned factors in wanting children and rules out the existence or importance of the former. The existence of some individuals or even an occasional whole culture where women do not want children still would not eliminate the possibility of innate mothering needs. For the believer in innate factors could argue that learning has suppressed an innate tendency (Mead, 1949; Kroger & Freed, 1962). Psychologists are among those who at least leave the door open to the possibility of innate factors (e.g., Beach, 1948; Centers & Blumberg, 1954; Newton, 1955; Rabin, 1965b; Sears et al., 1957). We shall not attempt to review the extensive and often controversial relevant research with animals. But there is the possibility that certain innate factors make motherhood—including pregnancy and the childbirth process—rewarding.

Having said this, we note a number of qualifications and comments. Even those needs that seem definitely to be unlearned—such as hunger—are subject to amazing modification through learning. If there are innate needs associated with biological motherhood, they are undoubtedly subject to similarly extensive moulding through learning. Even Mead (1949), who believes that women who do not want to be mothers have learned this, rejects the idea that women must necessarily suffer somehow if they learn to want to be childless, and are childless. The problems often found in women who choose to be childless are seen by Mead as being the result of learning that childbearing is expected, and then going against that learning—rather than as a result of frustration of innate needs.

If we grant the presence of innate needs for motherhood, it seems to this writer that we must either argue that these needs are satisfied by having one child, or that they persist and prompt a woman toward continual reproduction. In the former case one child is as satisfying as six. In the latter case even the women with six or eight children—while she has more need satisfaction than the woman with a small family—must leave her needs somewhat unfulfilled, since she might have reproduced even more children.

If research from comparative psychology and anecdotal observation of animal life are cited to try to show innate tendencies toward parenthood, in fairness we should note that some animals, including mammals, will eat or kill their own offspring.

We conclude that very little is known for sure about possible innate needs to be a mother. If such needs exist they have been heavily overlaid by cultural learning. Their very existence is extremely difficult to isolate and demonstrate, making them impossible to use as an independent variable in systematic research relating to family size. A best guess would be that if such needs exist they are probably relatively unimportant in making the difference between a family of two and four children, and population problems usually hang on differences of this magnitude or less.

B. Psychoanalytic Hypotheses

Freudian psychology has suggested a number of possible reasons —often unconscious—for wanting children. In most cases they are supported by no systematic research evidence. Some of these ideas may be used, perhaps with different terminology, by those who do not accept the Freudian speculations involved.

Virility

Producing a child is a conspicuous evidence of having sufficient virility, potency, sexual maturity, and adequacy to reproduce; successes in the sexual bed are not so clearly visible. If working class people live their lives closer to biological experience than the middle class, this may be especially important to them. Large families, or children born at a very young or a very old age or soon after marriage, or sons may be desired to show sexual adequacy and potency. Adopted children may, in some cases, be a sort of substitute demonstration of potency, like a bald man's wig. Two or three children may not suffice to reassure some people. Curtailing family size might be interpreted as a curtailing of sexual adequacy, although this should be less threatening if many people in one's sub-culture are following a similar pattern.

Male potency, involving a sort of rugged animal maleness—machismo—has been thought to be especially important in some Latin American countries, including Puerto Rico, with possible influences on men's family-size desires. Hill, Stycos, and Back (1959, 100–106) were not able to find empirical evidence that this factor had importance in birth planning.

Competition with One's Own Parents

In psychoanalytic theory, competition with one's parent of the same sex is thought to be customary. Having a baby is a way of competing, a man with his father and a woman with her mother. A woman's first baby may involve a hostile desire to replace the mother; having a larger or smaller family may be an attempt to outdo the mother. For example, a smaller family may say, "I'm smart enough to plan my family wisely"; a larger one, "I can handle more responsibilities and still run my life smoothly and well." A Puerto Rican couple who had lived in America for four years had eight children, wanted more, and seemed to be a very happy family. The wife said,

> "My husband's father had 15. We want to beat him with 16. I'm only 35, but we lost 2 years when my husband came to the United States." (GAF, 1959).

Sometimes family size may be used to compete with the husband's or wife's sibling in a very similar way, especially if the sibling was preferred over the individual. The Biblical Rachel and Leah, and the two daughters-in-law of "Big Daddy" in Williams' *Cat on a Hot Tin Roof,* wanted children to help in their sister-like competitions.

Children, and especially a first child, stand as a sort of evidence of adultness and independence from parents. Possibly in some American families marriage is no longer a sufficient symbol of independence, especially since many young married couples are financially or otherwise dependent on parents. Possibly having a baby takes on special symbolic value (LeMasters, 1957).

The American moving picture *Bambi* ends with the hero deer producing offspring. Early in the picture when the then hornless hero was born, his father was shown on an elevated, glorified rock. At the end Bambi fathers twins—not merely one baby deer at a time—and is shown, with his newly grown horns, standing beside his father on the same glorified rock. The father walks off into the forest, leaving Bambi alone on the rock, horns aloft, as the picture ends.

Other Sex-Related Hypotheses

Freud and many of his followers have held that girls normally have "penis envy"; some women are thought to want a child, especially a male child, as a penis substitute. The Oedipal attachment thought to exist between parents and opposite-sex children may be a basis for wanting children. A parent may desire a child to provide a lover. Mothers whose husbands pay them insufficient attention might be especially prone to this sort of unconscious influence. The mother may also be attracted toward a larger family because she unconsciously feels that having more sons lessens the threat of losing Oedipal gratification through the death of any given son. Also, if her Oedipal interests are divided among many sons this reduces the intensity of any one relationship;

thus she may feel less guilty over her own forbidden interests, and less guilty about the possibility of damaging any given son through one intense relationship.

Children may be seen as a punishment for sex. Some individual Roman Catholics seem to support their church's stance against most contraceptives because birth control devices remove the natural penalty for sex. Flugel (1947b) opines that husbands may want their wives to suffer with pregnancy, childbirth, and child care to atone for their own guilt. Likewise, people in a society may want others to become scapegoats and suffer with children. Children might be wanted because a parent has a need to be punished for specifically sexual behavior by a penalty that is closely tied to the guilt-producing act. More generally, people with "masochistic" needs—needs to be punished—may want children as punishment.

Extending the Ego

Psychoanalytic writers and others speak of the child as an "extension of the ego" or the "self" of the parent. The love that a person has for himself or herself (narcissism) is invested in the child. Having more children may be somewhat like building up a big business, or annexing another country to one's kingdom, or building another room onto one's house, or buying a car. Some of the same pride and defensiveness that a person feels toward himself, including his body, can be extended to children. Children are part of oneself. Both Tennessee Williams' *Cat on a Hot Tin Roof* and Faulkner's *Long Hot Summer* show powerful father figures who push their children toward producing grandchildren. Faulkner's character Varner says he wants to cover the countryside with Varners.

An investment of the self in such an extension may be a sort of reincarnation. Thus it may lead to a sort of immortality which is an extension of the ego not only into a broader area but into the future. The emphasis among the Hebrews on many "seed," especially before the time when belief in a personal after-life was formalized, may have been related to this need. In some contemporary cultures there is incentive to have large numbers of descendants who will honor and remember and perhaps worship one. In the Indianapolis Study (Swain & Kiser, 1953) about three-fourths of both the husbands and the wives answered affirmatively the question, "Is one of your greatest satisfactions in being a parent knowing that, after you are gone, some part of you will live on in your children?" Both Rainwater (1965) and Clare and Kiser (1951) found more husbands than wives emphasizing the carrying on of the family name as a reason for wanting children.

C. Conformity to Social Norms

Attempts to see whether people have been influenced in family-size desires by the specific opinions or recommendations of their parents, siblings, or friends have not provided convincing evidence of important relationships. But social conformity to much more pervasive cultural and sub-cultural norms is almost certainly a factor influencing the initial desire for children and the number of children desired. This influence is hard to research. Potter and Kantner (1955) used measures of "conformity" to group norms and tried unsuccessfully to show that the more conforming individuals were different from others in family size or contraception variables. Within any given culture at any given time, any given study may be dealing with a relatively homogenous set of family sizes, with a great deal of conformity to cultural norms being present as a constant for the sample as a whole. Thus even if there were some good way to measure conformity to "fashions" in family size, such studies probably would not reveal it to be as important an independent variable as it is. Somewhat more promising are approaches that look at different cultures or different periods of history.

Variations in family size in the United States since the depression are noteworthy and can be explained only partially on the basis of economic factors. The perceived ideal family size in America appeared to change from a mode of two to four children between 1941 and 1955 (GAF, 1959).

> The rapidity with which new standards of family size have spread throughout the whole society since World War II indicates how quickly a population may now adjust its values about such vital matters as reproduction. Apparently our population is now so closely linked together in a single system of communication and interdependence that . . . new values can be developed, diffused, and put into action on a massive scale very quickly (GAF, 1959).

In a similar vein, authors of the successor to this study tend to discount the reasons mothers gave for family-size preferences. They stress the probable importance of

> . . . family-size norms or 'fashions' of the religious, social and economic groups with which they and their families were closely associ-

ated. Most wives wanted to have about the same number of children as they said they thought their married friends of the same age would have (GAF, 1966).

There seems to be agreement among a number of writers that the family is in style in recent America. One British father complains:

> "The child is the Sacred Calf of the modern world, and the High Priests of the Child Cult are always bidding us bow down and worship the Sacred Calf, and reminding us of all the happiness it brings us . . ." (Balchin, 1965).

Bernard (1964) speaks of the "idolatry of reproduction" and asks whether marriage and family specialists' writing and research have helped produce the "mania for childbearing" seen among contemporary youth. He wonders if a fetish has been made of motherhood, so that it has become practically compulsive, and asks whether all women are capable of mothering so many children. In a hasty examination by the present writer, only three or four pictures in one prominent marriage and family text (Duvall, 1962) showed unhappiness, and one of these was a widow and another a woman alone. A couple of dozen pictures showed smiling people predominantly; a like number showed people interested in what they were doing, apparently creatively involved; a dozen gave no clues one way or another as to the happiness or sadness of family members.

Family activities and family values are exalted in the popular media and in the design of homes, communities, and a variety of facilities. Gurin et al. (1960) opine that the importance of parenthood in giving an adult an identity had probably been more exaggerated in the decade just before they wrote than ever before in America.

From his data, Rainwater (1965) abstracts one central norm: ". . . one shouldn't have more children than one can support, *but one should have as many children as one can afford*" (italics his). In this study, people who had large families were viewed as somehow "good," and those with small families as less laudable, often as selfish. This may imply some pressure to have larger families. Rainwater interprets some of the answers given by his middle class respondents as meaning

> . . . simply that some people have large families not so much because they really want them as because they feel social pressure to do so (Rainwater, 1965).

Rainwater concluded that his respondents as a group were aware of trends in family size. Note this response:

> "My Lord, my impression is that bigger families are more fashionable now. Almost as fashionable as 50–60 years ago. In the 1930's it was indecent to have a lot of children, now it's fashionable" (Rainwater, 1965).

If standards of family size differ according to social classes, the higher classes may set a model in proper number of children, just as they often do in other areas. Either larger or smaller families might be copied by those aspiring to "move up" or those who had recently "moved up" socially. Since contraception and smaller families have tended to come to the higher classes in any society first, small families would be the usual model in this hypothesis. But in some cases the higher classes in a society might favor large families. FGMA authors (1961) reviewed the rationale for this last possibility, together with some suggestive earlier evidence, but their data did not support this hypothesis (FGMA, 1961; 1963).

A similar hypothesis was advanced by Stycos (1958), in an attempt to understand the empirical evidence of ambivalence provided by the study of Hill, Stycos, and Back (1959). Stycos phrases his discussion in terms of differential norms and reference groups. On a variable such as social class or sex or age or marital status, a given individual may occupy a particular position. In addition he may aspire to the norms and values of some other position on that variable, since that position is perceived by him as desirable.

Stycos (1958) says that

> The same individual may have a number of conflicting attitudes, the salience of any one at any one time dependent on the situation. In the presence of a middle class interviewer the respondent may voice attitudes she feels more acceptable to that class; in the presence of her husband still another attitude might be voiced; in the presence of her peers still another.

He quotes Ryan's (1952) report concerning Sinhalese women:

> The sample of mothers . . . offered evidence that many women are torn between the community valuation of the large family and a personal desire for restricted numbers . . . It was sharply evident to the interviewers that infinite numbers of children were an unqualified blessing in situations where several women were present.

In trying to decide whether a child was wanted, the present

writer would tend to interpret what Ryan calls a "personal desire" as the "true" feeling, and a conflicting publicly expressed viewpoint as a facade or false front. However, the public view may be a very real part of the ambivalent feeling. Writing with an emphasis on the factors which affect family size rather than on parents' "wanting-unwanting" feelings, Stycos (1958) says:

> In the light of present knowledge, it would be fallacious to assume that a privately held attitude is more 'real' than a publicly held one. There is no reason to believe that one attitude has less consequences for behavior than the other. Indeed, since the number of one's children is a public phenomenon, it might be argued that the 'public' attitude is more significant for fertility than the 'private' one.

Hypothetically, people might arrange their fertility in keeping with the public attitude, even though that public attitude was at variance with what they privately wanted. For example, it is often considered abnormal for a married couple to want no children, and hence some people may want and have children in order to prove their normalcy when they "really" do not want to have any.

The preceding paragraphs highlight the possibility that an individual and his social group may be in conflict—perhaps even consciously—over whether conception is desirable. But, perhaps more typically, social groups influence an individual's family-size desires more quietly and with no conflict. They simply shape his thinking imperceptibly.

D. "Liking for Children"

One of the most common reasons people give for wanting children is that they like children (Rainwater, 1965; GAF, 1966). This may be a particularly easy rationale to give when asked. But to "like" and to "want" children are not mere synonyms. Many of the reasons for wanting children, suggested in this chapter, have little to do with liking them. It would seem to be better for children's mental health if parents actually did want them because they liked them, rather than for other reasons. Rainwater describes a father he interviewed as follows:

> . . . one gets the impression that he is more interested in his large family as a symbol of something than he is in relating to them individually (Rainwater, 1965).

Those who want larger families tend to reveal more "liking for children" (as inferred from interview statements), but this is true primarily when we compare those who want no children and those who want at least some. Among those who want at least some, the positive correlation between "liking" and desired number of children is smaller, if it exists at all (Pratt & Whelpton, 1955; Westoff & Borgatta, 1955; FGMA, 1961; 1963). Thus this may be more of a factor influencing people to have some children than a factor influencing variations in family size. It seems probable that liking for children can be expressed qualitatively instead of quantitatively.

Why do parents "like" or "love" children; what is meant by these terms? Psychologists are often accused of becoming so involved in looking at the hidden and dark motives for behavior that they overlook the obvious. Most of the present chapter might be used to support this criticism, and it is possible to dissect even "liking for children" into fragments, some of them sinister. But some of the open, common-sense "Mothers' Day" reasons for liking children are important. Children provide action and stimulation and change, some of the factors that attract adults to raise pets or watch a television program. Children are "entertaining." Many parents get a feeling of accomplishment and pleasure in watching children develop, and feel that children provide a generally happier atmosphere. Most people, whether they want children or not, agree that children provide a feeling of pride.

Children are, after all, human beings (despite parents' occasional doubts on this point), and many humans seem to find the company of other humans pleasant. People may want children in part because they enjoy the company of children, enjoy interacting with them. Many of the attractive things that other humans can do for a person, that person's children can also do. They can love a parent and provide someone to love. They can be talked with, played with, dominated and controlled. They provide an audience before which a parent can show off; they admire his accomplishments, and make a hero of him.

Some have speculated that in times of war or other broad social crisis and shock, people withdraw into the home, turn to children, and have more of them (Anonymous, 1945; GAF, 1959; Landis & Landis, 1963). In view of the prevalence of small families during the traumatic depression years in America, one might need to modify this hypothesis by adding the stipulation "if they are financially able."

Perhaps as the United States has changed in recent decades, there is somewhat less emphasis on, and opportunity for, upward social mobility and hard work as a way of "getting ahead." Perhaps many suburbanites are somewhat satisfied with their lot and have no great expectations of advancing. Promotion in many large organizations is based more on tenure and less on over-time, ulcer-producing work than was true in an earlier America. There is an increase of leisure time. Perhaps ours is a society that is relatively rich and bored. The frontiers of the West and even of upward social mobility and financial advancement are possibly less promising. Meanwhile the impersonality of many interactions between people in a complex urban life remains. Perhaps such factors combine to help make family life, including the three- or four-child family, popular. Children provide a do-it-yourself, build-your-own source of meaning at home instead of on the job; they have endless capacities to absorb time; they provide at least small challenges and upsets and crises in a culture that may be bored with its pleasant sameness; and they provide exceedingly personal interaction in contrast to the impersonality of many other contacts.

Westoff et al., (1961) tested a hypothesis that was related to some of the above ideas, although it was not posed as providing any comprehensive check on them. The study compared families where fathers were employed in small businesses or self-employed with those where fathers were employed by "bureaucracies." As predicted, on the dependent variables the former group tended to place in ways that relate to smaller family size. But this relationship disappeared when controls for religion were used, largely because Jewish parents were found disproportionately in the former group and also tended to have smaller families.

Liking to Help Others, and Dependency Needs

In a sense, everything a person does is done to meet his *own* needs; the psychology of motivation really has no other way to explain behavior. But this may include meeting one's own altruistic needs. Thus we might distinguish between self-serving which meets others' needs in the process and self-serving that is more directly "selfish." Some parents want and like children in part because children meet their needs to be giving and generous and helpful. At the other extreme, some parents are almost completely self-centered in their reasons for wanting children. Swain and Kiser (1953) tried to tap this distinction between more and less selfish motives for having children. What they called an "ego-centered" interest in children was assumed to be a more selfish basis for wanting children. However, there was no validation of the questions that purported to measure this variable (e.g., "Could anything give you as much satisfaction in life as having children of your own?"). The questions and parents' answers are of interest in themselves, but cannot be assumed to measure a particularly self-centered, as versus more generous, basis for liking children.

Many people seem to have needs to help others—including children—by providing for them, telling them what to do, and taking responsibility for them. This often makes men and women feel that they are important to someone. A psychoanalytic hypothesis holds that if an adult has strong dependency needs, one way to meet them is to have someone else take care of you, but another is to take care of someone else. At an obvious level, the person with strong dependency needs may enjoy the company of children and feel responsible and important. More deeply, a parent may be thought of as projecting his own needs onto whoever he cares for, identifying with the helped person, and thereby in a sense taking care of himself. If the person being cared for is one's child, an extension of one's ego, then this sort of identification would seem to be especially easy.

The FGMA authors (1961) hypothesized, in contrast to the reasoning above, that mothers with strong unsatisfied dependency needs and immature concerns with themselves and their problems would want fewer children. These variables were measured by both a modification of the Nurturance scale of the Edwards Personal Preference Schedule and an unpublished measure of "generalized manifest anxiety." The former asks questions about a person's desire to help others (not to be helped), so that it is a measure of dependency needs only if projection is assumed to operate. The correlations were not significant. Sears et al. (1957) noted some tendency for wives manifesting lower self-esteem at the interview to be those who recalled that the pregnancy had been unwanted.

E. Financial Gain

In many Western nations including the United States, children are not a financial asset for most people. But in many countries of the world children are still either an economic asset, even when they are young, or an investment in a sort of insurance for when parents are old, or both. Particularly where agriculture or home industry is the family's economic base, children can become economic producers after only a short "investment" period. In some cultures an individual believes (perhaps correctly) that his economic resources in old age will depend largely on the number of living children or related dependents that he will have at that time. Even if an additional birth means a net economic loss for the economy of the nation as a whole, it may mean an economic gain for the individual parent. In such a case, government programs to provide some other basis for old age security would seem to be important.

Some governments with pro-natalist policies have offered financial rewards for producing larger families. On a small scale the current program in the United States, whereby a parent is exempted from income taxation on an additional $600 each year for each additional child, may have the effect of permitting or facilitating larger families. In Roumania, pregnant women are granted a long leave from work with full pay (Mehlan, 1965). In a small experiment, couples with at least two children were offered a college scholarship for an additional child if he were born within the year 1940 (Flanagan, 1942). Couples had significantly more children than would otherwise have been born during 1940, and still other couples tried to take advantage of the offer but had fecundity problems. It is not clear whether these extra efforts involved children who would not have been born otherwise, or merely an earlier scheduling of conceptions that would have occurred later.

When public financial assistance is provided to poor parents according to the number of their children, with the intention of helping care for whatever children exist, in some individual cases this may provide a reason for wanting children. This writer knows personally of some women who have announced their intention of conceiving another child for this reason. This possible factor is sometimes greatly exaggerated by critics of the public assistance programs. Lower class mothers, whether on public assistance or not, tend to have many births that they do not want but do not know how to stop effectively (Meier, 1961). Although critics may exaggerate the above-mentioned factor, it is also possible that those professionally involved in administering public assistance programs may have unconscious tendencies to minimize it. In any case, a more positive program of influencing these families than cutting off their public assistance is to offer them birth control help, as an increasing number of communities in the United States are now doing.

Economist J. William Leasure has outlined a program of payments to poor mothers with several children, payments made for each year when they did *not* have an additional child. The state could afford such payments because of the money saved tax-payers by each non-birth. Mothers would thus be helped to break the vicious cycle of poverty by having more money and fewer children. The possible financial incentive to welfare families to produce otherwise unwanted children would be removed, if both births *and* non-births earned income.

F. A Role for the Woman

In Chapter 7 we discuss changes in the roles of women and men, and suggest that one of the costs of children to some women is in keeping them from other, more attractive roles out of the home. But some women do not want out-of-home roles, and find the mother role highly desirable. Lower class women, especially, tend to feel that motherhood is what life is all about; no other option really exists (Rainwater, 1960). Motherhood is a woman's destiny; it validates her existence; it makes her life complete. Middle class women may have more options. But a young woman of any class may be uncertain of her identity, role, importance, and meaning in life. Having a first baby may give her a role.

Hoffman and Wyatt (1960) present a hypothesis to account for American women's desires for larger families. This was elaborated and partially checked by Rainwater (1965). Housework and cooking have become less demanding, challenging, time-consuming, financially profitable and creative. Women in America are somewhat condemned by conscience and by others if they are idle; being bored with nothing to do presents psychological problems; they must be busy doing something. As the first two or three children begin to demand less time and care the mother must find other activities. If she tries to occupy herself completely with home, garden, or social activities she runs some risk of seeming selfish to herself and others. A job or some non-paid equivalent is attractive to some women, but not to others; for many women having another child may be a preferred alternative to out-of-home roles, and to idleness. "Labor-saving devices" may make it possible to have a larger family with less work. Also, the emphasis on child psychology and the challenges of being a good parent may make parenthood a more inviting option.

If the above rationale corresponds to reality, Rainwater argued (1965), middle class women who think of themselves primarily as interested in children should want larger families than women oriented primarily to husbands or to outside interests. There was a marked correlation of the type expected. In the data, the cause-effect relationships are hard to disentangle. Although most women who wanted larger families had not yet had them, it is possible that the desire for larger families affected the way they talked about themselves. Or the desire for large families may have kept interests restricted to home. Or the person with interests that veered away from out-of-home roles and toward home may have wanted more children.

Data from the longitudinal FGMA research (1961; 1963) are directly relevant to the Hoffman-Wyatt hypothesis reviewed above, but provide no clear support for it. There was no overall evidence that women who have better "adjustment to mother role" want and hence have more children. The FGMA researchers also studied women's participation and interest in employment and non-paid organizational activity, in relation to birth planning. While it may seem logical that out-of-home activities and having more children are in competition and conflict, this sample of women gave little evidence of acting in terms of this logic. Women who wanted more children were as liable as others to want out-of-home activities, for example. The choice of the FGMA population probably minimized strongly career-oriented women, and gave no check on the hypothesis that having some children gives a woman a role. But FGMA data are directly relevant to the Hoffman and Wyatt (1960) hypothesis reviewed above. The FGMA authors raise far-reaching questions about the whole conflict-of-roles hypothesis as a way of explaining mothers' family-size desires. Whatever the pattern showing up in group and even sub-group data, some individual women undoubtedly experience some competition between roles.

Also relevant to the Hoffman-Wyatt (1960) hypothesis are data that Rainwater (1965) tabulates for answers middle class women gave when asked to name some of their bad points. Of those whose primary concern centered around selfishness some two thirds wanted what Rainwater (1965) tabulates for answers middle class women centered around being somehow psychologically or physically unfit to do her job, only a fifth wanted a large family. This is consistent with the hypothesis that women who are worried about their selfishness, trying to minimize or overcome this fault, and perhaps to prove that they are not merely idle parasites, tend toward larger families. Meanwhile, women who are somewhat overwhelmed with the work involved in a small family, who do not experience the boredom and guilt over idleness and ease of housework mentioned by Hoffman and Wyatt (1960), would not be prompted toward large families. In the small sample of middle class women Rainwater used in this tabulation, 20 were placed in the "selfish" and 29 the "unable to do job" category. This balance may imply that the increased ease of housework and childcare must not be over-estimated.

There is still much room for the emphasis we make in Chapters 5 through 8, that children provide heavy costs to many parents, and that some women find the role of motherhood burdensome. Perhaps a "grass-is-greener-on-the-other-side-of-the-fence" phenomenon operates to some extent, so that both women tied to the mother-at-home role and those newly freed from it may be somewhat dissatisfied and envious.

G. Factors Involving Husband-Wife Relations

In both FGMA surveys (1963), better marital adjustment was correlated (.10 and .12) with the desire for larger families. But the correlation between marriage adjustment as measured in 1957 and the number of pregnancies between then and the 1960 re-survey was zero. The complex causal relationship between marriage adjustment and number of children will be discussed in Chapter 5. There is little doubt that among some individual couples happy marriage goes with wanting children, or more children (Sears et al., 1957). A person may wish to express happiness and love felt toward a spouse by sharing with her or him in procreation. In large part, however, the existence of an already happy marriage would not provide a "motive" for wanting a birth, but would provide a "nest" so that other motives for wanting a birth could be free to operate. It is also probable that in some individual cases parents do not want their happy marriage relationship interfered with by children or additional children (Greene, 1963; Rainwater, 1965).

The majority of respondents in two surveys (Centers & Blumberg, 1954; Christopherson & Walters, 1958) say they believe children are necessary to a happy marriage. Some couples want children because their marriage is in trouble and they seek to hold it together by children (Sloman, 1948). In one unusual case of the writer's acquaintance, a wife whose marriage was in frequent danger of breaking up said that she was seeking a fourth pregnancy to make the burden of alimony and child support heavier so that her husband would be less likely to leave.

Closely related to the preceding section on women's roles is what Rainwater (1965) discusses as "conjugal role organization." Where husbands' and wives' interests and concerns and lives are more inter-related and inter-dependent, Rainwater predicted that wives would want smaller families. Wives whose lives were more segregated from their husbands, so that their interests and activities and concerns were more isolated, would want more children. A significant relationship as predicted emerged as one of the most important findings of the study. Possibly some wives who feel that they are not free to participate extensively in the lives of their husbands have a tendency to want more children to fill a gap that would not otherwise exist. Blood and Wolfe (1960) make a similar interpretation of their similar findings.

However, such findings might also be related to a broader hypothesis. This holds that family organizations involving more rigidity in male and female roles and more male dominance tend toward larger families (see our Cha. 23). This hypothesis has been applied across cultures (Lorimer, 1954) and within cultures (Hill et al., 1959; FGMA, 1961; 1963); the correlation found across cultures is subject to varying interpretations, and the correlations found within any given culture are very small and are present only inconsistently. The hypothesized relationship is thought to spring in part from a greater emphasis, in "traditional" family organization, on factors already mentioned. These factors include the desire for a large family and male offspring as demonstration of male potency, the desire for male children because of their greater economic value (if parents are determined to have boys they may have more total children in the process), and the limited opportunity for women to know any other role than motherhood. In a male-dominated family there may be less husband-wife communication, less use of contraceptives, and less chance for the wife to stand up to the demands of her husband.

Men threatened by equalitarian roles, who want to increase male dominance, may desire larger families so that their wives will stay home and be submissive (Rainwater, 1960). Rainwater observes that in the eyes of lower class men, there are two classes of women, "good women" and those who do not stay home but run around. Children who keep mothers at home may help keep them "good" as well as submissive. These attitudes may be expressed in the statement, "keep 'em barefoot and pregnant."

Trying to understand the extremely low correlations between husband-wife dominance and birth planning variables, Westoff et al. (1961) suggest that researchers may have erred in treating husband-wife dominance as a fixed and unvarying entity. They suggest that several events in the wife's life, including both employment and the having of another child, may enlarge her sphere of activity and her power and authority. The degree of male dominance may be a result, as well as a cause, of birth planning variables. Hoffman and Wyatt (1960) and Rainwater (1965) suggest that both spouses may be attracted toward another birth because it will make each spouse feel more independent and autonomous. The pressing needs of children may make the wife feel more important, in comparison to her spouse, and may be used as a justifiable excuse for paying less attention to the needs and demands of her husband. At the same time, her very involvement with children may mean that the wife demands less of her husband. Paradoxically, these authors also suggest that having additional children may be attractive as a means of increasing the dependency of the wife on her husband, for this may be flattering and reassuring to him, help her meet some dependency needs, and reassure her of her femininity.

H. Factors Involving Existing Children

One boy whose parents refused to get him a puppy was advised by a friend, "Ask for a baby brother; they'll be glad to settle for a dog." The Indianapolis Study did not find evidence that many parents were influenced, in their desire for a baby, by the specific requests of existing children (Solomon, Clare & Westoff, 1956). Several of the mothers in another sample reported pressures from older children, particularly girls, to have another baby; some said this was the main reason for deciding to have another (Sears et al., 1957).

Much more commonly, parents report having additional children because of their belief that big families are somehow better for existing children. This is one of the most important rationales parents give (GAF, 1966; Rainwater, 1965; Sears et al., 1957), although this may be an easy answer. Many of the parents Rainwater studied suggested that bigger families develop in a more healthy way, and produce more generous, sharing people. The selfishness-kindness distinction noted earlier concerning parents of small and large families is extended to views about children. When parents say they have had conceptions for the sake of older siblings, sometimes this is true specifically because parents were worried about how an older child was developing.

> "I became pregnant with Steve, because we thought the other one needed a brother or sister, as he was such a devil. I don't think that anyone should have another child thinking it might help the first one—it doesn't" (Sears et al., 1957, 41).

Not all mothers are as displeased with the outcome. Having conceptions "to avoid an only child" may simply mean that parents wanted to have another child; but it may reflect a concern that a one-child family would be unhealthy.

The picture of the large happy family appeals to many parents as good not only for children but for themselves; when they say it makes children happier they mean that everybody is happier—"one big happy family." Some parents claim that large families are easier on the parents because of the relations set up between siblings; they "sort of raise themselves" (Rainwater, 1965).

> "I suppose there would be less discipline problems with three or four children; they would work out their problems on their own" (Rainwater, 1965).

Parents who lose a child through death sometimes try to replace the child with another conception.

Although some parents have larger families for the sake of existing children, some parents keep their families small with the same objective in mind. The rationale is different: conserve the finite supply of money, time, attention, love and opportunity for the maximum good of a few children. In the past, Protestants and Jews have heard more about the "responsible parenthood" theme than Catholics.

I. Factors Involving Sex of the Child

Parents in the United States and probably many other Western cultures have preferences for at least one child of each sex, and for male children (our Cha. 2). In the FGMA research (1961), when the first child was a boy the interval before a second child was conceived averaged three months longer than when the first was a girl. There was no support for the hypothesis that this might be because first boys created more problems for mothers (FGMA, 1963), as Sears et al. (1957) suggested. Instead, sex preferences are probably responsible.

Mothers' reports suggest that they were more pleased when they discovered their pregnancies, and were warmer in their relations with their children, when the sex composition of their existing families followed certain patterns than when it followed others (Sears et al., 1957). In some countries the preference for males is very strong. A common wish expressed to men in some Moslem countries: "May you have 100 sons" (Soddy, 1964). Turks with no sons are more likely to want additional conceptions than Turks with at least one son (Population Council, 1964b). Such preferences are not merely verbal; they tend to drive parents to have an additional conception if the desired sex composition has not already been achieved. Hence over-all family size is larger.

Preferences for males may be explained in part by the greater proof of virility thought to come from producing sons, the greater economic value of the male, and the fact that in some cultures he carries on the family name. Psychoanalytic thinkers contend that a boy child may be a greater consolation to a mother for her missing penis. The Mundugumor, especially the Mundugumor men, preferred daughters (Mead, 1935) for reasons somewhat idiosyncratic to that particular culture. Mundugumor men thought of sons as competitors in an especially fierce sense.

Desires for children of both sexes may be explained in part by resort to the psychoanalytic hypotheses of identification and Oedipal interests. If parents want children as extensions of themselves, extensions with whom they identify, this extension and identification may be especially possible with children of the same sex. In the Oedipal doctrine, it is important to a parent to have a child of the opposite sex as a special love object. Parents often feel especially kindly and flirtatious and permissive with children of the opposite sex, it is argued, and want someone to make this possible. Having both sexes of children may represent completeness and be tied in with virility in a way less important than, but separate from, concern with having male offspring. At another level, the same theme of "completeness" in a family with children of each sex may be important to the individual if the culture has exalted that theme. In the popular media in the United States, the happy family is almost invariably portrayed as having at least one child of each sex.

J. Influence of Parents' Family of Origin

There is often some correlation between the size of one's family of origin and of one's family of procreation (Berent, 1953; FGMA, 1963; Flanagan, 1942; Kantner & Potter, 1954). Even though religion and social class are held constant, the observed correlations may result in part from factors having little to do with how many children one wants. For example, customary age at marriage, or knowledge of contraception, or an "impulse control" that makes it easier to use certain kinds of contraception might be transmitted socially from one generation to the next. But when Kantner and Potter (1954) singled out couples where the husband and the wife had the same number of siblings, and were "efficient planners" of births, the correlation between generations was .29. To some extent people from larger families may have more children because they *want* more children (FGMA, 1961).

Itkin (1952) included a measure of the degree of acceptance or rejection felt toward children in general, in the set of scales he gave to some 400 unmarried college students and their parents. For female students there were low but significant positive correlations with both fathers' and mothers' scores; for male students, with mothers' but not fathers' scores. Data are consistent with the possibility that parents who like and accept children may tend to transmit this attitude, by precept and more pervasively by their entire relationship to their children.

A man or woman's parents or siblings may explicitly recommend that he or she have a given number of children, although this factor has not been shown to be too important (Potter & Kantner, 1955; Rainwater, 1965). In Tennessee Williams' *Cat on a Hot Tin Roof,* the older brother of the "prodigal son" tells the "Big Daddy," in effect, "You told me to have lots of kids so I did." Children may seek to identify with their parents by producing the same kinds of families their parents did, including the same number of children. People may seek to set up a replica of their childhood home, including the number of children there, as a source of comfort and security (Rainwater, 1965). The FGMA research (1961) found no consistent support for the hypothesis that mothers who had more happy childhood memories would be more likely to re-create the family size of their homes of origin than those with less happy memories. Possibly there is something of a swing from one generation to the next, even among "happy" families, so that extremely large or extremely small families prompt a reaction toward the other extreme in the next generation (Bossard & Boll, 1956; FGMA, 1961; GAF, 1966).

> "Three's aplenty. We don't want no big families like we came from. Life is too hard for the kids that way." She had 11 brothers and sisters (GAF, 1959).

Several studies have tried to show that people who recalled having happier childhoods were more likely to want and have at least some children, or larger families (Centers & Blumberg, 1954; Flanagan, 1942; Potter & Kantner, 1955; Westoff, Sagi & Kelly, 1958). No consistent pattern has emerged.

K. Religious Factors

Religion may affect the number of children one has because one's church has an ideological stand for or against certain contraceptives, or abortion, or sterilization; or because religion serves as a label for some such factor as "traditionalism" or national background or family structure. But our interest in this chapter is in more direct ways whereby religion leads people to want children, or more children. Roman Catholic ideology has shown a strong tendency to encourage large families. This is shown in papal statements, editorials in Catholic publications, marriage manuals and the like (Blake, 1966). The small family (sometimes caricatured as the one-child family) has often been portrayed as selfish and emotionally inferior. Even when using the approved "rhythm" method of family planning, Catholics are not free to avoid having another child merely because they want to; they must have more weighty reasons (GAF, 1959).

One sample of Catholic wives—a relatively young, urban group—was asked: "As far as you know does your religion take any stand on size of family? What?" About a fourth thought there was encouragement toward a large family, only one or two percent thought there was encouragement to limit family size, but approximately two thirds thought the Church took no stand (FGMA, 1963). These two thirds seem to have been unaware of the ideology which Blake (1966) finds expressed by Catholic leadership. These figures provide no evidence that Catholic respondents were aware of any movement to emphasize "responsible parenthood," although some Catholic leaders have recently stressed this theme (Rock, 1963).

The "responsible parenthood" emphasis among Protestants and Jews has stressed that contraception should be used as a means to avoid children that parents cannot afford (emotionally or financially), and to hold population growth in check. A fifth of Protestant wives in the second phase of the FGMA study (1963) thought their religion did have some teaching on birth control; presumably this was usually a teaching approving of its use. Perhaps because of the difference in Catholic and non-Catholic ideology just noted, the FGMA study (1961; 1963) found some evidence that more devout Catholics tended toward larger families and less accurate contraception than less devout Catholics, while for Protestants a somewhat opposite pattern might hold true.

Blake (1966) has argued that American Catholics are more "American" than "Catholic" in birth planning; their actual and desired family sizes are much closer to those of other Americans than to the ideals held forth by Church leadership. The differences between Catholic and non-Catholic views, however, though they are small, are among the most important, consistent, and well-documented differences among Americans in number of children wanted (GAF, 1959; 1966; FGMA, 1961; 1963). In Rainwater's study (1965), nine out of ten middle-class Catholic men who wanted large families suggested religious tradition as a reason. More generally, other respondents often mention religious tradition as a factor (GAF, 1966; Rainwater, 1965). It seems likely that some Catholic couples are subject to social pressures from their Catholic friends. Too small families may be conspicuous evidence of using questionable contraceptive procedures or "selfishly" avoiding conception, or both.

A few religious groups have encouraged members to minimize their involvement in some of the activities in the world around them. The pursuit of a high standard of living or "success," and certain forms of recreation have been discouraged. In some cases these are specifically tagged as "worldly" activities. If less time and energy are spent on the activities of the world outside, parents may be more likely to devote themselves to having children.

According to some religious teachings, children must be born in order to reach heaven, or to free souls from bondage, or to permit souls to go on their way in a cycle of transmigrations. Roman Catholic, Hindu and Latter-Day Saint (Mormon) teachings have suggested something of this emphasis.

Rainwater (1965) writes concerning Negro lower-class mothers with heavy interests in church activities that

> . . . the fundamentalist religious orientation of these women emphasizes the moral virtue inherent in motherhood, a virtue that is believed to increase as the number of children increases. The family can become a battleground for the struggle between Satan (in the form of male acting-out) and God (in the form of motherly virtue and love).

In the Judaeo-Christian tradition, barrenness has often been regarded as a curse and a full womb or children as a blessing (our Cha. 3). Some parents regard a birth as a token of heaven's favor:

> "We've done everything we can to have one. . . . We'd like to have three or four children—with the help of God. I can't believe that all our prayers will be unanswered. I think we will have children when God feels we are worthy of them" (GAF, 1959).

> "When we wanted a child we prayed. I really don't think I would have become pregnant except for prayer" (GAF, 1959).

L. Motives in Wanting Pregnancy Only

Some motives in wanting pregnancy or delivery have little to do with wanting the presence of a child later on. Some mothers also seem to want young babies but not older children (Wengraf, 1953). Obviously this often involves a short-sightedness with tragic consequences for parents and children. Some women act as if they want a "full womb" all of the time (Meier, 1963). Some women seem to feel better physically while pregnant, although this seems not to be the case for the majority of women (our Cha. 6). Some believe that feeling better is a physiological result of the pregnancy. One physician reportedly advised a woman to become pregnant as a way of curing her backache (Sloman, 1948). A lower-class mother who had no husband thought she would like to get pregnant to ease her rheumatism.

Pregnancy can be a conspicuous way of being noticed, inescapably. There is a certain holiness and tenderness with which others sometimes treat a pregnant woman. Husbands are likely to respond this way. Rainwater reports (1960),

> . . . many women indicated that the only time they really felt their husbands close to them and deeply interested in them was when they were pregnant.

Note these examples:

> "Having children has never been too bad for my wife. She isn't sick very much, and when she is I take better care of her than ever" (Rainwater, 1960, 84).

> "He babied me a lot especially towards the last part of pregnancy" (Duvall, 1962, 166).

> "He thought and acted as if I were now a woman, no longer a child" (Duvall, 1962, 166).

Although the last two statements contrast, both women seemed pleased. Pregnancy brings improved sexual relations among some couples (Landis et al., 1950; Rainwater, 1960). One possible reason is that the greater consideration and attention of some husbands improves sex relations. Of course, not all husbands are more considerate nor do sex relations improve for all couples during pregnancy.

Some of Rainwater's working class subjects (1960) reported that a nice thing about pregnancy was that this was the one time they could quit worrying about becoming pregnant. Some offered this as a rationale for the improved sex relations reported during pregnancy.

In some cultures, a first pregnancy is a way of showing fitness for marriage.

Pregnancy has deep symbolic significance, according to psychoanalytic writers. The woman identifies with the fetus; it is seen as a growth of her ego. This is narcissistically gratifying. The pregnancy may indicate that she has something that no one else can take from her; she may have half-conscious fantasies of a "secret companion," a friend that is hers alone. Women imagine the child as a reproduction of the father so that they can be his mother. After a girl loses some love object (through death or a family break-up, for example) she may become somewhat depressed and may seek pregnancy as a way of making up the loss.

Delivery may be unwelcome because it involves the loss of this precious part of the ego; post-partum depression, prolonged labor, and some childbirth difficulties have been interpreted as springing from sadness or ambivalence over this loss. Some writers contend that there is an unconscious equation of vagina with mouth, penis with breast, and semen with milk, so that pregnancy may be gratifying to oral needs. Some have suggested a "pregnancy envy" among men. Masochistic women may need the negative aspects of pregnancy and delivery.

For some women delivery brings rewards, not the least of which is the accomplishment of successfully producing a baby. Flowers, cards, gifts and visitors may attest to the admiration and appreciation of relatives and friends.

Sometimes a very hostile element is involved in the desire for a conception. This may occur either inside or outside of wedlock. In *Gone With the Wind,* the hero-villain Rhett Butler tells a friend how he got his wife pregnant to hurt her. Husbands may see the presence of children as a hostile way to chain their wives down and make their lives less pleasant. Often, however, the angry desire focuses on pregnancy itself, and relates to an angry, hurting view of sex relations. The crude expression "knocked up" as a synonym for pregnancy has a hostile flavor. Many of the synonyms used for sex relations are also used to describe a damaged, confused, generally "messed up" state that may occur to an automobile, enemy outpost, budget, or vacation plan. Men, especially, who have much hostility toward the opposite sex in general may want the pregnancy as a way of hurting that sex group. Less frequently women may feel that their becoming pregnant will somehow embarrass or hurt male partners, or men generally.

M. Special Motives in Out-of-Wedlock Conceptions

In cultures or sub-cultures that forbid conception out of wedlock, most such conceptions are unwanted contraceptive accidents, but this is not true in all individual cases. Out-of-wedlock conceptions may be desired for many of the reasons listed elsewhere in this chapter; there are also some motives peculiar to this circumstance (Kroger & Freed, 1962). Girls sometimes desire pregnancy to "catch" a man by forcing a marriage. Girls, especially, may seek pregnancy as a way of showing hostility to parents—both because this is precisely what they have been so often warned against, and because parents are humiliated by the public scandal often created among their acquaintances. Conception may be a way of getting parents to grant permission for a marriage of which they would not otherwise approve, or more generally of establishing independence. Hostility toward the opposite sex generally or to the sex partner specifically may lead either partner to want to hurt or trap the other with pregnancy. Shame and other disadvantages of out-of-wedlock pregnancies may meet masochistic needs. Kroger and Freed (1962) contend that some girls want pregnancy because of an unconscious desire for a father figure, perhaps because they had none in childhood.

N. Some Other Motives

Many of the ideas below are borrowed from Hoffman and Wyatt (1960), who give additional detail. In some cases we have elaborated and extended their ideas.

Parents may want children as a way of living life over again vicariously in children's lives (Swain & Kiser, 1953). They may seek to repeat pleasant aspects, and to avoid some of the mistakes and limitations of their own lives. The mother may rear her daughter as she wished her mother had reared her. Children may provide vehicles for fulfilling parents' own childhood fantasies. Later children may be desired as part of parents' attempts to recapture the happy times they experienced when earlier children were small. If mothers feel they have failed in the rearing of earlier children, they may want additional children to correct their former errors with a "new draft" that may also atone somewhat for their mistakes.

Children may be perceived as part of living a "whole," "complete" life; one should taste as many of the possible experiences available, and parenthood is one of them. A baby is the prerequisite ticket for initiation into a special club, the club of motherhood; baby showers and ceremonies may be viewed as initiation rites. Each additional birth may permit one some advance in the secret order and some added status: "Yes, it was that way with my first two too, but when you have four . . ." For women who feel they are aging, having another baby may permit them to play the role of young woman. In a society that puts a special value on youth, the whole pregnancy and young baby routines may serve as props, like dyed hair or youthful clothes.

Much as a record sprint is even more impressive if it is done with a severe headache or when carrying extra weights, children may be valuable as "handicaps" to make one's accomplishments more dazzling. The wife who can complete an education or work outside the home and manage her household at the same time may feel that she will be judged more remarkable if she does this while managing children.

Mothering children may be important as a token of femininity, especially since men's and women's roles are in such rapid transition and seem less far apart than formerly. The woman with some sex role confusion, homosexual tendencies, or doubts about her femininity may be impelled by this motivation.

Rearing children may involve some of the same creative, artistic needs that make some people enjoy painting or writing. The physical creation of babies in the uterus, feeding them and watching what happens, and the design of lives through child-rearing procedures probably appeal to some. The study of child psychology may have exalted creative child-building, sometimes almost as a "hobby." Others watch the process, and if the work of art "turns out" well, parents are gratified.

Children may provide relief from boredom; they bring novelty and change. Being idle or bored may threaten a mother with the possibility that dangerous impulses will get busy in the "devil's workshop." Children may provide welcome escape from freedom. They may enforce a regime of hard work, a ritual that safeguards and brings security.

Some motives for wanting conception occur only in one or two cultures, or occur so rarely that we may characterize them as idiosyncratic. To try to list all of these would be impossible; some examples may suffice. In the United States people sometimes want children so that the father may avoid the armed forces. In Mundugumor society as reported by Mead (1935), after a couple had a girl it was desirable to have a boy without too much delay, so that he could be exchanged in the customary marriage negotiations. In Jamaica there is a belief in a fore-ordained or "due" number of children which a given woman must bear in order to fulfill herself (Stycos & Back, 1964), although this may serve more as rationalization than real motivation for wanting children.

Meier (1959) contends that when a group of people from some country is displaced and put in refugee camps or concentration camps, they may have a stronger than ever desire to reproduce.

Despite the apparently hopeless conditions of life, children may provide a kind of defiant assertion that the group has a right to continue in existence and that its way of life is right. It is possible that after the extermination of thousands of Jewish people in Nazi Germany, some Jewish parents wanted children as a way of showing that the Jews were too hardy or virile to be eliminated, even by such drastic measures.

Some individuals or couples feel that they have few friends; that others are not greatly interested in them; that somehow they are being politely shunned or ignored or tolerated. It seems possible that having children or having a larger family may be a way to grapple with this feeling of rejection. Being busy with children provides a basis for rationalization ("people don't invite us to their homes because they know we've got our hands full helping raise this family the right way"). It also keeps time so occupied that there is less left to fret over social rejection. Third, having a family sets up a sort of microsociety which is under the control of parents. Peers may reject or ignore a parent, but children, at least while they are young, simply cannot refuse to interact with parents.

O. Summary

Major studies have sought without much success to show empirical relationships between psychological independent variables and dependent variables related to family size. For several reasons these generally negative findings should not force a discarding of the hypotheses tested. Nevertheless the ideas presented in this chapter (and in Chapters 5–8) must be viewed, at best, as either assumptions or hypotheses for further testing.

(A) It seems possible that certain innate factors make some aspects of motherhood rewarding. However, "maternal instinct" has been greatly over-worked in explanations of why humans want children. Our guess would be that, at most, unlearned factors would constitute only a minor role, and are relatively unimportant in making the difference between a family of two and four children. (B) Psychoanalytic theory contributes hypotheses involving proof of virility, competition with and independence from parents, Oedipal needs and masochistic needs, and the quest to extend the ego in space and time.

(C) Desires to be a parent and to have a family of a particular size are heavily influenced by social pressures. Family size seems to have aspects of "fad" or fashion within a given culture. At present the family seems to be "in style" in America. (D) Enjoyment of interaction with children constitutes one reason for wanting them. Reasons for liking children include parents' needs to help others and parents' dependency needs. (E) In many cultures and subcultures children are an economic asset even when they are very young, or a sort of insurance policy for old age, or both. Perhaps some American mothers on "welfare" aid have children as a means of increasing their income.

(F) Motherhood provides a role for the woman; it may be the chief means of establishing her identity. In the United States, as a mother's first two or three children reach the stage where they are perceived as needing slightly less care, the mother may face a choice between an out-of-home role and having more children in order to continue the mother role. (G) A person may wish to express happiness and love felt toward a partner by sharing in procreation. Children may be sought to force a marriage or to hold a faltering marriage together. In one study wives who felt their lives to be more separated from their husbands' lives wanted more children than other wives. In other ways, the marriage relationship may influence the desire for children.

(H) Parents sometimes report having additional children because of a belief that large families are somehow better for existing children. (I) Many parents have preferences for at least one child of each sex, and for male children. There are other factors, in turn, behind such preferences. These desires may influence parents to have additional children.

(J) People may seek to identify with their parents by producing the same general size of family as did their parents. They may seek to set up a replica of their childhood home, as a source of comfort and security. (K) Roman Catholic ideology has encouraged people to have children and to have more than small families. In other ways religious beliefs may influence parents toward wanting children. (L) Some motives lead people to want a pregnancy or delivery, specifically, whether or not they want the child that results. (M) There are certain distinct motives that may make people want conceptions out of wedlock. (N) Some miscellaneous reasons for wanting conceptions have been discussed.

11
Wrong Reasons

PLANNED PARENTHOOD

Storyboard for TV spot advertisement, 1972

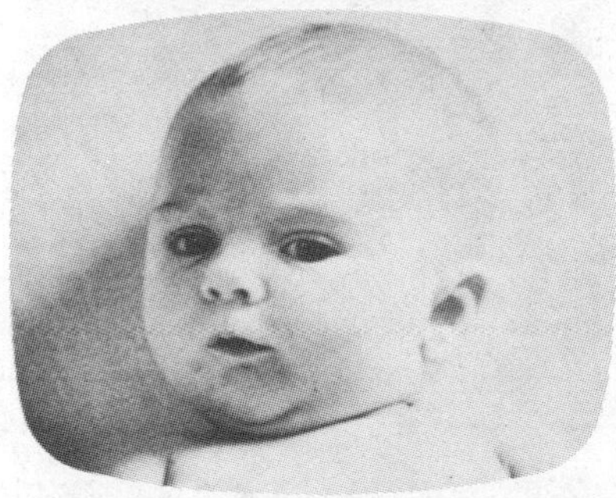

ANNCR(VO): A lot of people have children for the wrong reasons.

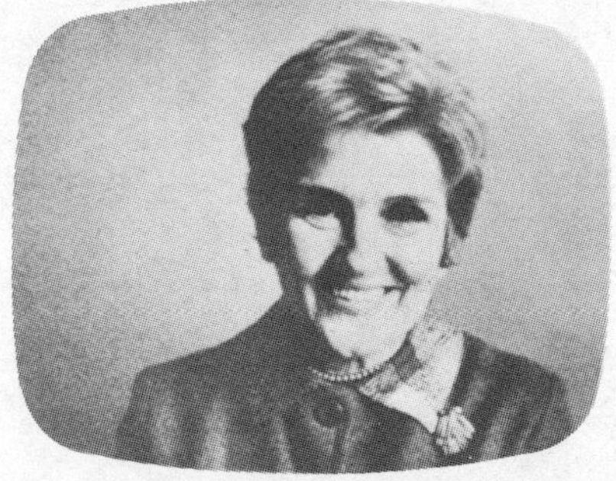

GRANDMOTHER: You've been married a year now. When are we going to see some grandchildren?

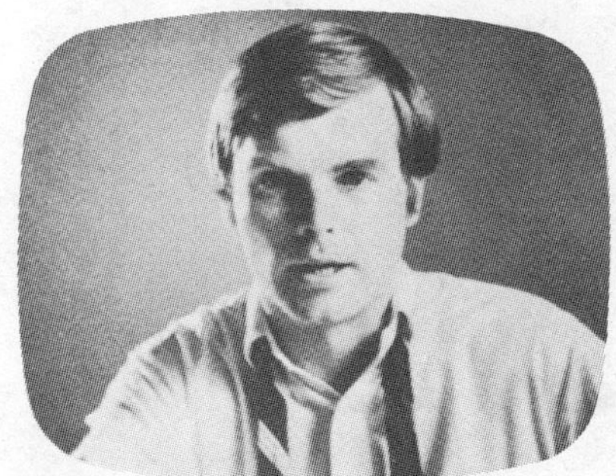

YOUNG MAN: You want to have a baby, Evelyn? All right, we'll have a baby! Maybe that'll patch things up!

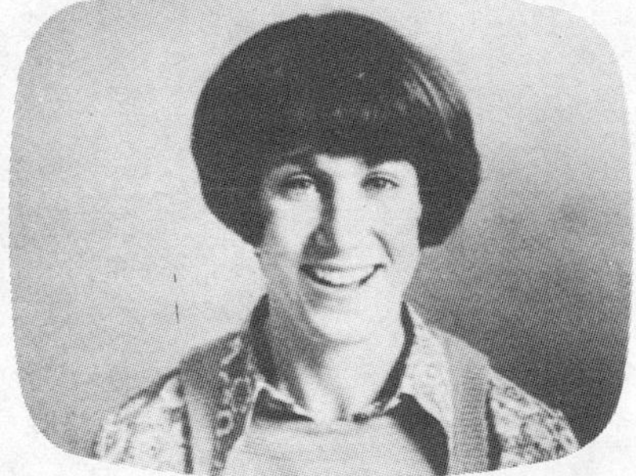

YOUNG WIFE: We only want two children. But if one of them isn't a boy—we'll keep trying.

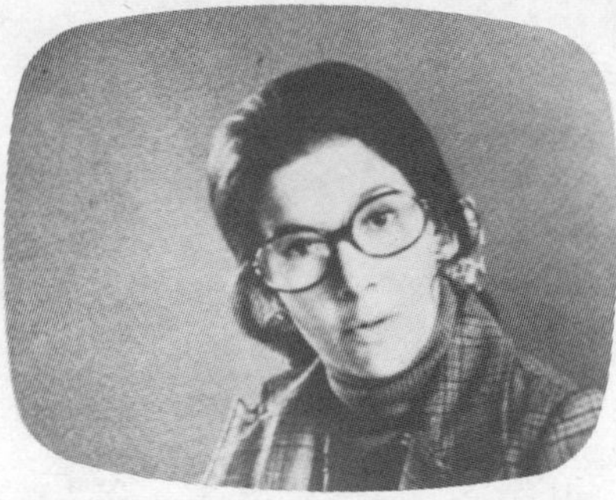

WOMAN: Why knock myself out working when I can have a baby.

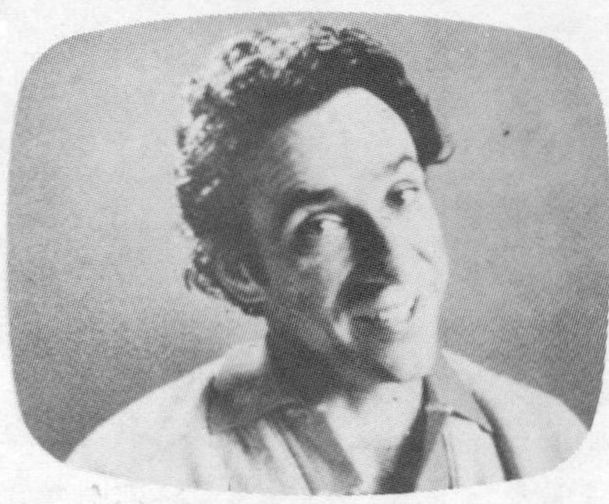

MAN: Heh-heh, hey Harry. What are you and Marge waiting for—huh?

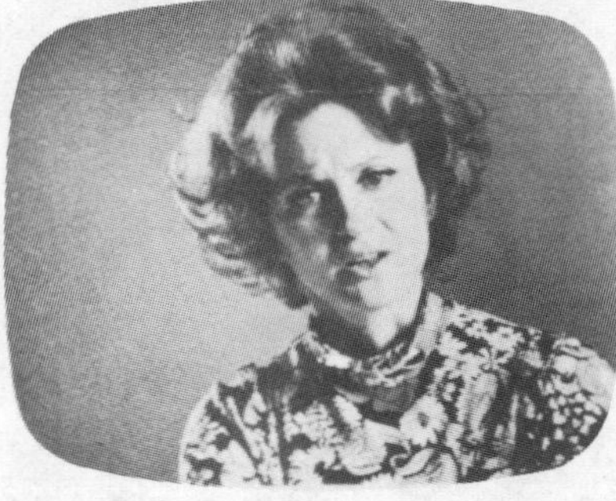

YOUNG GIRL: Sure I want another baby. What else is a woman for?

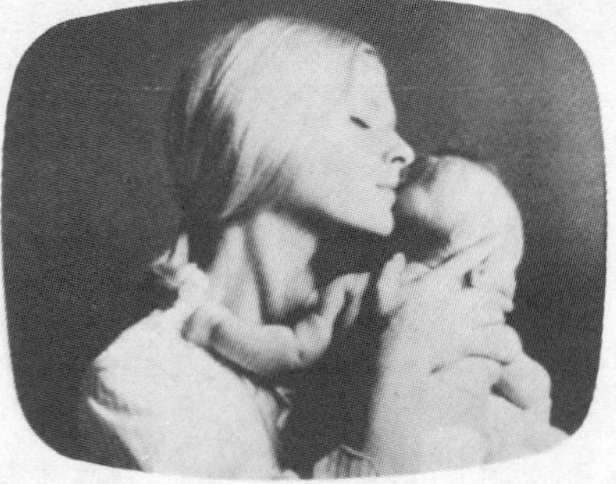

ANNCR(VO): As we said, there are a lot of wrong reasons to have a child —but only one right reason: because you really want one. And that takes planning.

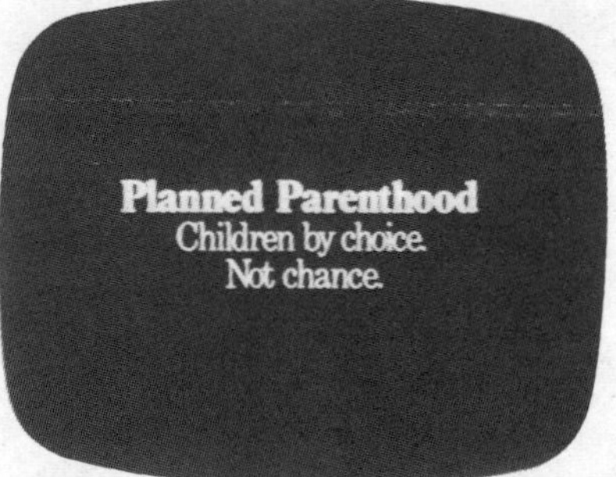

ANNCR(VO): For more information, write Planned Parenthood, Box 840, New York, 10019.

12

The Wrong Reasons to Have Children

ROBERT E. GOULD, M.D.

Associate Professor of Psychiatry, New York University Medical Center

Once upon a time, when children helped work the land to assist in supporting the family, every child was an economic necessity. This situation no longer exists. Neither does the need for procreation to insure survival of the race. Social scientists, in fact, are saying in louder voices and larger numbers that survival of our species now is dependent on *decreasing* the birth rate.

So it is pertinent to ask whether or not a couple should plan to have any children at all. The fact is that we no longer automatically need to have children. And many of us who choose to have them do so for the wrong reasons. It is time we recognized these reasons so that we can stop having babies who seem to be wanted, but are in fact only expected.

Wrong reason #1: "Our parents want grandchildren."

How common, how pathetically common, it is for parents who are beginning to feel useless, or bored, to push for grandchildren, through whom they may rekindle an interest in life or a sense of importance.

Love for one's parents should not have to be shown by bestowing on them the role of grandparents. This pressure can be relieved if you can persuade your parents to develop new interests and to keep up some of their old ones—such as sex. Masters and Johnson, in their studies of sexual behavior, found that older couples are quite capable of engaging in and enjoying sexual relations. The ease with which they give up sex as well as many other ac-

The New York Times Magazine, May 3, 1970

tivities seems again the result of cultural expectation rather than physical or intellectual limitation.

Wrong reason #2: "We can afford to have a baby."

Traditionally, the young couple scarcely clears the economic hurdle of "Do we earn enough to get married?" before rushing to the next one: "Can we afford to have a baby?" To convince neighbors and friends—and sometimes each other—a couple will scrimp to produce an heir. Keeping up with the Joneses' birth rate, however, is hardly a sensible motive for having children.

Wrong reason #3: "If I'm somebody's mother (father), then I'm Somebody."

The hope of enhancing one's image by adding an important new role—"father," or "mother"—is that, by assuming this new role, which holds responsibility and importance, one gains automatic status. Again, the need to increase self-esteem would be better answered if one addressed oneself to the real or imagined shortcomings. A child is neither a substitute for, nor an extension to, one's self.

There is another reason for having children, which is closely allied to becoming Somebody; this reason is a need for power, a chance to exercise control over someone. And a baby is the perfect helpless victim.

It is unfortunate that so many adults have spent their lives on the receiving end of orders and insults. The need for a scapegoat who will take *their* orders and abuse all too often results in the production of children to fulfill that desire.

Few parents are aware of this power-hungry motivation, but it is a tragic commonplace. The child-abusers and the bullies who inflict both physical and emotional harm on their youngers are members of this unhappy parent group.

Wrong reason #4: "I need to be needed."

Having a baby in order to feel worthwhile, important, and needed, is closely but not identically related to wrong reason three. The basic motivation is a sense of inadequacy, which the parent attempts to compensate for by having another individual wholly dependent upon him.

Such a parent is likely to have a difficult time letting the youngster grow up and achieve independence.

Wrong reason #5: "A baby will give me something to do."

The feeling that life is empty, that one is going nowhere and achieving nothing, is frequently the main impetus for the wonderful idea of having a baby. There is little doubt that it provides one of the easiest ways to achieve a dramatic change. A baby will certainly fill the day with new duties, but it cannot fill the parent's inner emptiness. A child conceived as a cure for boredom will cause more problems than he can possibly solve.

Wrong reason #6: "We thought it would help our marriage."

One of the worst, but by no means the rarest, reasons for becoming parents is the desperate hope that a baby will magically bring husband and wife closer together. The expectation is inevitably unfulfilled, since the cause of the trouble is not being treated, but is rather being camouflaged by the addition of another complication—the baby. The stress of this new responsibility can only cause further deterioration of the marriage. A marriage in trouble is a good reason to delay having a child until or unless the trouble is worked out.

Wrong reason #7: "It is the only way to prove you're a man (woman)."

This is a throwback to the old line that boys once used to persuade girls to "go all the way." (This tactic does not seem so necessary in today's more accepting sexual climate.) But belief in the extension of the argument is still with us: to "prove" sexual maturity and effectiveness, the wife "must" bear a child, thus fulfilling her female role, and the husband "must" be able to impregnate her, as a sign of his virility.

Wrong reason #8: "We don't want to be different."

In a society where there are general, subtle and specific pressures to be like everyone else on the block—pressures applied to adults as well as adolescents—there are many communities and groups that make a childless couple feel uncomfortable, if not peculiar, just as a single person is made to feel slightly unacceptable in a world full of married couples. The discomfort forces people to conform by having babies (or marriages) they don't really want. It's hardly a promising start.

Wrong reason #9: "I want my child to get the things I never had."

A child seems to offer a second chance to have your own ambitions and dreams vicariously satisfied. This offers a powerful temptation to many people who have not had the courage to follow their convictions or who have otherwise wasted their lives or failed to realize their potential. As parents, they will attempt to mold their children into the ideals they had for themselves. This is one more way of misusing a child. If you can't do your own thing, it's hardly fair to expect a baby to do it for you.

Wrong reason #10: "A child is my only claim to immortality."

Many of us can't bear the thought of dying and leaving nothing behind by which we can be remembered. We may see having a child (an extension of ourselves) as our only tangible legacy. Thus the baby provides a means to gratify vanity—and an excuse for not achieving much else. A constructive, useful life, good work and good relationships are other ways to leave a mark on the world. A baby is not a substitute for any of these.

Wrong reason #11-A: (men only): "A baby will keep a woman in her place."

The simplest way to prevent a wife from exploring the world outside was always just to keep her "barefoot and pregnant." In the current revival of the Women's Liberation Movement, it may seem terribly old-fashioned to mention the philosophy of Kinder, Kirche, Küche (children, church and kitchen) but there still are men who expect and demand that their wives stay housebound; such husbands still find that pregnancies and babies are effective methods of achieving that result.

This kind of husband seldom faces the fact that his own insecurities are the basis of his "old-fashioned" philosophy. He fears that his wife may find the outside world of work (and other men) too desirable.

Wrong reason #11-B (women only): "A baby will keep my husband attached to me and less likely to stray from home."

This wrong reason is not quite so bad as the one which encourages having a baby to save a rocky marriage. This old-fashioned notion simply represents a woman's insecurity over her own legitimate hold on her husband, or it may reflect a lack of trust in him. In either case, having a baby is no solution to such insecurity in the relationship between husband and wife.

These eleven reasons are a sampling of the important motives that drive couples to parenthood, often to the detriment of their children and themselves. When any of these reasons is the predominant motivation, then I believe parenthood is a mistake.

Unfortunately, becoming a parent takes little effort and even less intelligence. I say unfortunately, because this leads people to think that becoming a *good* parent must also be easy. To make the point more pointed: To be a *good* parent is to achieve one of the most difficult goals of modern life. There are outstanding individuals in all the professions who have failed miserably at the task of raising their children well. Often the very quality that made them successful—as scientists, artists, or politicians—also caused them to fail as parents. The same ambition and dedication necessary to succeed at a demanding career are also necessary to succeed as a parent. Time, effort and skill must be devoted to the art of child-rearing. And, as with any other art, talent is also required.

It is much more difficult to present the case for becoming a parent. Good motives are not as clear-cut as poor ones, especially when they involve a decision so charged with emotion.

It is presumptuous, I believe, to try to set standards for parenthood. If every couple had to meet such standards, there would be too few children to perpetuate the race. A couple very much in love, wanting to create a living image reflecting their love, should probably go ahead and have a baby, provided they are not being pressured by any of the "bad" motives that might keep them from raising the child in a healthy manner. True, it may be somewhat narcissistic to want to produce a baby of your own, when you could as easily adopt one of the many unwanted children already alive; but none of us can be totally altruistic and generous. The urge to have one's own cannot be denied. Nevertheless, every couple should examine all their motives carefully, and then examine themselves as prospective parents. Do they have what it takes to raise healthy and happy children? How can they tell?

Very few people are graced with the ability to excel in several diverse areas simultaneously. This is probably why so many outstanding statesmen, writers, scientists and psychiatrists fail as parents. They spend so much time attaining success that, even if they are not emotionally spent from their exertions, they lack time to meet the needs of a child. Love, of course, may be there; but if a parent does not have the time or energy to communicate that love, his child cannot develop a feeling of security and the sense of positive identification with that parent which is necessary for healthy development.

I am not saying that the gifted artist or ambitious businessman or politician should not have children, but that if he does, and if he expects to be a good parent also, then he must not allow his work, hobby, or recreation to shut out his children. He cannot resent the time that it takes to be a parent, for then even if he puts in his "time," he will telegraph his resentment and ambivalence to the child.

Before leaping into parenthood, each couple should try to work out the life pattern best suited to them. Even if the wrong reasons for having children have been eliminated, they should have positive reasons for proceeding.

There are many couples whose preferred way of life makes parenthood undesirable. Their interests and goals may be incompatible with parenthood. One couple I know, both psychiatrists, live a fulfilled and happy life without children. They enjoy travelling and do so four months a year. They work together and publish many articles and books. Some of their research is so demanding that they could not conduct it without months of selfless dedication—a commitment that would interfere constantly with good parenthood. And the months of travel that serve as an antidote for these excessive work pressures, would not be feasible if they had children. Their temperaments and chosen style of life would not have permitted the constant mothering and fathering that every child needs. Some writers and artists become so intense in their work that they have nothing left to give emotionally. They seldom make good marriage partners, let alone good parents. To them the production of books, the completion of scientific experiments, the winning of public office may be psychologically equivalent to producing a baby—and incompatible with raising a happy child.

These illustrations indicate that there are many constructive, fulfilling and happy ways to live without being parents. It is time to retire the old-wives' tale that life without children is not complete. After all, no one lives a "complete" life. One makes choices: if you choose one thing, you give up another. Those who do not become parents *are* missing something. But there are balances and compensations—as every parent knows, there are things he cannot do, simply because he is a parent.

Many of the qualities that make a good teacher also make a good parent—patience, understanding, the desire to share what you know, a genuine concern and interest in helping youngsters grow strong and independent, the ability to enjoy children and the skill to communicate with them.

Contributing to the growth and welfare of the young should be so rewarding that one is willing and able to give up other pursuits without feeling resentment.

I do not expect anyone to get 100 percent on such a test in order to be admitted into the order of parenthood, but it is at least a guideline and a standard against which one's hopes, ambitions and goals can be measured. There are undoubtedly cases where an individual may surprise everyone, including himself, by rising to the demands of parenthood and revealing a natural talent for the role. And there is no shame in failing to achieve high parenthood marks. The shame and tragedy in people's lives is choosing wrong ways to live in order to suit others or to live up to a false picture of themselves.

There are many honorable ways to live; the whole secret in living is to find the right way for you—and follow it.

13

Parenthood as Crisis

E. E. LeMASTERS
Beloit College

Introduction

In recent decades the impact of various crises on the American family has been subjected to intensive analysis. Eliot,[1] Waller,[2] Angell,[3] Komarovsky,[4] Cavan and Ranck,[5] Koos,[6] Hill,[7] and Goode [8] have published what is perhaps the most solid block of empirical research in the field of family sociology.

In all of these studies of how the modern family reacts to crisis, it appears that the shock is related to the fact that the crisis event forces a reorganization of the family as a social system. Roles have to be reassigned, status positions shifted, values reoriented, and needs met through new channels.

These studies have shown that crises may originate either from within the family itself or from the outside. It has also been demonstrated that the total impact of the crisis will depend upon a number of variables: (1) the nature of the crisis event; (2) the state of organization or disorganization of the family at the point of impact; (3) the resources of the family; and (4) its previous experience with crisis.[9]

These studies report a sequence of events somewhat as follows: level of organization before the crisis, point of impact, period of disorganization, recovery, and subsequent level of reorganization.

This study was conceived and designed within the conceptual framework of the above research.

Marriage and Family Living, November 1957

The Present Study

In the study being described in this report, the main hypothesis was derived through the following line of analysis:

A. If the family is conceptualized as a small social system, would it not follow that the *adding* of a new member to the system could force a reorganization of the system as drastic (or nearly so) as does the *removal* of a member?

B. If the above were correct, would it not follow that the arrival of the *first* child could be construed as a "crisis" or critical event? [10]

To test this hypothesis, a group of young parents were interviewed, using a relatively unstructured interviewing technique. In order to control socio-economic variables, couples had to possess the following characteristics to be included in the study: (1) unbroken marriage; (2) urban or suburban residence; (3) between twenty-five and thirty-five years of age at the time of the study; (4) husband college graduate; (5) husband's occupation middle class; (6) wife not employed after birth of first child; (7) must have had their first child within five years of the date interviewed. Race and religion were not controlled.

Using these criteria, forty-eight couples were located by the device of asking various persons in the community for names. As a precaution, the exact nature of the study was not stated in soliciting names for the sample—the project was described as a study of "modern young parents."

Once a name was obtained that met the specifications, every effort was made to secure an interview. No refusals were encountered, but two couples left the community before they could participate, leaving forty-six couples for the final study group. The couples, then, were not volunteers. All of the interviewing was done by the writer during the years 1953–1956. Both the husband and wife were interviewed.

Typical occupations represented include minister, social worker, high school teacher, college professor, bank teller, accountant, athletic coach, and small business owner.

Various definitions of "crisis" are available to the worker in this area. Webster, for example, states that the term means a "decisive" or "crucial" period, a "turning point." [11] Koos specifies that crises are situations "which block the usual patterns of action and call for new ones." [12] Hill defines as a crisis "any sharp or decisive change for which old patterns are inadequate."[13] This is the definition used in this analysis.

A five point scale was used in coding the interview data: (1) no crisis; (2) slight crisis; (3) moderate crisis; (4) extensive crisis; (5) severe crisis.

The Findings

The essential findings of this exploratory study are as follows:

1. Thirty-eight of the forty-six couples (83 percent) reported "extensive" or "severe" crisis in adjusting to the first child. This rating was arrived at jointly by the interviewer and the parents.

In several cases there was some difference of opinion between the husband and wife as to what their response should be. In all but two cases, however, the difference was reconciled by further discussion between the interviewer and the couple. In the two cases, the wife's rating was recorded, on the theory that the mother makes the major adjustment to children in our culture.

For this sample, therefore, the evidence is quite strong in support of the hypothesis. The eight couples (17 percent) who reported relatively mild crisis (values 1–2–3 in the above scale) must be considered the deviants in this sample.

Stated theoretically, this study supports the idea that adding the first child to the urban middle class married couple constitutes a crisis event.

2. In this study there was strong evidence that this crisis reaction was *not* the result of not wanting children. On the contrary, thirty-five of the thirty-eight pregnancies in the crisis group were either "planned" or "desired."

3. The data support the belief that the crisis pattern occurs whether the marriage is "good" or "poor"—for example: thirty-four of the thirty-eight in the crisis group (89 percent) rated their marriages as "good" or better. With only three exceptions, these ratings were confirmed by close friends. By any reasonable standards, these marriages must be considered adequate.

4. There is considerable evidence that the crisis pattern in the thirty-eight cases was not the result of "neurosis" or other psychiatric disability on the part of these parents. Judging by their personal histories, their marriages, and the ratings of friends, it seemed clear that the vast bulk of the husbands and wives in the crisis group were average or above in personality adjustment.

5. The thirty-eight couples in the crisis group appear to have

almost completely romanticized parenthood. They felt that they had had very little, if any, effective preparation for parental roles. As one mother said: "We knew where babies came from, but we didn't known *what they were like*."

The mothers reported the following feelings or experiences in adjusting to the first child: loss of sleep (especially during the early months); chronic "tiredness" or exhaustion; extensive confinement to the home and the resulting curtailment of their social contacts; giving up the satisfactions and the income of outside employment; additional washing and ironing; guilt at not being a "better" mother; the long hours and seven day (and night) week necessary in caring for an infant; decline in their housekeeping standards; worry over their appearance (increased weight after pregnancy, et cetera).

The fathers echoed most of the above adjustments but also added a few of their own: decline in sexual response of wife; economic pressure resulting from wife's retirement plus additional expenditures necessary for child; interference with social life; worry about a second pregnancy in the near future; and a general disenchantment with the parental role.

6. The mothers with professional training and extensive professional work experience (eight cases) suffered "extensive" or "severe" crisis in every case.

In analyzing these cases, it was apparent that these women were really involved in two major adjustments simultaneously: (1) they were giving up an occupation which had deep significance for them; and (2) they were assuming the role of mother for the first time.

Interpretation of the Findings

There are, of course, various ways of interpreting the findings in this study. It may be, for example, that the couples obtained for the sample are not typical of urban middle class parents. It might also be true that the interviewing, the design of the study, or both, may have been inadequate. If we assume, for the present, that the findings are reliable and valid for this social group, how are we to interpret such reactions to parenthood? It is suggested that the following conceptual tools may be helpful.

1. That parenthood (and not marriage) is the real "romantic complex" in our culture. This view, as a matter of fact, was expressed by many of the couples in the study.

In a brilliant article some years ago, Arnold Green [14] suggested as much—that urban middle class couples often find their parental roles in conflict with their other socio-economic commitments. If this is true, one would expect to find the reconciliation of these conflicts most acute at the point of entering parenthood, with the first child. Our findings support this expectation.

2. Ruth Benedict has pointed out that young people in our society are often the victims of "discontinuity in cultural conditioning." [15] By this she means that we often have to "unlearn" previous training before we can move on to the next set of roles. Sex conditioning is perhaps the clearest illustration of this.

Using this concept, one can see that these couples were not trained for parenthood, that practically nothing in school, or out of school, got them ready to be fathers and mothers—*husbands* and *wives,* yes, but not *parents.* This helps explain why some of the mothers interviewed were actually "bitter" about their high school and college training.

3. One can also interpret these findings by resorting to what is known about small groups. Wilson and Ryland, for example, in their standard text on group work make this comment about the two-person group: "This combination seems to be the most satisfactory of human relationships." [16] They then proceed to pass this judgment on the three-person group: "Upon analysis this pattern falls into a combination of a pair and an isolate. . . . This plurality pattern is the most volatile of all human relationships." [17] This, of course, supports an earlier analysis by von Wiese and Becker.[18]

Viewed in this conceptual system, married couples find the transition to parenthood painful because the arrival of the first child destroys the two-person or pair pattern of group interaction and forces a rapid reorganization of their life into a three-person or triangle group system. Due to the fact that their courtship and pre-parenthood pair relationship has persisted over a period of years, they find it difficult to give it up as a way of life.

In addition, however, they find that living as a trio is more complicated than living as a pair. The husband, for example, no longer ranks first in claims upon his wife but must accept the child's right to priority. In some cases, the husband may feel that he is the semi-isolate, the third party in the trio. In other cases, the wife may feel that her husband is more interested in the baby than in her. If they preserve their pair relationship and continue their previous way of life, relatives and friends may regard them as poor parents. In any event, their pattern of living has to be radically altered.

Since babies do not usually appear to married couples completely by surprise, it might be argued that this event is not really a crisis—"well adjusted" couples should be "prepared for it." The answer seems to be that children and parenthood have been so romanticized in our society that most middle class couples are caught unprepared, even though they have planned and waited for this event for years. The fact that parenthood is "normal" does not eliminate crisis. Death is also "normal" but continues to be a crisis event for most families.

4. One can also interpret the findings of this study by postulating that parenthood (not marriage) marks the final transition to maturity and adult responsibility in our culture.[19] Thus the arrival of the first child forces young married couples to take the last painful step into the adult world. This point, as a matter of fact, was stated or implied by most of the couples in the crisis group.

5. Finally, the cases in this sample confirm what the previous studies in this area have shown: that the event itself is only one factor determining the extent and severity of the crisis on any given family. Their resources, their previous experience with crisis, the pattern of role organization before the crisis—these factors are equally important in determining the total reaction to the event.

Conclusion

In this study, it was hypothesized that the addition of the first child would constitute a crisis event, forcing the married couple to move from an adult-centered pair type of organization into child-centered triad group system. Of the forty-six middle class couples located for this study, thirty-eight (83 percent) confirmed the hypothesis.

In all fairness to this group of parents, it should be reported that all but a few of them eventually made what seems to be a successful adjustment to parenthood. This does not alter the fact, however, that most of them found the transition difficult. Listening to them describe their experiences, it seemed that one could compare these young parents to veterans of military service—they had been through a rough experience, but it was worth it. As one father said: "I wouldn't have missed it for the world."

It is unfortunate that the number of parents in this sample who did not report crisis is so small (eight couples) that no general statements can be made about them. Somehow, however, they seem to have been better prepared for parenthood than was the crisis group. It is felt that future work on this problem might well include a more extensive analysis of couples who have made the transition to parenthood with relative ease.

If the basic findings of this study are confirmed by other workers, it would appear that family life educators could make a significant contribution by helping young people prepare more adequately for parenthood.

14

Changes in Marriage and Parenthood: A Methodological Design

HAROLD FELDMAN
Professor, Department of Human Development and Family Studies, Cornell University

In the field of marriage research we are plagued by the notion that any finding is an obvious one. However, had we found the opposite, it too would be accepted as obvious. In this paper I will quite regularly state and build a case for mutually exclusive hypotheses and will confront them with the findings as we proceed. The findings will be presented mainly from my own studies on marriage and parenthood. The findings will be based on statistically significant differences although actual data will not be reported in this paper. The first of these is a cross sectional study of 852 middle and upper-middle class couples in an urban setting. The second is a short-term longitudinal study with cross sectional controls about the transition to parenthood—the effect on the marriage of the couples' being parents for the first time. This study was designed in order to explore further one of the salient findings of the cross sectional investigation and to expand the findings using a panel study with cross sectional controls.

The cross sectional study focused on middle and upper-middle class couples, using the concept of socio-geographic area developed by C. Willie at Syracuse University. Each census tract was placed into one of six classifications according to the composite score based on five criteria derived from census data. These were:

1. percent of single family dwellings
2. average monthly rental

Study supported by National Institutes of Mental Health No. 2931 under the rubric "The Development of the Husband-Wife Relationship."

3. average market value of owned homes
4. median school years completed
5. percent of operative service workers and laborers

Every third dwelling unit was selected as a target and final data from both husband and wife were collected on 85% of the eligible target sample. This procedure resulted in there being 88% of the sample classified as white collar. Eighty-seven percent of the sample were married only once. Thirty-one percent were working wives, 84% had the husband's educational level about the same as the wife or somewhat higher, and 79% had husband and wife the same age or the husband somewhat older, and the religious distribution was both Catholic (21%), both Protestant (35%), both Jewish (27%), and mixed or no religion (17%). In general, the sample appeared to be quite similar to that expected on an upper-middle class, urban community.[1]

Data for the second study were gathered in a similar fashion to the cross sectional one, i.e., subjects were contacted by letter, a personal call made, the questionnaire explained and left and personally picked up several days later by appointment. Follow-up letters and gifts were sent to all participants, resulting again in a very high (85%) rate of return. Here, subjects were studied three different times. Samples were selected from areas where they would be indigenous, i.e., blue collar from Flint, Michigan, students and white collar from Ithaca, New York, upper white collar and lower class from New York City.

In order to make the hypotheses more theoretically interesting, I will try to state hypotheses which would result from, on the one hand, trait theory and on the other hand, role theory.

Trait theory assumes a consistency of personality which transcends the situation and predicts no special change of the person over time. Traits are fundamental "foci" of the personality, formed in childhood and continued throughout life, being consistent over marriage and not influenced by the addition of parenthood.

Role theory, on the other hand, predicts changes in behavior as a function of the social position a person fills and would predict that a person's behavior or expectations for behavior would change as a result of marriage and parenthood. This is a very condensed treatment of a very complex issue, but it will suffice for the present.[2] One more word about an additional plague—the confusion by social scientists about the use of the term role. I shall use it to include both expectations and behaviors associated with a social position and occasionally shall also use it in the vernacular sense of the role of parenthood or marriage when I really mean social position.

The first set of hypotheses deal with marriage, while later ones will focus on the relationship between parenthood and marriage.

1. Hypotheses About Marriage through the Family Life Cycle

These hypotheses will concern the changes in marital satisfaction and changes in aspects other than marital satisfaction through the life cycles. Two different groups of hypotheses will be examined.

Trait theory hypotheses

There are no differences in stated marital behaviors throughout the marital life cycle.

A pattern once established will tend to continue, regardless of circumstances. Persons establish a relationship based on their traits and tend to continue in this fashion. We change very little as adults, since our patterns of relating to others were established early.

Role theory hypotheses

There are significant changes in relationships of marital partners over the marital life cycle. We will begin first with the change of marital satisfaction.

A. Change in Marital Satisfaction through Family Life Cycles

Starting with the variable of satisfaction with marriage, the following are some of the logical possibilities for ways in which marital satisfaction may change over the marital life cycle.

1. Linear relationships

a. The longer couples are married, the happier they are with each other. After all, it takes a while to know another, and those not compatible have dropped out of marriage. This hypothesis implies a linear and positive relationship between stage of marital cycle and marital satisfaction.

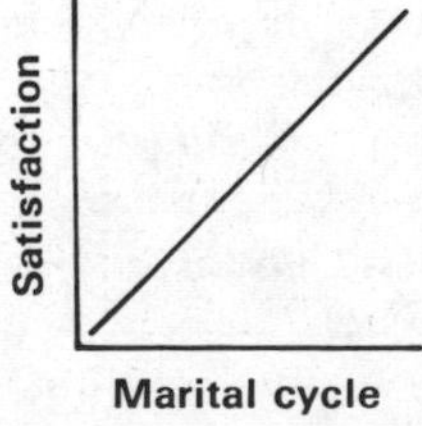

b. Marital satisfaction declines throughout the cycle. There is the heat of early marriage, followed by increasing disillusionment and boredom. This nihilistic view finds major support from some contemporary viewers of marriage, i.e., the longer one knows another, the less one likes the relationship with the other.

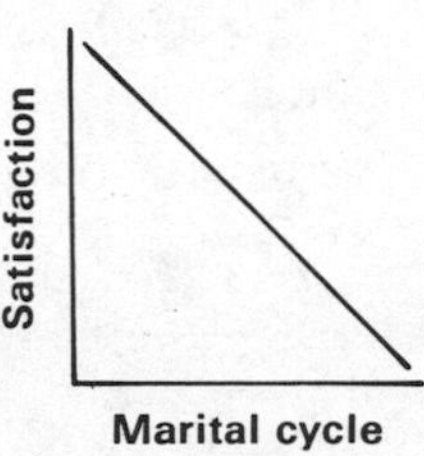

2. *Curvilinear relationships*

a. Negative and then positive. Early love is followed by disillusionment, since inordinately high expectations for marriage are not met. Children come and add to marital difficulties. There is later, then, an acceptance of the other as the other is, an imperfect person. This change in expectations, coming as children grow older, is accompanied by a more positive affect for the other and for marriage.

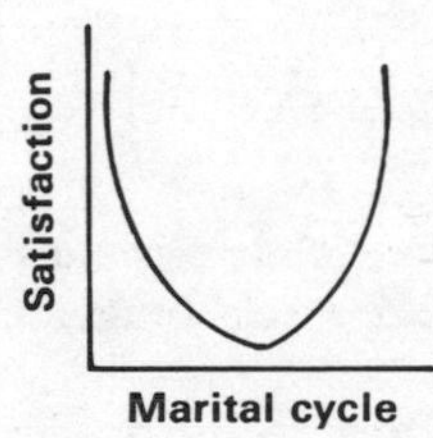

b. Positive then negative. The obverse of the above curvilinear relationship is the myth that marital conflict is high at the beginning when many adjustments need to be made. There is an elimination of some persons from their first marriage through divorce. The remainder are drawn together by their common interest in children. After the children leave, only the couple remains with an accompanying lowering again of satisfaction.

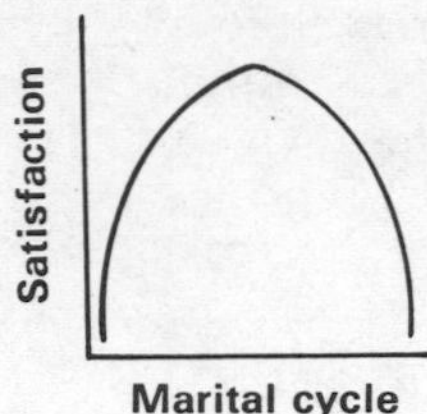

METHOD

In the cross sectional study of 852 couples from a middle and upper-middle class, urban setting, the couples were classified into four general marital life cycle groups.

1. beginning marriage (1 group)
2. child bearing (3 subgroups)
3. child rearing (8 subgroups)
4. post child rearing (2 groups)

Satisfaction was measured by five different sets of indices. Four of them derived by factor analysis and the fifth, the response to the single question about stated marital satisfaction. The four marital satisfaction factors were:

1. overall satisfaction over the stages of marriage
2. satisfaction with independent child stages of marriage
3. satisfaction with the earlier stages of marriage
4. marital stress composed of 9 items

The fifth component, stated marital satisfaction, was derived from a single direct item about the amount of time things were going well in the marriage.

F tests were computed for testing the significance of the difference among the 14 marital life cycle means, and correlations were computed between life cycle stage and marital satisfaction scores.

FINDING

The present study found a significant F value for all five marital satisfaction factors for differences among life cycle groups and a curvilinear relationship over the cycle as predicted in 2a above. Couples were as happy in the later post childbearing years as they were in the early years of marriage, with the low points being in the middle of marriage when the last child went to school and when the family had teenagers.

DISCUSSION

There are changes in attitudes about m of marriage to another, lending some suppo behavior tends to change in adulthood, t theory. The conclusion was that if a couple long enough the satisfaction level increases to b marriage. The major limitation of this conclus based on a cross sectional study, so that differen lated to a number of factors attributable to the c of the groups, such as the social setting when marrie ., war, depression, affluent period, and nonchance differences among the groups' religious, educational factors.

B. Change in Aspects of Marriage other than Marital Satisfaction through the Family Life Cycles

The next question was to explore the nature of marriage beyond marital satisfaction. Was marriage at the beginning and late stage similar, since level of marital satisfaction was the same? What was marriage like at the low points? What was the shape of the curve over the marital cycle for other factors? Note we could make predictions about these trends over marriage and that mutually exclusive ones might seem to make good sense, but then nothing so slays a beautiful hypothesis like the ugly facts.

The first question is whether there were more differences in marital factors other than marital satisfaction over the cycle than would appear by chance.

METHOD

The data from the precoded questionnaires were factor analyzed and yielded 44 principal components, tested for cycle differences.

FINDING

Twenty-seven of these factors had statistically significant F values for comparisons among the 14 life cycle groups. Chance would result in less than three of these being significant at the sacred 5% level—so we may conclude that there are more changes in marriage than expected by chance.

The 44 factors were combined conceptually into three categories: the socio-emotional, the objective and power symmetry.

There was a linear decline in the socio-emotional aspects of marriage, e.g., have gay times together, feel close to the spouse is talk about sex, the importance of sex to a satisfying ...ge, frequency of conversations about affective topics, such ...personal feelings. There was an increase in objectivity such as the frequency of marital conversations about the house, news, cultural topics and sports and also an increase in symmetry regarding the power relationship. The wife had more power in the beginning in most aspects of marriage except for decision making about sex, which the couples felt became vested more in the husband as the marriage progressed.

DISCUSSION

Even though there were more changes than would be expected by chance, we still have to consider the alternative that the components were not independent. Actually, most of the factors were quite independent of each other.

Several alternative explanations are suggested for the stated increase in husband power about the frequency of sex.

Perhaps, as Kinsey suggested, the wife becomes a more willing sex partner as the marriage progresses and her children take less of her libido so that her sexual performance may depend more on her husband's initiative. Perhaps her increased power in other areas of marriage may make her more willing to give up her authority potential about sex. Perhaps as they grow older the wife may have learned more about how to have her husband feel he has more to say about sex. It may be that all three explanations are valid, since most behavior is multicaused.

Pineo suggests, as marriage increases in length there may be some disengagement but it may be accompanied by a more realistic assessment of the other. With the lowering of unrealistic aspects of romanticism, couples may accept the other more realistically as persons with human failings, so that the increase in marital happiness late in marriage may, in part, be a function of lowered expectations. In any case, if one stays with marriage long enough, satisfaction appears to be quite high, although the relationship is quite different than at the beginning. It's not quite that dull either—the couple in late marriage said they laughed together about once a day.[3] These hypotheses need more findings. In any case, role theory has received further support.

The next set of hypotheses relates parenthood to marriage, i.e., what is the influence of being a parent on the marital relationship?

2. Hypotheses about the Relationship Between Parenthood and Marriage

The hypotheses here will concern the relationship of parenthood with marital satisfaction and other aspects of marriage than marital satisfaction.

A. Relationship between Parenthood and Marital Satisfaction

There are no differences in marital happiness between those with and without children (trait theory hypothesis).

Attitudes toward marriage are a function of intra personal factors and are not affected by extra personal factors, such as having or not having children.

Hypothesis 2B

Couples with children are happier in marriage than those without children (role theory hypothesis).

Children have a cohesive influence on the marriage by drawing the couple together and giving marriage a central focus.

Hypothesis 2C

Couples with children are less happy in marriage than those without children (role theory hypothesis).

Children bring out latent feelings of hostility which tend to become displaced against the spouse. Conflicts about child rearing cannot usually be resolved by compromise, i.e., when he cries the baby cannot be picked up one time and left to cry it out the next.

METHOD

In the cross sectional study of marital satisfaction, comparisons were made between all those couples who had a child in the home and those who never had children. There was no statistical difference in the length of marriage for the two groups.

FINDING

Those with children had a significantly lower level of marital satisfaction than did those without children.

DISCUSSION

This serendipitous finding was not the major focus of the original study but the next step in logic was to discover whether the finding would hold for those just entering parenthood.

METHOD

Comparisons on marital satisfaction were first made for those in early marriage who were without a child with those who had an infant as their only child.

FINDING

Those with an infant had a significantly lower level of marital satisfaction than did those who were childless. However, those with a child were married longer.

METHOD

Comparisons on marital satisfaction were made for those with and without a child, controlling for length of marriage.

FINDING

Those with an infant had a significantly lower level of marital satisfaction than did those who were childless, when the length of marriage was controlled.

DISCUSSION

The comparisons made, however, were cross sectional ones and perhaps there were other factors differentiating the two groups, such as the unpleasant possibility that unhappier people have children, or that the two groups differed on some obvious or obscure demographic factor. The decision was made to follow up the cross sectional study with a more complex design. Armed now with a stack of IBM cards, an additional grant of money from NIMH, and a larger, more hostile computer, we began the next study. A somewhat clearer question could now be asked. What is the effect of becoming parents on the marriage?

The Short Term Longitudinal Study with Cross Sectional Controls

Hypothesis 3A

When a couple become parents, there is no change in their marriage (trait theory hypothesis).

Hypothesis 3B

When a couple become parents, their marriage improves (role theory hypothesis).

Hypothesis 3C

When a couple become parents the marital satisfaction declines (role theory hypothesis).

METHOD

The design for this second study is found in the table below.

TABLE 1

Design of Study Illustrating Longitudinal Panels with Cross Sectional Controls [4]

Number of Children	*Time* A	B	C	N
0	0A	0B	0C	40
1	1A	1B	1C	400
2	2A	2B	2C	40

The design attempted to combine the assets of both the longitudinal and cross sectional approaches. The main study group was the primipara, a set of couples having their first child (1), while the primary control group, nullipara, was those not having a child (0). In addition, there was a group to test for the replication of parenthood effect, multipara—those having their second child (2).

There were three time intervals: time A when the primiparous mother was five months pregnant, time B when the first child was about five weeks old, and time C when the child was about five months old.

The first comparison on marital satisfaction was made for the primipara during pregnancy (1A) and after the child was born (1C).

FINDING

Since it is unlikely that a decrease in marital satisfaction yields a baby, the cause and effect relationship is more probably in the opposite direction, i.e., having a baby causes a decrease in marital satisfaction. The mean change score was significantly greater than zero—with the postpartum couples being less satisfied with marriage than they were before the child was born.

DISCUSSION

Since it is unlikely that a decrease in marital satisfaction yields a baby, the cause and effect relationship is more probably in the opposite direction, i.e., having a baby causes a decrease in marital satisfaction.

Since some couples increased in satisfaction with the addition of parenthood, while others did not, it was decided to explore the hypotheses about the reasons for improvement in marriage with parenthood.

Hypotheses Concerning the Relationship Between Companionate Versus Differentiated Prepartum Marriage and Change of Marital Satisfaction After the Birth of the First Child

Hypothesis 4A [5]

Increased marital satisfaction after the birth of the first child will be positively correlated with the extent to which the marriage was *companionate* prepartum.

Couples who have found a close relationship with each other during pregnancy would be better able than would more differentiated couples to cope with the crisis of having a baby. Being accustomed to relying on each other, they are brought even closer together by parenthood.

Hypothesis 4B [5]

Increased marital satisfaction after the birth of the first child will be positively correlated with the extent to which the marriage was *differentiated* prepartum.

Those who are more differentiated have a void, and these couples, finding a focal point for companionship in the first baby, will be drawn closer together in marriage with addition of parenthood.

METHOD

The procedure to test these hypotheses was to compare marital satisfaction scores during mid-pregnancy (1A) and after the child's birth (1C) and then to correlate these changes in satisfaction scores with the attitudes about marriage during the pregnancy period.

FINDING

In each case, the finding confirmed the hypothesis that an increase in marital satisfaction after becoming a parent was positively correlated with having a more differentiated, rather than a more companionate, marriage before becoming a parent, i.e., those whose prepartum marriage was characterized by a lower level of verbal communication with each other, lesser use of spouse as an interpersonal resource, less likely display of emotionality toward spouse during conflict, and a belief system precluding husbands' participation in household tasks were more likely to increase in marital satisfaction when the couple became parents.

DISCUSSION

An additional datum may help to clarify the finding. There was a positive relationship between an increase in satisfaction with parenthood and several indices of maternalism, i.e., concern for the child's crying, preference for breast feeding, being child centered in plans for feeding.

The relationship between maternalism and an increase in marital satisfaction is part of the pattern which may reflect the fruition of the wife's hopes and aspirations regarding family life. She wants the baby because, besides being a highly valued object in its own right, the baby may likewise serve to create a less differentiated, more companionate marriage. Evidence for this latter perceived cohesive effect of the child is exhibited in the relationship between rise in satisfaction and expectations that the husband will take part in many of the child-caring tasks. Wives who increase in satisfaction tend to expect that the husband will not only change diapers, put the baby to sleep, and quiet the baby when it cries, but will also care for the child when the wife is not present. Furthermore, although the amount of attention received from the husband during pregnancy was not related to changes in marital satisfaction, expectations about the amount of attention the wife will receive from her husband in the postpartum state was positively correlated with satisfaction shifts. It appeared that the woman who increased in satisfaction felt that being a mother would draw her husband closer to her.

For the companionate marriage, one explanation may be that if the marriage satisfaction level tends to decrease with the coming of the child, then it could be postulated that the child is an interference factor in an otherwise closely knit marital relationship. Perhaps a triad is a more unstable relationship when contrasted with a closely knit dyad. If the new mother must cope with a child for which she finds less maternal feelings within herself, the demands of her husband for companionship may be too much for her and, she is disappointed with herself for not coping with the in the kitchen. He is disappointed in the loss of attention from her and she is disappointed with herself for not coping with the baby or her husband. If she were less dependent on him or he on her, then the marriage might not be so vulnerable. It would be very interesting to separate out all those cases of closely knit couples where the wife is maternal. Perhaps this combination may also result in a positive change.

Hypotheses Concerning the Relationship Between Attitudes Toward Pregnancy and Change of Marital Satisfaction after the Birth of the First Child

The next set of hypotheses concerns the relationship between attitudes about pregnancy, an early stage of parenthood, and changes in marital satisfaction.

Trait theory states that the best prediction of a subsequent event is the antecedent one: Studies of school performance have shown that academic success in college may be predicted by performance in high school. Studies of marriage have shown that marital adjustment is related to experiences in the family of orientation. Similarly positive attitudes toward pregnancy should be associated with positive affect in the postpartum period.

On the other hand, negative attitudes toward pregnancy may be associated with positive attitudes toward marriage if pregnancy was viewed as an unpleasant state or as a necessary chore which must be endured antecedent to the positive state of actually having the baby in the family.

The two mutually exclusive hypotheses concerning attitudes toward pregnancy and marital satisfaction are:

Hypothesis 5A

Increased marital satisfaction after the birth of the first child will be positively correlated with the extent of satisfaction with pregnancy—a trait theory hypothesis implying consistency from pre to postparental attitudes.

Hypothesis 5B

Increased marital satisfaction after the birth of the first child will be negatively correlated with the extent of satisfaction with pregnancy—a role theory hypothesis implying that situational factors may be of greater influence.

METHOD

Several factors about attitudes toward pregnancy itself were correlated with changes in marital satisfaction, pre and postpartum, for the primipara.

FINDING

Improvement in marital satisfaction after the birth of the first child was associated with such negative attitudes toward pregnancy as concern about appearance, feeling uncomfortable in public and feeling that one's appearance was more attractive before pregnancy. Also associated with improvement in satisfaction were prepartum feelings of fatigue, nervousness and "depression" and a tendency to state explicitly that one did not enjoy pregnancy.

A rise in marital satisfaction after the birth of the first child was correlated with viewing pregnancy as a negative experience, a finding which supports the hypothesis based on role theory.

DISCUSSION

Positive changes in satisfaction with marriage have been shown to be related to attitudes during pregnancy—being more differentiated from spouse, being maternal toward children, expecting the husband to take an active interest in children, and having a negative attitude toward pregnancy itself. Another line of evidence contributing to an understanding of the parenthood effect on marriage is that there is a direct relationship between length of acquaintance prior to marriage and the increase in satisfaction with the birth of the first child. Perhaps each spouse has had an opportunity to become an identity somewhat separate from the spouse so that the more differentiated couples are more likely able to cope with parenthood.

B. Relationship Between Parenthood and Other Aspects of Marriage than Marital Satisfaction

The next step was to explore the nature of changes in marriage, other than marital satisfaction, and to attribute these changes to the advent of first-time parenthood. We have already demonstrated that, in general, marital satisfaction declines with parenthood and have explored the earlier correlates of this decline. Now let's look in at the other changes. No specific hypothesis will be promulgated, although it should be noted that alternative findings would be quite logical.

METHOD

Our design allowed us to contrast the marriages of those becoming parents (1C–1A) with those not becoming parents (0C–0A). The difference scores of the marital factors for primipara (1C–1A) had to meet the statistical tests of being significantly greater than zero and also be significantly different from childless, allowing us to hold constant the effect attributable to length of marriage.

FINDINGS

The overall results indicated that, of the statistically significant differences from pregnancy to postpartum period, about 40% of them were unique to the primipara. This number is well above the number of differences one might expect by chance and the conclusion is that having a first child indeed has a unique effect on the attitudes of marital partners.

Some of the unique consequences are:

1. The primipara seemed more overwhelmed than when they were pregnant. They had even less time to use as they wished than before the child was born.

2. They admitted to more problems about sex than before parenthood. The wife had more concern about the sexual relationship and the husband was more dissatisfied.

3. Attitudes about the self were different from prepartum. As parents the husband was rated with a lower sense of humor, though being less self-centered. The wife was perceived as less moody, less selfish, less egocentric, and getting angry less easily but she felt nervous and "blue" more often.

4. The husband took a greater part in decisions about the home than before.

5. The wife had a gain directly attributable to parenthood. She felt needed now more than before, but to some extent at the expense of the marriage. She stated she was more satisfied with marriage before pregnancy and felt as a parent she couldn't express her feelings to her spouse as well as before.

6. The focus of marital conversation had shifted toward the wife's interests. However, areas of potential conflict increased when they were parents in the areas of their parents, money, and his job. Of course, conversations about the new baby were now proceeding, even more by the primipara than anticipated by the nullipara.

7. The primipara had a change in life values. Emotional and financial security were more important and, interestingly, so was the importance of developing their own interests.

8. They were more confident about their ability to care for their child as parents. The difference was greatest for the comparison between the primipara and the anticipated level of confidence about child care by those without children. In other words, when anticipating the event, the situation appeared more serious than actually being there and facing it.

9. The primipara expected that their situation would improve as the child got older. The child would interfere less with the

marriage, the house would look better, they would feel less tired, have more and better sex, would feel less nervous, "blue" and have more free time for themselves.

DISCUSSION

In general, the finding by LeMasters that parenthood is a crisis seems to be substantiated.[6]

Although marital happiness may be lowered, as shown here, and a crisis exists—still it is possible that the wife's total happiness may be higher. Feelings of being needed more may make the sum of happiness higher. It is important to note that we are referring here only to marital satisfaction, not to satisfaction with other areas of life such as satisfaction with parenthood, with work or self in general.

The next set of hypotheses have to do with replicated child effects—those factors which showed commonalities attributed to those having children whether for the first or second time.

C. Relationships Between Marital Satisfaction and Successive Parenthood

Hypothesis 6A

The influence of parenthood on marriage is unique for the first experience with parenthood and there is an increase in satisfaction the second time.

Hypothesis 6B

The marital crisis experience continues for second-time parents.

METHOD

Comparisons were made where the change scores from pre to postpartum for the primipara were greater than zero and not different from the multipara. These scores were then compared to those during the same time intervals for the childless.

FINDINGS

More effects than expected by chance replicated when couples had their second child. If anything, there appeared to be an even greater negative effect for the multipara.

These child effect changes found for both primipara and multipara were: lowered satisfaction in marriage, perceived negative personality change in both partners, less satisfaction with home, more instrumental conversation, more child-centered concern and more warmth toward the child, and a lowering of sexual satisfaction after childbirth.

DISCUSSION

Thus far, we have demonstrated a marked effect of parenthood and children on the marriage. This effect occurs in both the cross sectional and longitudinal studies and for those having their first and second child, but to what extent are the differences found attributable to attitudes about children?

D. Relationship Between Marital Satisfaction and Consensus Between Spouses Toward Child Rearing

Hypothesis 7

Differences between husband and wife on child rearing attitudes were more predictive of marital happiness than differences on attitudes about the wife's career orientation.

METHOD

Child rearing items included overall attitudes toward support and control of children as well as preferred practices about weaning and toilet training. Career orientation items related to the motivations for women's working and the time for working.

FINDING

Consensus between husband and wife on child rearing attitude was more significantly related to marital satisfaction than was consensus about the wife's career orientation.

DISCUSSION

Perhaps we need to focus even more on attitudes about children than on other premarital factors in parent education programs.

The next question to be explored is whether the child has to be physically present for this effect to appear.

Attitudes Toward Child Rearing of Childless Couples and Couples in which the Wife Is Pregnant

Hypothesis 8A

Pregnancy period is essentially the same as the nonpregnancy period of marriage (trait theory hypothesis).

Hypothesis 8B

Pregnancy is a unique period with its own marital consequences (role theory hypothesis).

METHOD

Cross sectional comparisons were made between those who were pregnant and those married for the same period of time, not pregnant but answering as though they were pregnant. The groups were matched on demographic factors.

FINDING

1. Couples with pregnant wives talked more about children and felt children were more important to success in marriage.

2. Those actually expecting had lower confidence in their ability to cope with the event. The nulliparous husband estimated he would have more confidence in changing the baby, getting the baby to sleep, in quieting the baby and in caring for the baby when the wife is away, than did the husband with a pregnant wife.

3. The childless couples expected that the wife when pregnant would be more irritable and more concerned about her appearance during pregnancy than were those with the wife actually pregnant. The reality of money problems attributable to parenthood was greater as a source of concern to the couples with a pregnant wife. In general, the closer to the event the more tension regarding performance or its consequences, particularly on the part of the husbands.

4. Neither pregnant wives nor their husbands viewed the wife's situation as very delicate. Childless husbands, when responding as if the wife were pregnant, stated they felt that the husband should and would help the wife with housework somewhat more than before she was pregnant, compared to the level of only slightly more by husbands of the pregnant wives. Pregnant wives concurred by stating that the husband should help less than those who were childless.

5. Husbands were less apt to take a sex typed stand about their participation in child care and housework than were the wives. The wives felt that the husband should take a less active part than did the husband. This sex difference was greater for the pregnant.

6. Romanticism was higher in the pregnant, rather than in the nonpregnant, and there was a generally more optimistic feeling toward the future on the part of pregnant wives.

DISCUSSION

Interesting differences are brought out by these findings. It appears that nullipara viewed pregnancy as more debilitating than it actually is. Perhaps the wife in the actual situation of pregnancy felt that she must begin to perform the roles expected by society.

She may be unaware that her husband prefers to take a more active part.

One might predict that romanticism, a naive, unrealistic, inflexible, but very love-oriented attitude toward marriage, might be more prevalent in nonpregnant couples for they are the carefree ones, unencumbered with the approaching responsibilities of parenthood. It would be reasonable to predict that the pregnant are more aware of the realities of life and, consequently, of marriage as well. It was revealing that this was not so.

We see that pregnancy is a time of tension and anxiety for those actually experiencing the situation and it may be that anxiety about performance resulted in a lowering of confidence but also an increase in romanticism—possibly as a way to deal with the anxiety—an hypothesis to be tested.

Trying to take on the role of another without really experiencing the situation appears to produce different outcomes from those in the situation, thus again supporting role theory. Generally, pregnancy elicits new role behaviors.

Conclusions

1. Parenthood has a pervasive influence on the marriage. This effect appears at pregnancy and continues during the life cycle when children are at home.

2. Differences in child rearing attitudes between the husband and wife appear to have a marked effect on marital happiness. After the child is born these differences may be latent to other heterogamies the couple may have, such as differences between the husband and wife on religion, social class, educational levels and ethnic origin.

There is the need for parent education prior to and shortly after couples have a child in order to minimize the influence of differences of opinion about child rearing and its influence on marital satisfaction. Couples should explore their attitudes about children before they have them, since these differences may be more deep seated than couples may believe they are.

3. A longer period of acquaintance with the spouse prior to marriage, having a more differentiated marriage, having a lower satisfaction with the pregnancy period but being maternalistic and expecting that the husband will be more interested in child care are associated with an increase in marital satisfaction with the coming of the first child. These findings were not of such a magnitude to be predictive for any specific instance and the study needs

further large scale replication, but they do suggest that couples may want to evaluate their marriage and preparation for parenthood prior to having children.

4. There are a number of misconceptions held by the childless about the pregnancy and the postpartum period. Family life education could help in teaching the young the hypotheses which seem to be most like reality.

5. There appears to be some support for role theory as opposed to trait theory as these two theories have been defined. Trait theory assumes that persons are consistent over time, that traits are fundamental foci of personality continuing unchanged regardless of change in social position such as the addition of parenthood to marriage.

Role theory assumes that behavior may change as the individual moves from one social position to another and that the addition of a new social position to a person's repertoire would have some influence on his behavior in another.

The dichotomy regarding these two theories may not be as clear as we have posed it to be. Cottrell[7] in an earlier paper attempted to integrate these two theories and proposed that personality may be defined as the "organization of the roles the person plays in life," while "role is the organization of habits and attitudes of the individual appropriate to a given position." According to these definitions, then, roles are a function of organized traits, while traits are a way of organizing roles.

Perhaps the intra and inter role consistencies of a person are his traits while his cross role inconsistencies are best described by role theory. In any case, this classic issue is out on the table again as it may apply to parenthood and marriage.

6. The generating of hypotheses and confrontations with the finding have proven to have a very heuristic function. As a result of this exercise in posing alternatives and seriously considering another point of view, many new hypotheses about the nature of marriage and the family are suggested even by the tightest research design. The brighter the light shed in one area, the clearer the contrast with what is yet to be known.

One of the needs of the family field is to have studies done on a large scale so that the results can be cumulative. We need to join together with other universities and interested persons in order to test hypotheses on a large enough scale to have a national effect.

7. The cross sectional study has identified crucial points to be investigated more intensively. Some of these points in the marital life cycle are associated with significant changes in the child's life—

his birth, entrance to school and leaving home. The panel study with cross sectional controls seems to overcome some of the disadvantages of many other designs and combines some of the advantages of the short term longitudinal study with the cross sectional one.

As a longitudinal study, the design allows for studying the effects of a natural intervention, i.e., the child's being born, going to school or leaving home. Before and after measurements can be made of the marriage, the design becomes even tighter with the addition of cross sectional controls to hold constant other effects, such as length of marriage for those families who do not experience the natural intervention, i.e., do not have a new child, or do not have a child leaving home. The natural intervention group and the control group can be matched on factors crucial to the study, i.e., family composition in addition to the standard factors such as social class, religion, employment of wife and length of marriage. The design was illustrated in the present report where data from the cross sectional study contributed to the selection of the problem and the suggestion of areas to be investigated more intensively by the panel study.

15

The Implications of Motherhood for Political Participation

NAOMI B. LYNN and CORNELIA B. FLORA

Department of Political Science, Kansas State University, Manhattan, Kansas; and Department of Sociology and Anthropology and Population Research Laboratory, Kansas State University, Manhattan, Kansas

Political scientists have largely ignored women as participants in political life. Most of the studies mentioning women use them as a basis for comparison with the more relevant actor—the male. In this study, we will focus on women and their political activity with particular emphasis on the effect which motherhood has on their self-image and its relevance for women's political participation.

Sociologists have long stressed the primacy of the role of mother in the identification of the adult female. Lopata [1] describes and analyzes the changes in a woman that take place during the life cycle, stressing the importance of becoming and being a mother. LeMasters, Dyer, and others [2] have pointed to the crisis accompanying initiation to motherhood. For young women, in particular, absorption in the care of young children is the norm.[3] As the "self" of an individual can be seen as emerging "through the internalization by the individual of social processes of experience and behavior," [4] the new set of interactions and experiences prescribed by the role of mother can be seen to give a woman new criteria for self-evaluation and to remove many of her previous interactions which reinforced her old identity.

Prepared for delivery at the 1972 Annual Meeting of the American Political Science Association, Washington Hilton Hotel, Washington, D.C., September 5–9.

Motherhood and Self-Image

Many sociologists see the role of mother as the crucial one in limiting female behavior, and, by extension, her resulting self-image. Ginsberg points out that "although a husband may broaden or narrow a woman's margin of choice, children almost always narrow it." [5] While the nuclear family dyad is expanded into a triad, doubling the types of potential sets of interactions, the emphasis on the mother as the sole or primary guardian of the child's everyday needs limits to a large degree any other kind of interaction she may experience. Lopata points to two types of self-modification that occur with motherhood: an "identity crisis," "the feeling that the whole personality is affected by constant physical work and contact mainly with infants in a small confined space," and "an increase in maturity, in capacities, and abilities." [6]

Past research has seemed to agree that motherhood is the major role of women, particularly young women, and that motherhood is a confining role. But the results of the saliency of motherhood among young women have not been systematically analyzed for their political implications.

Motherhood: The Political Self

Political socialization does not end with adulthood; it is a continuing process which may be affected by any major change in the life of the individual. Dawson and Prewitt point out that "acquiring a political self is a natural corollary to general social maturation." [7] Almond and Verba have concerned themselves with the relationship between non-political roles and the political role and suggest that there is a "tendency to generalize from one social sphere to the other." [8] Bell has described parenthood as "the most significant and demanding new role that most individuals encounter during their lifetime." [9] If motherhood does indeed have such a tremendous impact on women and their self-image, what implications does it have for their political self?

Radical members of the women's liberation movement have linked woman's lack of political activity to her role of wife and mother. As pointed out by Linda Gordon, "one of the institutions of this society that the women's liberation movement has been particularly vocal in condemning is the nuclear family." The method of child care of the nuclear family is seen as destructive to both adults and children, turning the mother's "adult mind into mush" [10]—a prosaic way of describing the changing self resulting from a new set of interactional processes.

The nuclear family, with stress on the child-rearing function of the adult female, is claimed by members of the movement to separate people into small, isolated units which distrust outsiders. This distrust, according to Gordon, "is one of the forces making it difficult for people to join together to act politically." But it is the family as an institution, rather than the mother-child relationship, which is identified as the anti-political force.

Children serve as one of many factors that add to the devaluation of women, contributing to women's low self-esteem that hinders them in attempting to participate in politics.[11] The myths surrounding motherhood then entrap women into false consciousness. The political self never has a chance to develop in mothers.

Are mothers actually less political than non-mothers? If so, this would definitely have the conservatising influence pointed to by Gouldner in his study of labor leaders, where he found that motherhood increases the wife's demands on the husband and further "depoliticizes" him.[12]

National Data

To compare the degree of political participation of mothers to non-mothers we used data from the 1968 study of the American electorate conducted by the Survey Research Center, University of Michigan. Political participation can be defined as the "use of resources (including time) to influence political outcomes." [13] Since there was no single indicator of total political participation, we approximated it through a measure of political efficacy. Studies have indicated that individuals who are efficacious politically are more likely to become politically active.[14] Political efficacy is also highly related to voting turnout.[15] DiPalma states that "political efficacy is the orientation dynamically closest to participation, for in a way it asks the individual whether he feels he can participate." [16] In addition, we wanted to compare the national data with our own sample of young mothers. We also wanted to look beyond the short-term and perhaps fluctuating levels of political participation to a measure with more long-term implications.[17] We decided to use as our measure of political efficacy the question: Would you say that voting is the only way people like you can have any say about the way government runs things, or that there are lots of ways that you can have a say? [18]

Women between 20 and 40 were selected from the 1968 National Election Study. This was felt to be the group most under the pressures of child-bearing and child-rearing. Presence in the household of one or more children under 18 was chosen to indicate that a woman had assumed the role of mother. It is possible for a biological mother not to have her offspring in her own home due to a number of causes, and it is also possible for a woman who is not the biological or legal mother of a child to have that child in her household. However, we felt that the role behavior required by the child's presence would justify this indicator, in the absence of any other measure of a woman's past fertility.

Political Participation and Motherhood

Of the total group of 343 women who responded to both questions of presence of children and to ways of political participation, 48.1 percent said that there were many ways of political participation (high political efficacy), and 51.9 percent said that voting was the only way for someone like them to have an influence on the government (see Table 1). Those without children under 18 were statistically significantly more likely to reply that there were more ways than voting than were the women who were mothers (58.3 percent compared to 45.4 percent). This relation between childbearing and political efficacy held when we controlled for region of the country, rural-urban residence, and labor force participation. When controlling for indicators of socio-economic status (income, education, and class identification), we found that among groups of low SES, political efficacy was generally low and motherhood made no difference.[19] However, among women who are of the SES more usually associated with a high degree of political activity, presence of children under 18 made a significant difference.

When women between 20 and 40 with a high school education or less are compared according to whether or not they feel that

TABLE 1

Ways of Political Participation

By Presence of Children Under 18 and Under 5 Women 20–40, SRC 1968 American National Election Study

Ways of Political Participation	*Presence of Children*				
	No Children Under 18	*Children Under 18*	*Children Between 5 & 18*	*Children Under 5*	*Total*
Many	58.3	45.4	41.7	48.1	48.1
Only Voting	41.7	54.6	58.3	51.9	51.9
Total	100.0	100.0	100.0	100.0	100.0
	(72)	(271)	(114)	(159)	(343)

voting is the only way someone like themselves could influence the government, 41.7 percent replied in the negative: that there are more ways than voting. Among women of the same age group with some college education or more, 63.1 percent replied that there were more ways than voting, a difference of over 20 percentage points. This difference by educational attainment is expected, in accordance with a large number of studies linking political participation and political efficacy to educational attainment.

When each group was broken down into mothers and non-mothers, political efficacy was not affected for the lower educational category. The same percentage of mothers and non-mothers—only 42 percent—said there were more ways than voting to influence the government (see Table 2). This result suggests that for the women of high school education or less, motherhood does not result in a change in their political self-image. Their life has been aimed primarily at gaining the status of mother and thus the birth of the first child is not deviant from their previous life but resulting from it. There is probably better anticipatory socialization for motherhood which Lopata suggests is missing for middle class women.[20]

Among those with at least some college education, however, the differences between mothers and non-mothers was marked and

TABLE 2

Ways of Political Participation and Presence of Children by Age by Education of Respondent Women 20–40, SRC 1968 American National Election Study

Education: High School or Less

Ways of Political Participation	*Presence of Children*				
	None Under 18	*Some Under 18*	*Some 5–18*	*Under 5*	*Total*
Many	42.4	41.5	39.8	43.0	41.7
Only Voting	57.6	58.5	60.2	57.0	58.3
Total	100.0	100.0	100.0	100.0	100.0
	(33)	(207)	(93)	(114)	(240)

Education: Some College or More

Many	71.8	57.8	50.0	61.9	63.1
Only Voting	28.2	42.2	50.0	38.1	36.9
Total	100.0	100.0	100.0	100.0	100.0
	(39)	(64)	(22)	(42)	(103)

statistically significant. Nearly three-quarters of the non-mothers (71.8 percent) responded that there were more ways than voting to influence the government, compared to only a little over half (57.8 percent) of the mothers in the sample.

Anticipatory socialization for the role of mother means that actual achievement of the role does not create as great a disruption, both psychic and physical, in the life of a woman. Previous self-image is probably reinforced, rather than changed.[21] Thus the minority of women with high school education or less who are politically efficacious are able to maintain this degree of efficacy even as they become a mother. Having been socialized to see their main life-goal as motherhood, and having previously learned some of the skills connected with it, a woman with high school education who is politically efficacious maintains that view at various points in her life cycle.

Political Participation and Number of Children

We have linked the change in a woman's self-image to motherhood as a single event. We thus suggest that the change in self-image is due to the change in interactional processes that occur with the advent of a child, due to the increased activity in the home, the increased repetition of tasks, and the increased social isolation demanded of a woman in a society where infant care is the responsibility of a single individual female.[22] However, we also argue that these changes, first engendered by the material reality of a woman's changing interaction patterns become internalized and continue to exist once the material necessity has lessened.

If the decreased political efficacy were merely a result of the increased amount of work a child brings, we would expect an incremental decrease in political efficacy with the advent of each additional child. However, examination of the SRC 1968 data shows no linear relation between total number of children and our measure of political efficacy. Beyond the initial decrease in political efficacy that occurs with the first child, there is no systematic impact of additional children on political efficacy. Those with additional children continue to have a lower percentage who are politically efficacious than those who have no children at all.

Political Participation and Age of Children

Another way of determining if it is the burden of increased work of young children that is accounting for the decreased political efficacy of mothers 20 to 40 is to compare those women with children under 5 to those who have children five or over. If it is only the added work of young children, we would expect mothers with pre-schoolers to have lower political efficacy than mothers who have all their children in school. However, when we look at the national sample, we find there is no significant difference between the women who had children under 5 and those with older children. Of the 271 women with children under 18, 159 had at least one child under five, while 114 had children only between 5 and 17. The mothers with children under five actually had a higher, but not statistically significant, percentage who were politically efficacious than those mothers who had no children of pre-school age—48 percent compared to 42 percent. This tendency for the mothers of pre-school children to be slightly more efficacious than mothers of older children held when controlling for education, income, age, rural-urban residence, and region of the country. Almost always, the difference by age of child was not significant.

An explanation for the general lack of difference by age of child could be the immensity of the change in female self-image that takes place in motherhood. Once a woman is defined in terms of child and household duties, it may be difficult to diversify her interaction circle to allow for the development—or redevelopment—of a political self. This suggests the primacy of the role of mother in female self-definition even when the immediate demand of child care is not present.

Implications of the National Data

In summary, examination of women 20 to 40 in a national sample shows the importance of presence of children on our measure of political efficacy. Presence of children, which we have utilized as a measure of taking on the role of mother, is especially important in explaining political participation among those elements in the population who tend to be most politically efficacious. Among upper middle class, college educated women presence of children makes the greatest difference in political efficacy. Examination of the data suggests that it is the role of mother, rather than total number of children or age of child, which is important.

Our analysis of the SRC 1968 American Election Study suggests that there are differences in the political participation of mothers and non-mothers. However, we know nothing about the causal direction involved, although we have argued deductively that motherhood is the causal variable. Furthermore, the process by which the self as mother acts to retard the self as political actor needs further study.

The Local Sample: An Examination of Process

In order to get a better understanding of the process involved in becoming a mother and how it is related to political participation, we decided to do in-depth interviews of a small sample of women who had recently become mothers and who, at least legally, had had the opportunity to be politically active previous to the birth of their first child.

We felt that women with a child between one and a half and two had been mothers long enough for the role to be somewhat normalized. At the same time with a child this young it would not be too difficult for the women to recall and discuss their life before they became a mother. Our interview schedule was modeled after a life-history technique, in order to get the women's own insight into their changing roles.

To determine our universe, we got a listing from the two Manhattan, Kansas, hospitals of all mothers who had their first births in 1970. The mothers were listed by age at birth of the child. A random sample was taken of all the women on the lists between 21 and 29. Initially, we rejected all the names which were no longer listed in a variety of current city directories. Our working sample was composed of 50 women who appeared to be currently living in the Manhattan, Kansas, area. Each woman on the list was sent a letter describing our project and asking for her cooperation.

In first contacting a respondent there is always the problem of how much to tell a potential interviewee. We stated our topic quite explicitly in our initial letter, thus perhaps sacrificing those potential respondents who felt most inadequate as mothers or least involved politically. We followed up each letter with a phone call, and in phoning, found that another nine of our potential respondents had left the area. Another respondent was eliminated because her first baby had died. Three had telephones in service, but were apparently on vacation the month during which the interviews took place. Three respondents refused to be interviewed for a variety of reasons, but agreed to respond to a mailed questionnaire. Only two women refused completely to participate.

Our final result was 32 usable interviews. We do not claim to have a representative sample of all mothers, nor all mothers who had their first child in 1970, nor even such mothers in Manhattan, Kansas. Our aim was to try to get a perspective on the process and interaction between motherhood and political participation.

Description of the Sample

Our sample was homogeneous in that all the women had their first births after the age of 20. Thirty-one were white and one was oriental. For whites in the United States in 1965, the median age of mothers at the birth of their first child was 22.2 years. Presser reports the same median age at first birth for whites in 1967.[23] The median age for our sample was 23.5, and the mean age was 24. Pohlman, citing Ryder, mentions as results of delaying the age of mother at the time of first birth: 1) increased education, 2) increased employment of women, 3) increased capital formation, 4) increased geographical and social mobility, 5) individualism instead of familism, and 6) loosening of ties to traditional patterns, by delaying the time when young people are tied down. All of these results also have consequences for political participation.[24] Presser suggests that the timing of the first birth is an important determinant of subsequent role behavior among women. She suggests that if a woman has her first birth early, the nature of her options in non-familial roles may be limited.[25] Conversely, by postponing the first birth, non-familial role options may be multiplied.

Our sample, by the definition of the universe, seems to be biased toward potentially political participants, to women who might actually develop a political self, given the right conditions of what Burstein calls formal roles and network interaction.[26] However, their potential as political participants is somewhat restrained by the fact that political participation generally reaches its peak at a later age, and that breaking away from the traditional pattern may initially present cross-pressures discouraging political participation.[27]

Socio-Economic Characteristics of the Sample

The thirty-two women in our sample were relatively well-educated, again increasing their potential as political actors. They all had at least high school education, and averaged over three years of schooling past high school. Only four had no formal schooling past high school. One had a Ph.D. and several are currently working toward advanced degrees.

The age at marriage of our sample varied between 16 to 27. The mean age at marriage was 21.32. The mean length of marriage was 5.1 years, varying between 3 and 9 years. All the women were currently mated, although one woman in our sample had a husband absent due to overseas military service. None had been previously mated or had any conceptions previous to their first birth. The period of time between marriage and first birth varied between slightly under one and seven years. The mean was three years. None of our sample was pregnant before marriage.

Thirty-one of the women had had only one birth, although five were currently pregnant. Only one had had a second child, two months old at the time of the interview. Most have stated family size preferences—only three are unsure of their total desired family size. One woman wants one child, 10 women want two, six want "2 or 3," 12 want three (with one couple planning to adopt the third child). Twenty-eight plan the spacing of their children. This fertility data indicates high personal efficacy which has been found to predispose one to political participation.[28] In terms of seeing herself as an effective person, and thus capable of making an impact on the larger world, an effective family planner can gain the self-confidence to act politically. However, the impact is lessened somewhat by Ibrahim's finding that the identification of the wife with community-oriented roles of women in society had no effect on the degree of effectiveness in family planning.[29] However, by looking at fertility as the dependent variable and identification with community-oriented roles as the independent variable, he is focusing on women as breeders and contributers to over-population, and not looking at what being an effective family planner contributes to a woman's self-image.

Manhattan, Kansas, is a community of 27,600, located in the northeastern part of the state, about two hours west of Kansas City along Interstate 70. Kansas State University and Fort Riley, a large Army base, account for a major part of the economic structure of the town, although Manhattan does house a few small factories and a major pattern factory. Of the persons employed in Manhattan in 1970, four percent were in manufacturing industries, 64 percent were in white collar occupations and 41 percent were government workers. It is also the marketing center for an agricultural hinterland.

Our sample reflects the economic structure of the community. Currently ten of their husbands are students, although most of them hold other jobs on the side. Three are in the Armed Forces, six are teachers, elementary to college level, while the other men are in lower level white collar or skilled blue collar jobs. One is currently unemployed.

Thirty-one of our thirty-two mothers have had some labor force participation. Thirty wives were employed before marriage. Eight were students, with odd jobs to help support themselves. Ten had secretarial or clerical jobs before marriage. Two were nurses and three were nurses aides. Six had other jobs requiring specialized training, including teaching. Interestingly, one in our sample had been a nun. One of the women had worked primarily as a waitress.

Labor force participation continued for the women we interviewed after marriage but before the baby was born. Fifteen were in secretarial jobs. Six were technicians of various sorts. Three were graduate assistants or instructors at the university. Four were registered nurses and one was a nurse's aide. One was a beauty operator. The wages varied between $100 and $800 a month, with a mean of $360. The relatively high level of their occupations (for women) can be related to the postponement of childbearing among our sample.[30]

Six of the women worked right up to the birth of their first child. Eleven quit their jobs between six weeks to a month before the baby was born. Three quit two months before, and the rest quit working from 3 to 12 months in anticipation of child bearing.

At the present time, with the child between one and a half and two and a half, fourteen of our respondents are no longer in the labor force. Eight are working part time and nine are working full time. Those that continue full time employment are in professional or technical fields, and relatively well remunerated. Thus we are able to assess the process of becoming a mother and its interaction with political participation for workers and non-workers as distinct female types.

Political Characteristics of the Sample

Our sample was not highly political, although 25 out of the 32 replied that there were more ways than voting for a person like them to influence the government. Ten identified as Republicans (Kansas is a strongly Republican state—55 percent of the presidential vote went to Nixon in 1968, although currently a Democrat, Dr. William Roy, is the Congressional Representative from the district which includes Manhattan), eight are Democrats, 12 classify themselves as Independents, and two frankly stated they did not know what their political leanings were.

Sixty percent of our respondents voted in the 1968 presidential election, 43 percent voted in the 1970 congressional election, and 39 percent of those eligible voted in the 1971 city-wide election. (Five of our respondents were living in university housing, which is not part of the city, or in mobile home parks outside the city limits at the time of the city election.)

By combining each woman's recent past political behavior, we divided our group into low, medium and high political participators. Twelve women were in the low category, twenty-two in the medium category, and eight in the category of high political participators.

The Development of the Mother's Political Self

Motherhood, Time, and the Political Self

Lack of time is the first major objective change resulting from motherhood. The demands imposed on the motherhood role limits the opportunities women have to develop their political selves. Their daily time-consuming tasks leave little energy for developing political skills. An individual has to have more than minimal free time if she is going to engage in doorbell ringing, writing letters, circulating petitions or joining political groups. For the young mother who is feeling the constant pressure of taking care of her child, the time just doesn't seem to be there. Lane mentions lack of leisure time in explaining why lower class women are not politically active, but the same may be said for the middle class young mothers.[31]

Many of our respondents mentioned lack of free time as their major frustration from motherhood. "Lack of privacy, lack of time . . . I can't think . . . It takes so much effort to just sit down and say 'Now I can think.' " "Getting free time to do things for myself or with my husband." "Physical exhaustion . . . constant interruptions."

The tasks of childrearing seem never ending. "Once you get everything all done up (laugh) and you sit down and you think 'Ah! It's all finished' and you turn around and here they've got a pile here and pile here and you about pull your hair out."

The Self and Interaction Networks

The importance of the other in the formation of self-conceptions has been theoretically stressed by Mead, Katz and Lazarsfeld and others.[32] Woelfel and Haller[33] present evidence that the relative influence of "significant others," as opposed to ascribed attributes, can be quantified. The network interactions of mothers, the voluntary behavior conditioned by their formal roles, is crucial to understand when explaining the development of their political selves.

Prewitt has pointed out that it is an individual's location in a network of social-political relationships that determines whether family background, educational experiences, occupational choices, leisure time activities or community conditions "expose him to political stimuli in very unequal amounts." [34] Milbrath writes about locating individuals in terms of political participation along a central-peripheral dimension. Those most likely to be active are persons located near the center of the relevant communic actions network, and those with high rates of social interaction.[35] The formal roles of young women are highly related to their exposure to a variety of networks.

Child-Centered Networks

Non-working mothers living in close proximity to neighbors with small children tended largely to limit their social interaction to these neighbors. Although there was much visiting back and forth, this social interaction did not necessarily mean they were not politically isolated. The women mentioned that most of their conversations with their neighbors were about children and the problems of child-rearing with a minimum of political discussion. One mother described her personal contacts in these words, "I also found that I made new friends and most of our neighbors had children which gave me something in common with them." Another stated: "Now that I have a child, there's more to talk about with my friends since they also have children."

Under these circumstances where interaction is determined by geographic location, it would be expected that cross-pressures would be minimized by avoiding topics which might put a strain on the friendship. Political views in such circumscribed social options were never the basis of friendships. For the apolitical, the problem of disagreeing with their child's friend's mother would never arise. For the potentially political, ambiguity was avoided by not thinking in political terms.

Child-Centered Networks and the Political Self

Thus the personal interactions of these young mothers still left them politically isolated. Their interpersonal channels of information were restricted and they were exposed to few politically knowledgeable people. Heiskanen has observed that "through differential accessibility and participation in different opportunity structures females are given less opportunities for exposure to phenomena that are here suggested to be indispensable components of effective political participation." [36] These mothers have social interactions but they are not the kind likely to lead them to Milbrath's center and away from the periphery. They more closely resemble those described by Miller as living "within a restricted life space without much sense of restriction and without great affect toward the outside world." [37]

The depoliticalizing influence of friendships with neighboring mothers is best illustrated by a negative example, a woman outside the child-centered networks and highly politically active.

Mary Ann has no close friends with small children. Lacking social interaction with young mothers, which tends to satisfy the social needs of most of the non-working mothers we interviewed, she feels especially tied down with the birth of her daughter.

" . . . once you get to feel tied down that's when you want to get out and do something else." Previously concerned about social issues but not active toward them, she joined the League of Women Voters and worked to elect McGovern people at the county-level delegate caucus.

Although her husband is a student, she lives in a single-family home in an older section owned by her in-laws. She and her daughter are very close to their nearest neighbors, a retired sociology professor and his wife. She hates being at home and avoids all day-time television but "Sesame Street" (which she claims as her favorite program). As a result of her determination not to be tied down, she goes out every day and always takes her daughter with her. Her best friends were in her college sorority and, although married, have no children. She doesn't discuss politics with them very much, however, nor with her husband, who is much more politically conservative than she is. The main "significant other" for her political self is the media—but she selects *Time, The Saturday Review,* and television news rather than soap operas and women's magazines. She reacted to relative social isolation by forming new political networks.

Child-Centered Networks and Mass Society

The political isolation of the child-centered neighborhood means that some of these mothers exist not in a pluralist society but one more closely resembling the mass society described by Kornhauser and others.[38] The typical housewife interacts primarily with her family and others in her neighborhood. She has no personal and direct ties to the intermediary groups which intervene between citizens and the larger polity.[39] Living as one in a mass society, she assumes the characteristics of mass "man." She carries out the duties and responsibilities of motherhood as prescribed and demanded of her by society and all its manipulators. Society has so specified the perimeters of the role of mother that she no longer feels free to behave in an autonomous manner. One of our respondents lamented, "I'm just a mother, more than a person." She behaves like Kornhauser's mass man who "substitutes an undifferentiated image of himself for an individualized one; he answers the perennial question of 'Who am I?' with the formula 'I am like everyone else.' " [40]

Work Networks vs. Child-Centered Networks and Political Participation

We had expected the working mothers to be the ones with high political participation, although our analysis of the SRC data showed that motherhood was more important than labor force participation in explaining women's political efficacy. That this differed from other studies might be because non-mothers, the more politically active group, are also more likely to be in the labor force.

Labor force participation in the mothers we sampled did expand their interaction network and increase their amount of political discussion. However, only those that explicitly stated that their husbands helped with the child actually carried the increased political saliency into action. Even with the non-working mothers, those that could count on their husbands to help with the child were the ones more likely to engage in politics at any level. For other working mothers, the job just meant that their household tasks dominated a major portion of their non-working time.

For most of the working mothers, their reactions to motherhood and its concomitant demands were surprisingly similar to the non-working mothers. Although it was possible for both working and non-working mothers to be politically active, it was only when they found a reflection of an active self outside the work sphere or the neighborhood sphere, which was generally sought as a response to a feeling of isolation directly related to becoming a mother. And only geographic and organizational separation from the comfortable young mother network allowed the mothers—working or non-working—to actively seek the new roles.

The Mass Media as a Social Network

Besides these limited personal interaction networks, the major source for political identification among the sample was the mass media.

All respondents were exposed to the mass media in varying

degrees. Some spoke with pride about reading at least one newspaper daily and listening to the 5:30 news each evening. Although the news was on television, they were involved in meal preparation and thus could not concentrate fully. One would normally expect that exposure to the mass media would lead to increased political activity,[41] but since they felt they did not have the time to get involved, this preoccupation with the media served as a means for fulfilling their civic duty.[42] Although lack of time may make this displacement necessary, it may also serve as a "narcotizing dysfunction" with respect to activating political activity.[43] Some respondents were substituting the passive intake of information for the more demanding and active political activities which they denied themselves either through choice or necessity.[44]

Media Network and the Political Self

Although radio, television, magazines and newspapers were utilized by the women we interviewed, they were generally selective and preferred the non-political items. Although most of the women listened to the radio, as an accompaniment to housework, many did not listen to radio news. They enjoyed instead a musical background to their domestic activities. The social page, Heloise and Ann Landers were popular among the newspaper readers, although only one person said she purposely skipped the news.

One respondent categorized in the low participation group mentioned that she had written a letter to a Senator. When asked what motivated this letter, she answered that Ann Landers had suggested that a letter be written encouraging the passage of a health bill. This was the only time she had taken any political action other than voting. Another respondent, in expanding the political efficacy question, mentioned petitions as a way an individual could influence the government. She had read about a woman who had effectively used this tool in an article in *Good Housekeeping* magazine. This suggests that women are being politically socialized and activated by newspaper and magazine reading not normally associated with high political participation. For these mothers, their political "generalized other" were media figures rather than their immediate neighbors.

The majority of women, even those with minimal political participation, at least skimmed the front page, which, in the local paper, emphasizes local news. Many of the more politically conscious read local and national news quite thoroughly. Those who did not read a newspaper at all or who read only the non-political sections were also those who felt voting was the only way someone like them could influence the government and did not intend to get more involved in the community when their children were older.

Television viewing habits were similar to radio and newspaper consumption. The totally uninvolved did not ever see the television news or only seldom watched it. Those in the high participation group watched regularly, although one of these mothers mentioned that since the baby came she watched the news just as regularly, but "now with more interruptions."

The media was a form of relief from the isolation that motherhood imposed on many of the women. Some of our respondents had to be asked to turn off the television or the radio in order for the interview to be conducted. One woman, when asked how often she got to watch television, replied, "A lot. Lots of times I just leave it on. If I do have to sit down with the kids while they're just playing around, well then, I'll watch a game show or something. And then I have it on in the afternoons . . . I think it's force of habit—I leave it on and go about my work."

Respondents in the low participation and highly individualistic categories spend a great deal of their day watching soap operas. Tending to be the respondents least involved in political activity, they generally had no plans to get involved in community affairs when their children were older. Although differences in education and social class may account for this lack of interest in political activity, more attention needs to be paid to the effects which daytime TV viewing may be having on the housewife. Politics by definition is a group activity. If changes are going to be made in the polity they will have to come as a result of group effort. Life as it is portrayed by the TV actor is a series of personal mishaps. If there are problems, they are caused by individual weaknesses; if solutions are to be discovered the individual hero will have to do it. Personal tragedy resulting from social forces beyond the individual's control are largely ignored. The value of organizing and working with others to tackle the societal ills is virtually nonexistent. Women for whom life on the video tape may have become as real as their own will find little motivation for political participation.[45] The advantages of political solutions to life's problems may be more unreal to them than the complicated maze of plots upon which they focus their attention every day. That the women who were the most devoted soap opera fans were also the most apolitical and did not in the future plan to become more active in community affairs supports this.

Political Isolation and Attitudes Toward Political Processes

Both apathy and alienation are predicted results of these limited interaction networks. Interestingly we found very little in what our respondents said that indicated alienation—even the level of cynicism was slight. One woman had worked for a state agency and her experience there had led her to conclude that all politicians were corrupt. A lab technician who lived in a rather isolated trailer court replied when asked about her preference in a presidential candidate that she had none and did not intend to vote. She nervously laughed and added, "No, I have what you might consider a bad attitude. I feel that anyone smart enough to be president is smart enough not to run." Those more politically active also were quite cynical about the way the political system works. "Unless you have a lot of the money and the pull behind you and then as a single person you're going to have a lot. Sure, you're going to have a lot to say and people are going to sit up and listen. But me as a small person, I'm—if I said something, people are going to say you know, 'Look at that dummy sitting down there.' You know, I feel like this, I really do." But these cynicisms were unusual and generally a result of job-related political socialization. What was more common was apathy toward the political sphere.

Family Networks and the Political Self

Family life and passive use does not provide opportunities for inter-group interaction in the many activities and roles which would give women the opportunity to develop leadership skills. Studies have shown the cumulative effect of these opportunities. Those who are confronted with the larger problems of society, those who are called upon to play a variety of roles, are more likely to be politically aware and hence to participate more actively in the political process.[46]

More important, perhaps, is the fact that the political socialization which takes place in the small family circle may not be enough to meet the demands of the larger polity. There are basic differences between experiences in organizations and on the job and family living. Almond and Verba describe individual experiences at work and in voluntary associations as being different from those in the family because "they are closer—in time as well as in structure—to the polity." [47] The patterns of authority in the family are much more informal and implicit than the patterns of authority in work situations, organizations or even schools. The latter thus are closer to the political mode.

Role Behavior and Political Socialization

Nottingham, in analyzing the role and status of middle-class women, points out that in her role of mother and wife, a woman's success is based on harmonious balance of interpersonal relationships, rather than on individualistic achievement or even efficiency.[48] The role of mother is a very particularistic one, diffusing competition in the public sense of the term. The political role necessitates a universalistic frame of reference. It calls for cooperation and competition different from family-directed activity. Activity in the political sphere is geared primarily toward achievement and efficiency. Several of our respondents actually described themselves as less competitive after becoming a mother.

World Views and the Political Self

Among our young mothers, the tendency of a particularistic world view seemed for some to stand in the way of universalistic analysis of world and local affairs. While the completely inactive defined the country's problems rather vaguely, and the most highly politically active defined the problems in systemic terms, two distinct world views emerged among the moderately politically active respondents.

The moderately active women, so defined because they did feel there were more ways than voting to influence the government and who had attempted, generally through writing letters or signing petitions, to act on issues which concerned them, can be further classified as individualists or globals in their definition of problems and their actions toward them.

The Individualists

For the individualistic group, all questions relating to political, social, or community problems tended to be answered in personal terms. It was impossible for these women to look beyond personal experience and personal immediacy in our conversations with them.

Question: "What do you think are this country's main problems?" Answer: "Indecision on the part of youth . . . my brother, for example—he can't decide whether to go to college . . . He can't make up his mind on anything."

This individually oriented group acted in the public sphere solely in terms of immediate personal impact. "Things that bother us (her and her husband) immediately, we do things, we act on it."

Another respondent answered, "Guess it all depends on the magnitude—how much it would affect me personally. That's probably a selfish point of view, but I would . . ." Because they act on personal, individual level issues, they are basically content with the system. They have found that their personal difficulties, from being cheated on promised discounts to being denied Blue Cross-Blue Shield by the Air Force, can be solved through individual pressure. They are personally efficacious people, and their private lives they see as well organized.

"We don't like to get out on our high horse and yell and scream around because we don't feel that that's the way to do these things and we've found that—you know—it takes a little time but by working through the system—however long it takes—why, we usually get something done."

Motherhood for them means doing things that relate to their children's locally defined interest. Indeed, many of these women justified their previous activity in terms of potential benefits to their children or their husband. For instance, when asked if she thought she might get more involved in community affairs once her children were older, one of the individually oriented women replied: "No, I think the time to be involved in forming a community and in the building of a community is when your children are young and when you're building something for them. You're voting for a school tax bond because by the time your children are in school, that school will be built, or you're voting a new swimming pool or you're voting for the commissioners that will be in office during the period of time your children will be growing up—this type of thing." This group of women we have defined as moderately active individualists basically were not joiners. They belonged only to their church, which they took quite seriously. One young attractive mother spoke often about "Pastor Jim" and his futile efforts to spur them to social concern and political action. "He tells us we should get involved, but we just don't do it." Other women tended to object when the church got involved in governmental problems. One woman got so tired of the minister preaching against the war in Vietnam that she wrote him that he would get no more of her tithe—an individual protest against an institution acting on a public issue.

The Globals

The most politically active defined problems in institutional terms and saw the necessity of group participation.

"As far as the government, I don't know. I guess it would be nicer if we could all have a little bit more of a say as a person, but like I said, I think you have to get more in a group or do a whole lot of squawking . . . group action does a lot more than single . . . If I get into a group, I have more to say."

Both the moderately active globals and the highly active generally belonged to voluntary associations besides the church (and some were not church goers). Although one of the highly active women stated that she did not like to belong to organizations because she felt it made an individual's voice weaker by aligning oneself with an already biased organization, she had in the past mobilized groups to act on political issues of interest to her, particularly those involving women's rights.

For some of our young mothers, membership in voluntary associations was something they were postponing for the future. Even those who were not politically active might then become more global and more active once they joined an association which cultivated their political selves and provided them with a political "significant other." The League of Women Voters was mentioned by several of our mothers as a way other than voting by which someone like them could influence the government. Some of the women currently moderately active but who proposed more community activity in the future mentioned the League as the vehicle they would use to increase their participation. For these women, a reinforcement for a more politically active self was already latently present. However, these women who looked forward to League activity when their children were older were college graduates and not members of the labor force.

We asked the respondents if they had ever gotten concerned about a public issue. Most mentioned some issue, although they had not necessarily done anything about it. The typical reply sounded like this: "Yeah, I get concerned, but that's as far as I go." The issues two-thirds mentioned fell into the moral-religious category or dealt with social-welfare issues which political scientists have observed are of special concern to women.[49] One young mother commented, "I think the only thing that I was really concerned about, the only thing I remember I got a little motivated about, was probably liquor by the drink and that was just here in the state of Kansas. Some national issues have concerned me, but I've never worried . . ."

Many of our respondents, mentioning drug abuse, alcoholism, and education, went on to say that they had become especially concerned about these issues since the birth of their child, once again corroborating the observation that these women operate from a narrow periphery which limits their political observations to those of immediate concern.

Our globals were able to identify national level problems, even when talking about issues of special concern to women. One woman replied that she was concerned about "education, social welfare—the state of people on welfare—the large gap between the people who have it and don't—that bothers me." As with our other globals she went beyond these issues to other national problems. "The distribution of taxes bothers me a lot—like on both ends—where they get it and where it goes—that bothers me.

Conclusions

We have tried to show that motherhood structures the environment of young women in ways which for many retard the development of a political self. Our in-depth interviews supported our contentions, based on our national data, that among women with educations past high school, motherhood has a negative effect on self-image and thus political participation. This is especially true for those mothers who become part of child centered networks. The media as an interaction network can effect political participation in either direction. For some of the socially isolated women, it served to increase their political awareness and to mobilize them to action. For some it even served as a political "significant other." Unfortunately, for others it reinforced an individualistic, personalistic view of life or at best acted as a catharsis for civic duties not performed.

This study has emphasized how political isolation affects *women,* not their children or their husband. It is important to view women as political actors in their own right rather than as semi-mindless culture brokers. Clearly this study suggests more than it answers. The impact of fatherhood on a man's political self should certainly be examined. Furthermore, our national data suggests that the self imposed by the objective conditions of mothering young children carries over into the period when the children are of school age due to subjective self-definition. Similar in-depth interviews should be conducted with mothers whose children have recently entered school in order to see if redefinition and politicization of a woman's self occurs.

PART III

Childfree by Choice

Childfree. The word has not existed for long; and as yet it is found in no dictionary. The traditional term used to describe the nonparental condition has been child*less;* and both popular and professional tendency has been to equate the word with infertility—to presume that this state was a medical problem rather than a lifestyle choice.

Book and periodical titles such as *"Childlessness: A Study of Sterility"* illustrate this attitude well. These, as well as reception-room pamphlets which offer "Hope for Childless Couples" or "Help for the Childless" are rooted in the pronatalist presumption that everyone wants (should have) children, that childlessness is an undesirable condition to be escaped if at all possible.

Certainly there are individuals who view their inability to bear or beget children as a problem. But this may be, in part, because the word society has ascribed to their condition *(childless)* strongly denotes a lack, an incompleteness. It should be evident that the self-concept of persons or group*s can be* affected by words affixed to them. And there comes a time in the development of most movements aimed at raising the consciousness of a particular group, when certain members of that group reject prior terms of description and choose new ones. Thus, for example, leaders among the descendants of former slaves rejected an entire vocabulary (*colored, Negro,* and other ascribed terms) and chose instead *black, Afro-American,* etc. So, too, the feminists have pointed out, it is important that an adult female not be referred to as a "girl"—since that word's connotations of immaturity may handicap her ability to view herself as capable of independence and self-determination.

In similar manner, the word *childfree* has sprung up, in defiance of the idea that if one is without children one is "less."

Though the word indicates a new attitude toward parenthood on the part of some who are nonparents volitionally, it may eventually replace *childless* even when describing involuntary nonparents—both as an aid in promulgating the idea, now gaining currency, that parenthood is not a prerequisite to a full life; and simply as a psychological aid to both voluntary and involuntary nonparents. If *child*less suggested deficiency or evoked pity, *child*free by contrast, expresses self-respect and a new pride which results from a recent, growing acceptance of this lifestyle.

The word is not yet used consistently, however, even among those writers who have addressed themselves to this trend. And, keeping in mind that social approval of childfree adults is a very recent attitude, it is perhaps not surprising that a lack of full confidence in personally choosing childlessness is shown by one writer in this section.

Our first selections here are personal statements, two of which, "Why We Don't Want Children" by Lynnell Michels and "A Vote Against Motherhood" by Gael Greene, reflect the feelings of women who have approached the childfree decision in noticeably differing manners—one cautiously, one confidently.

The content of Lynnell Michels's article belies her title—for indeed it is not at all clear that she and her husband "don't want" children, merely that they are somewhat hesitant about it. Hints of the inevitability of children ("Some day, when Dave and I are parents . . .") recur.

Ms. Michels certainly approaches the possibility of having children with commendable prudence, viewing parenthood as a great responsibility and not something to be entered into lightly. But she does not even give herself full credit for this. Instead she labels her caution "fear," her intuited lack of aptitude for motherhood possible "inadequacy," and even wonders aloud if she and her husband are guilty of selfishness and immaturity. Her passive tolerance of pronatalist pressure from others seems to result from uncertainty, rather than from assurance that rejection of childbearing is right for her.

One has to wonder if Michels's contentment would be greater were she not confronted with pressures from friends and relatives or if her ambivalence might in fact be solely the product of such persistent social suggestion.

Gael Greene casts a much stronger "Vote Against Motherhood," refusing to be influenced by negative reactions to her decision, more clearly treasuring the positive aspects of her childfree life. Whereas Michels tolerates pressure, Greene takes an attitude of humorous condescension toward it. Accusations of selfishness have entered Michels's consciousness; but they have no such effect on Greene, who takes such accusations and throws them back at the accusers—pointing out that many are selfish in their reasons for *having* children (as, for example, when progeny are desired for manipulative purposes).

To some extent, these differences may be due to the contrasting career situations of the two women. As a professional writer, Greene has opportunities for wide travel, varied experiences, and an extraordinary range of acquaintanceships. It seems likely, too, that she has encountered other women who are childfree by choice; her career seems to offer more chances for support of her decision than would Michels's teaching situation.

Dedication to career seems a definite motivating factor for Greene; yet she also seems aware that motherhood can impinge on other *personal* roles, inhibit freedoms, and even affect identity. She expresses that she does not want to be ". . . the unhappy creature who is mother first, wife second, woman third, and human being last . . ." and quotes a mother who yearns for "just one hour a day to be me." Michels, by contrast, fails to perceive or discuss disadvantages to parenthood as fully.

Both papers describe pronatalist prejudice as experienced by the writers—perhaps the clearest manifestation of this prejudice is found in the simple fact that childfree women like them are required to explain themselves. (Mothers need not write tentative, half-apologetic articles on "Why I Want Children.")

The existence of such prejudice raises a vital question about nonparenthood as an option in our society: *to whom is the option available?* Some women, such as Greene, are strong enough to make the childfree decision and easily resist subsequent challenge. For other women, such as Michels, susceptibility to social pressure makes "childbirth by coercion" a serious possibility. One must ask: is nonparenthood to be limited to the strongly independent?

An independent voice reflecting a different motivational basis than that of either Michels or Greene was heard in 1969 when Stephanie Mills, as class speaker for the Mills College graduating class of that year, declared, "Our days as a race on this planet are numbered. . . . I am terribly saddened by the fact that the most humane thing for me to do is to have no children at all." The likelihood of an appalling future due to worsening population problems clearly emerges as Mills's reason for terming herself "an ex-potential parent."

Though several researchers feel that concern for overpopulation problems is more apt to be a convenient "excuse" for nonparenthood rather than a true motive, there can be no doubt that Mills's statement is sincere and deserving of respect and admiration.

Stewart Mott, in "Reflections of a Non-Parent," argues the need to accord greater overall social respect and admiration to those who forego childbearing, given social and environmental problems that have been exacerbated by population growth; he offers as well some personal thoughts on his own reasons for not becoming a father.

Mott's paper is of interest partly because of his prominent role as philanthropist, political activist, and social reformer—as well as an outspoken nonparent. (It is interesting to note, for instance, that although Mott is one of the wealthiest men of this generation, even he is not completely immune to social pressure to produce children.)

Mott's essay begins and ends with a reference to the newly established Non-Parents' Day, which the author regards as a holiday of symbolic importance.

"Changes in Views Toward Childlessness," an informal but revealing report by Edward Pohlman, documents a striking increase in acceptance of childlessness among the young. Over a five-year period, from 1965 to 1970, the study indicates a rise both in the number of college students intending to remain nonparents and a corresponding change in attitude toward others who hold this preference. Of course, opinions of college students might not fully correlate with attitudes among the general public; nevertheless these is some indication that overall public feeling is changing as well. Within approximately the same time frame as that of this study, voluntary childlessness in the adult population increased markedly, from 1.3 percent in 1967 to 3.9 percent in 1971, according to Census Bureau figures.

Three selections (Popenoe, Gustavus-Henley, Veevers) discuss characteristics of those individuals who choose not to have children.

The Popenoe article is something of a historical curiosity. Written during the depression decade of the 1930s, when nonparenthood in America became almost commonplace, this article points to several motives for childlessness *other than* economics. If Popenoe's underlying attitude is typical of the times, it may also be illustrative of a social climate which prevented the full development of the nonparenthood trend which then seemed to be beginning.

We should note two limitations to the author's approach. First, Popenoe's chosen method of research was not to ask childfree couples themselves about their motivation, but to ask a group of adult college students to submit histories of permanently childfree couples of their (close) acquaintance, and to *ascribe motives* which they (the friends and relatives) believed to be operative in these nonparent marriages. Second, since the "researchers" were university-educated, the childfree couples whose histories were submitted constituted a somewhat atypical sample. We should also note that one-third of the childfree couples were childfree involuntarily, rather than by choice.

With these limitations in mind, a few significant observations may still be made.

Though it is usually presumed that "hard times" and hard times alone gave rise to the unprecedented number of childfree marriages during the depression years, Popenoe reports two reasons here which ranked ahead of economics as a motivation for childlessness: these he calls "self-centered" and "wife's career."

At this point, we begin to perceive Popenoe's bias. He terms the most-noted motivation for nonparenthood "self-centered," explaining that he uses this term "for lack of anything better." An objective investigator, however, might have thought of a more neutral term.

His tone is sarcastic when he refers to the couple "so much in love with each other" that they do not want a child; he disdains "supposedly intelligent" people for admitting a dislike of children; (one fears his implication to be that even a couple who *disliked* children should *have* them), and classifies the woman who fears childbirth as neurotic or infantile.

When one reads this Popenoe selection after glancing once more at Leta Hollingworth's "Social Devices for Impelling Women to Bear and Rear Children," one is strongly tempted to identify Popenoe as representative of the "social guardians" of childbearing of whom she spoke.

It is instructive to compare Popenoe's methodological approach and underlying value system with a study conducted a generation later by sociologists Susan O. Gustavus and James R. Henley, Jr. The latter work is far superior in data collection and analysis; and, the attempt at objectivity which is to be expected of social researchers is obvious in comparison, though there remains some holdover of pronatalist assumptions.

The Gustavus-Henley sample is obtained without the complicating variable of personal referral, but because it involves couples who chose sterilization through a private agency, it remains a very select group, as the authors readily admit. They stress the difficulty in obtaining a more random sampling because of the small percentage of the population choosing this life-style. After claiming that childlessness is becoming rarer, they suggest there is a good chance that a reversal will occur given the increased availability of birth control methods and the emerging social concerns of recent years. (If the attitudinal data collected by Pohlman and others is a guideline for future behavior, this will certainly prove correct.)

The most common reasons here given by couples for their choice bear an interesting resemblance to Popenoe's, with one obvious and another provocative exception. Economic reasons would be expected to play a smaller role in comparison with depression-era statistics. However, the leading category in the 1930s study of Popenoe ("self-centered") is here replaced with "population concern" and now identified as a factor by the respondents themselves rather than observing parties.

"Population concern" however is held suspect by the researchers. Gustavus and Henley suggest that this intellectual concern might be a socially acceptable veneer for the "selfish" reasons ascribed to childfree couples by society in general.

Although they attribute this judgment to "society" rather than to themselves, the authors are apparently somewhat unconvinced that humanitarian motives are in fact operative.

Sociologist of the University of Western Ontario, Jean E. Veevers, who has studied voluntary childlessness more than any other researcher, feels that concern for population does not play a *primary* role in the decision, though it may reinforce a decision already made. She points out that childfree couples, who may be exceedingly capable in describing other matters, nonetheless find it difficult to articulate their reasons for their life-style preference (just as people *with* children would have difficulty explaining their motives for parenthood).

In part, the childfree couples' variance from the social norm can account for much of their uncertainty regarding their reasons. But the factors involved in this decision—i.e., factors relating to a developing self-image and choice of life-style—are so complex and interrelated, with no clearcut decision points, that it is all but impossible to coherently pull out *one* factor as an explanatory response.

Veevers has a deep sensitivity to the pronatalist pressures facing childfree individuals, and a corresponding sensitivity also to intellectual and emotional factors affecting their decision-making process. Whereas Gustavus and Henley find their data somewhat compromised by the response that couples "simply do not wish to have children," Veevers attempts to discover what characteristics might lead to such a point of view, and how this view evolves.

Veevers bases her paper "Voluntarily Childless Wives: An

Exploratory Study" on in-depth interviews with fifty-two such women; the interviews were unstructured and lasted an average of four hours each.

She begins by approaching the basic question of *how* these wives arrived at their unusual choice of life-style. Contrary to what might be expected, the clear majority assumed when they married that they would become mothers. Childbearing was postponed, however, until some future time—a "future which never came," Veevers comments.

The typical decision to remain childfree (if it can be called a decision) may not involve a conscious weighing of alternatives and may not even result from a direct conversation about the matter. Veevers identifies four stages through which a couple's thinking may progress: during these stages occurs a gradual shift from an unspoken assumption that there will "of course" be children someday, to an implicit mutual agreement that "of course" there will not be.

During the initial stages of postponement, childfree wives are indistinguishable from their sisters who are merely delaying motherhood. However, factors involved in the initial decision to postpone children seem different from those which influence a choice to remain childfree. The former relate merely to perceived disadvantages of parenthood at a particular time; the latter grow from direct experience of a life-style which has been found pleasurable.

Yet many couples do not find themselves in a childfree state long enough to examine this alternative as a permanent option: their view of self is implicitly that of "potential parents" rather than "presently childfree." At marriage, for example, most young people are primarily concerned with career options and finances. However, a child is often part of the future view: it is planned that a wife will work *until* a child comes; money will be set aside *for* the childbearing eventuality.

In marriages where parenthood is initially postponed, however, there is at least the possibility that aspects of the childfree state may be perceived as beneficial—and that this life-style will become a permanent choice.

Voluntarily childless wives are so because of a basic contentment with their situation; nevertheless, an almost universally expressed problem is the considerable social pressure they encounter to abandon their situation and become mothers.

This social pressure seems to reach a peak for both husbands and wives during the third and fourth years of marriage—after sufficient time has passed for children to be "expected" but before the couple has learned to deal skillfully with (or avoid) their social detractors.

Veevers mentions that many childfree couples arrive at a common strategy against social pressure: when questioned about their nonparenthood, these couples respond by saying that they are considering adoption. (This is deemed a social defense strategy rather than a real desire, since Veevers found that almost no couples who spoke of adoption had made any actual inquiries about the process.)

Though Veevers found that most of the childfree wives she interviewed eventually became "remarkably well defended" against social pressure, she was, of course, talking only of those who had met the criteria for her study and who had remained childfree for more than five years after their marriage. The possibility certainly exists that other voluntarily childless wives who were *less* "well defended" against criticism abandoned their life-style—and became mothers.

Further, even though the wives in Veevers's study may feel generally secure and unthreatened by social prejudice, many expressed a wish to know of *other women like themselves,* so that they might talk freely about their choice without fear of misunderstanding: in the opinion of Veevers, neither support from husbands nor from population and feminist groups was quite sufficient to meet this need to communicate with others of like mind.

In reporting on the characteristics of childfree couples, the two contemporary studies (Gustavus-Henley and Veevers) showed similar profiles: childfree couples tend to be in a relatively high socio-economic class; are highly educated; live in or near metropolitan areas; and are not strongly religious.

Yet there is a remarkable lack of other, similar reports from which to further check consensus on these points; and many areas of study remain completely unexplored. This may point to an extremely subtle occurrence of pronatalist bias which extends through the professional community and which could be viewed as somewhat purposeful in nature. In our final selection, "Voluntary Childlessness: A Neglected Area of Family Study," Jean Veevers charges that, thus far, researchers have subjected this field to "selective inattention," and further, that this neglect may not be purely a matter of oversight.

She presents evidence suggesting that scholars, in analyzing procreation, have focused almost exclusively on groups who do not pose a threat to conventional values. For example, couples who *want and have* children and couples who *want but cannot have* children are found to have received more research attention than have the voluntarily childless. And, some studies of family formation actually "design out" the possibility of a response indicating that no children are desired—respondents are asked, "How many children do you want to have?" and this query is not preceded by the equally logical one, "Do you want to have any children?" (Such simple questionnaire omissions should not be regarded too lightly; to deny or ignore the existence of any group, in this case those people who do not want children, is a significant indication of disapproval or discrimination.)

These and other evidences of research neglect support Veevers's contention. The dearth of surveys or hard data in the area of voluntary childlessness is something we have personally noted as recent students of the subject—and in fact this lack provides one reason why the following selections [presented] must necessarily emphasize personal statements, not academic investigations.

Several dangers are inherent in this situation:

First, dearth of knowledge about nonparents contributes to socialization for parenthood. For lack of information to the contrary, popular stereotyped views of childfree individuals as "selfish," "hedonistic," or "irresponsible" persist. This is obviously detrimental to the image of those who are confirmed nonparents; and may lead some who are wavering between the two alternatives to have children *merely to avoid* a negative stereotype. Our personal experiences lead us to view the negative nonparent stereotypes as false, but hard research which might support this view is nonexistent.

Second, researchers could better understand problems of those who *do* have children if investigation revealed more about the dynamics of those who do *not*. Valid information concerning motives for avoiding parenthood could help shed light on the nature of dissatisfactions and resentments of some parents. Veevers thus sees dual value to investigation of the polar types.

A third point is that an understanding of those who choose not to bear children could be a valuable aid in coming to grips with our continuing problem of overpopulation.

These are perhaps the most compelling reasons why this "neglected area of family study" should be neglected no longer; once such reasons are comprehended (and as the trend to childfree lifestyles becomes more visible) it is almost certain that nonparenthood will receive increased research attention—though thus far only one major researcher, Jean Veevers, has given this field priority. In part as a result of her pioneer investigations, however, more than a few other studies are now in formative stages and should be appearing with some regularity over the next few years.

A focus on the childfree phenomenon can be expected to contribute to the breakdown of pronatalist thought by increasing the visibility of this life-style option; and thus it should also aid the development of new family norms apart from that "traditional" pattern which has held both marriage and parenthood to be prerequisites to social approbation.

16

Why We Don't Want Children

LYNNELL MICHELS
Granada Hills, California

"Married nearly five years and no children yet? Don't be discouraged, my dear. My sister and her husband tried for nine years before she got pregnant. Just keep trying and I'm sure you'll succeed."

Some women might have been annoyed at receiving such unsolicited advice, but I wasn't. In fact, I was amused. However, rather than laugh and offend my mother-in-law's old friend, I merely nodded knowingly. Catching my husband's eye, I saw that he too was working hard to keep from grinning.

Why did we find such humor in the situation? I suppose it was because never once in the time we'd been married had Dave and I tried to have a child. In fact, I had been on "the Pill" since our wedding day. So it struck us as funny that this older woman had quite automatically assumed that since we didn't have a family, it was because of lack of success, not lack of desire.

This, of course, was not the first time others had spoken to us about our childlessness. My own mother headed the list. I still remember a particular scene on my wedding day. My mother, near tears, in one breath bemoaned the fact that she was losing her "little girl" and in another urged us not to wait too long before making her a grandmother. Mama's wish has not yet been granted —to her chagrin—and she faithfully and gently reminds us now and then that it's about time we "settled down."

I don't resent my mother's hints, nor does it bother me when other people tell us what we're missing by waiting. We believe they

Redbook Magazine, January, 1970

mean well and are really sincere when they try to convince us that children make life and marriage more worthwhile. I wouldn't be a bit surprised if they were 100-per-cent right; someday, when Dave and I are parents, I probably will look back and wonder why we waited so long.

What, then, is our problem?

That's a good question, one I'm not sure Dave and I can answer, even to ourselves. When we were first married I was 20 and still in college; Dave was 22, newly graduated and just beginning to work at his chosen profession, engineering. We had been teen-age sweethearts who had waited for marriage until we were in a position to be independent—four and a half long years.

Once our financial independence was achieved, we had too many other goals and ambitions to fulfill before considering the added responsibilities of parenthood. I wanted material security, a home and the opportunity to work as an English teacher. Dave wanted to earn his advanced degrees and have time to pursue rather costly interests—airplanes and cars. We both wanted to travel. Children would simply have to wait.

Now, five years later, we have reached nearly all our goals. We own a three-bedroom, completely furnished house; I have taught for more than three years in a junior high school; Dave has finished all his course work for his Ph.D. and holds a pilot's license. We spent six weeks in Europe last year and plan to travel to Mexico this year. We own stock and we have a respectable savings account.

Most important, our marriage is strong and loving. In nearly every way we present a picture of a couple ready for a family. But the picture is false. Some time has passed since my mother-in-law's friend made her remark, and frankly we have thought quite seriously about children lately. But something prevents us from making the final decision to go ahead.

I believe this "something" could be called fear. For one thing, life is so good right now that we hesitate to change it in any way. When we voice this fear to family and friends, they tell us that we're foolish, that having children doesn't mean giving up all else. Intellectually we agree, but emotionally we're not sure—we view children as an unknown risk.

All around us, we see young parents struggling with budgets, baby-sitter problems, measles, crayon-marked walls and other assorted annoyances too numerous to mention. These annoyances alone are not what bother us; we feel we'd be able to cope with them as well as anyone else. What does terrify us is the awesome, 24-hour responsibility of it all. Unlike our two dogs, who are put outside and forgotten until morning, children cannot be ignored; they are always there, needing attention and love. Children do not disappear when you have a headache or would like another hour's sleep.

The restrictions that children would place on our personal freedom worry my husband more than they do me. My main concern is that I have strong doubts about my ability to fit into the role of a mother. I've never been around small children much; I've never even changed a diaper. I feel very comfortable and warm with the junior-high-school children I teach, but they require so much less care than an infant would; and even with them, my responsibility officially ends at three o'clock each day.

The prospect of taking care of the physical needs of an infant, helping him to grow properly, providing him with values and raising him to be a well-adjusted, useful adult is a most rewarding one, true. But to me it is also a very frightening one. All along the way loom pitfalls and the possibility of errors.

What if, in spite of our best efforts, our child turned out to have severe emotional problems, to be a drug addict or a criminal? In my profession I frequently encounter earnest and well-intentioned parents to whom this has happened. I worry that just loving your children and doing your best may not be enough to prevent such a tragedy. So even though nowadays I frequently long to hold and cuddle a baby of my own whenever I see someone else's, my fears soon come to the surface to confuse me and make me hesitate.

As it happens, this past year, for reasons of health, I have stopped taking the birth-control pills. We have been using other means of contraception, none of them as reliable as the pills. To be honest, I think that subconsciously I almost hope I will conceive accidentally, so that the responsibility of a decision will be out of our hands. And realizing this, I become ashamed, because it is a form of cowardice. When we have children it should be because we really yearn for them and plan to have them.

This next year will be a real test. I have thought seriously about taking a leave of absence from teaching in order to go back to college for my master's degree. On the other hand, we have also thought seriously about having a family, as I have mentioned. When I told my mother about my indecision she said. "Do both. Have a family now, then in a few years go back to school." But I'm afraid that once I have children, I'll never again have the patience or ambition to take on the added pressures of scholastic life.

Another possibility exists, of course. I could go to school now and in a couple of years, when I have earned my degree, have children. However, this alternative serves only to prolong our indecision. And secretly I wonder if my desire for further education isn't just a cover-up for our self-doubts.

Are all these fears and doubts a mask for our own inadequacies? Are my husband and I really too immature or selfish to want children, as some may say? Perhaps the fact that we are reluctant to have a family is a sign that we are not fitted for it, and we should heed these fears as a warning. We have never thought of ourselves in such terms, but maybe it's true.

Or are our fears normal ones that many couples struggle with before actually starting a family? Are we typical of many young couples who later become happy, contented parents and wonder why they ever were so panic-stricken? It's so hard for us to know.

17

A Vote Against Motherhood

GAEL GREENE
Contributing Editor, New York *Magazine*

I don't want to have any children. Motherhood is only a part of marriage, and I am unwilling to sacrifice the other equally important feminine roles upon the overexalted altar of parenthood. Instead of condemning myself to the common syndrome of the unhappy creature who is mother first, wife second, woman third and human being last, I champion the wondrously satisfying love of a woman and her husband, two adults enjoying the knowledge and mystery of each other, tasting dependence, accepting responsibility, yet individual and free.

Femininity is the acceptance, appreciation and enjoyment of being a woman. Motherhood is only a part of it. The complete woman is also devoted wife, lover, playmate, buffer, a man's stimulant and tranquilizer, a creator (in the kitchen if not at the easel or typewriter), an active mind, an unfettered human being involved in activities and causes and battles beyond the boundaries of a particular plot of crabgrass.

The idea that a couple would deliberately choose to remain childless seems to strike sparks of uncontrollable indignation. The decision is not one we have been able to discuss calmly with friends. Occasionally visitors to our apartment—so obviously designed for two adults with no thoughts of family expansion—will ask, "But where do you plan to put a nursery?"

"We're not planning for babies, so we don't need a nursery," I answer.

The Saturday Evening Post, January 1963

The shock and disbelief could not be greater if my husband announced he had just accepted a job spying for the Russians and I was busy running a Communist Party cell in the basement boiler room.

Our decision not to have children was neither simple nor sudden. Both my husband and I come from families where children are a major *raison d'être* for marriage and each new grandchild is looked upon as a divine blessing. Under these circumstances it certainly never occurred to me that one might consider married life without children. Children were taken for granted as a part of marriage. Indeed, as a teen-ager I had rather ambitious plans for a huge brood, mostly boys. (I felt I had been greatly deprived as a child by not having an older brother and was determined no daughter of mine would be so underprivileged.) These were the dreams of an adolescent who had been captivated by the adventures of the Bobbsey Twins and the Gilbreth youngsters of *Cheaper by the Dozen* fame. I wasn't thinking what it might mean to be a Bobbsey's mother. I was thinking what fun it would be to be a Bobbsey twin. "Mother," beyond the warm, loving, gentle creature who was my own, was a vague, inconceivable concept.

Parenthood's Real Price

Then I began to have doubts. When I looked about at our friends—young couples with children—I was shocked and appalled at what I saw. Men and women floundered under awesome responsibilities, suffered total loss of independence and privacy. Frustration, tension and bitterness strained love. Most frightening of all, women appeared shredded, pulled apart by the demands of a dozen conflicting roles.

In the homes of my friends I received my first intimate and disillusioning insight into the meaning of motherhood. Too many of these mothers had made the supreme sacrifice to motherhood. They felt trapped. They simmered with resentment. For others it was a passive surrender, an automatic, often unthinking, response to a thousand pressures.

I refuse to be pressured into this state of parenthood just because society or some advice columnist tells me it is a noble, joyous state and my sacred duty. Everywhere I turn, there are the voices assuring me that a woman can only know fulfillment through motherhood. My experience tells me differently.

Recently my husband, leafing through one of the ladies' magazines, came across a paragraph in a column of marriage counseling that infuriated him. "In the early months of marriage," it read, "*when love is at its height,* each spouse is most generous and tolerant. . . ." The suggestion that love reaches a peak with the honeymoon and then begins to taper off as romance fades and reality intrudes is shocking. Implicit in the following paragraphs was the "reassurance" that when the glow goes, various other roles (parenthood) would take up the slack.

From this must follow that line, so often uttered in supposed jest, "Well, the honeymoon is over." Ours is not. Love only seemed "at its height" in the early months of our marriage. We keep discovering new peaks. We enjoy our life and the things we do singly and together. We appreciate the time and freedom to pursue potential talents (even if they should prove to be nothing more than minor skills). We treasure the freedom to pick up and disappear for a weekend or a month or even a year, to sleep odd hours, to breakfast at three A.M. or three P.M., to hang out the DO NOT DISTURB sign, to slam a door and be alone, or alone together, to indulge in foolish extravagances, to get out of bed at seven A.M. on a sudden whim and go horseback riding in the park before work, to become embroiled in a political campaign or a fund-raising drive, to devote endless hours to intensive research for a project that might lead somewhere or nowhere, to have champagne with dinner for no special reason at all, to tease and love anywhere, any hour, anytime we please without a nagging guilt that a child is being neglected. We take so small a privilege as privacy for granted; yet, to our friends with children, privacy is a luxury for which they envy us.

I have read too many articles by young mothers and heard too many of my own friends complaining that motherhood is a prison. It is plain that the creation of a child, its care and tending a home are not enough for many women. Some turn to a job or back to a career or lock the door of a spare room to make it a studio, trying to serve on three or four fronts at once and serving on none well. Money and a reliable baby-sitter free a mother to spend afternoons haunting museums or studying ballet or serving as a Gray Lady, but money apparently does not buy away a conscience that talks of child neglect.

Many women thrive on motherhood and never stop growing. I am thinking of a college dorm-mate who took her degree in archaeology and was hailed in the class yearbook as "the girl most likely to find the ruins of lost Atlantis." Well, the only digging she's done since has been in backyard sandboxes. She has a passel of kids—four, and one on the way, at last count. She obviously loves her life, wades happily through what others might consider sheer drudgery and approaches such tasks as brewing an infant's formula or umpiring a brood of toddlers with all the zest she once devoted to geology expeditions. She's a fine mother, a great wife and an exciting woman to be with.

Yet I see so many of our friends, some of them with children they hadn't necessarily planned on—bitter, frustrated, vacillating between devotion and despair, screaming at their youngsters, tearing into each other. The child is there. Never for a moment would they wish it away, but they seem to be fighting a furious battle as they watch themselves becoming people they never meant to be.

"All I want is just an hour a day to be me," I overheard a woman complain to her husband. "Not to be a chauffeur or a bandage dispenser or a screaming harpy in a torn muumuu. Me, glamorous, calm, funny, in lingerie that isn't held together with safety pins—remember?"

"I don't know why you even call me anymore," a former classmate said to me recently. "I haven't had an original thought in two years, and the only multisyllabic word that's come out of me all week was 'Toidy-seat.' And that's hyphenated, so I don't even know if it counts."

Envy of the Childless

Cara left her job as an interior decorator three years ago—reluctantly, in her eighth month of pregnancy. "You don't know how lucky you are," she said, gazing about our living room. "To have a stairway without a kiddy gate and a velvet sofa without stain-resistant slipcovers. If you'd told me three years ago I'd have slipcovers or plastic-laminated anything, I'd have laughed myself silly."

Betty reads medical journals whenever she can sneak the time —while the kids nap or at the Laundromat. "It took me eleven years to become a pediatrician, and I've never even practiced," she says. "I want to go back as soon as all three of the boys are in school, but it frightens me to think I'll be ten years behind."

The more we watch our contemporaries trying to cope with child-rearing, the more we see them bowing to its conflicting demands and surrendering their individualities and dreams, the stronger our decision to remain childless becomes.

Our resolve has been strengthened by the prevailing philosophy of child-rearing. They call it "permissiveness." But it emerges as total child autocracy. All decisions revolve around the child. Vacations are planned to suit the children. A mother who would not sacrifice a new winter coat to buy her son an English racing bike is looked upon as an unnatural animal. Never mind that mother's idea of a relaxing holiday does not happen to include camping out and cooking three meals a day on a portable barbecue—it suits the youngsters. Girls I met when I first came to New York, who vowed they would never leave the city, have moved to the suburbs: "It's so wonderful for the children." Papa becomes a commuter, and a man and a woman who once shared the world now occupy two separate and distant islands, meeting for a few hours each night.

Parents Become Children

To be less than the complete mother the community expects one to be leaves a woman racked with guilt. She becomes so much the mother that she may one day find herself treating that tweedy, commuting chap who was once her husband and lover as just another one of the brood—another runny nose to wipe, another mouth to pop a vitamin pill into, another finicky appetite to cater to—an overgrown and petulant child. He even calls her "mom." She calls him "dad," and that sums up their relationship.

"No you may not have another Martini before dinner," she will say in exactly the same tone in which she would forbid the six-year-old another slice of chocolate cake.

I have heard some women say they refuse to bring children into a nuclear-panicked world or into a civilization that has lost all morals. These are not the only legitimate reasons for remaining childless, and I suspect some couples have reached conclusions similar to those of myself and my husband, yet hesitate to express them for fear of being accused of subversion, immaturity or selfishness.

Why then do people have children? They should not be so quick to condemn us for selfishness without first examining their own motives. People have children because they want them. Fine—go to it. But what of those who use their children as pawns or as instruments of revenge or as amusing little pets or as glue to patch a floundering marriage? What of those who don't really like children but have them anyway? And there are such people—just as there are those who don't like cats or jazz or abstract painting. What of those who produce progeny and regard them as a sort of status symbol? What about couples who procreate because they're afraid of being criticized for not having children? And what of those who haven't the courage or interest to face squarely what parenthood will mean or what kind of parents they will make?

Too many men and women who don't really want children, who are selfish, immature, ill-prepared, hostile and baffled, are spawning youngsters with less thought than they would give to the purchase of a new car. These children must suffer.

Whom do I harm by not having children? The nonexistent child? The world—which already has too many? Surely having children for the wrong reasons or for no reason at all or bringing them into an atmosphere of resentment and neglect is the greater selfishness.

There is a choice. Couples should be permitted to make a decision, whether to have children or not, without social pressures. There is no reason why their choices should be regarded as shocking, evil or an affront to humanity.

18

The Future Is a Cruel Hoax

STEPHANIE MILLS

Class speaker, 1969 graduating class, Mills College

Our days as a race on this planet are numbered. And the reason for our finite, unrosy future is that we are breeding ourselves out of existence. Within the next 10 years we will witness widespread famines and possible global plagues ranging through famine-weakened populations. Soon we may have to ask ourselves grisly questions like, "Will I be willing to shoot my neighbor if he tries to steal my last loaf of bread? Will I be forced to become a cannibal?"

The hideous fact that we are reproducing so rapidly that it is conceivable our means of sustenance will be grossly inadequate within 10 years was foreseen nearly two centuries ago. In 1798 Thomas Robert Malthus said, "Population, when unchecked, increases in a geometrical ratio. Subsistence increases only in an arithmetical ratio." We have had nearly 200 years to think over the consequences of that projection, yet at the turn of the century, people were arrested in New York for distributing birth control information; and only last year Pope Paul VI issued an encyclical which forbade the members of his flock to use contraceptives.

One of the most depressing aspects of the problem is that we cannot escape unscathed. Dr. Paul Ehrlich and others say that immediate action must be taken simply to minimize the consequences. I AM TERRIBLY SADDENED BY THE FACT THAT THE MOST HUMANE THING FOR ME TO DO IS TO HAVE NO CHILDREN AT ALL.

As an ex-potential parent, I have asked myself what kind of world my children would grow up in. And the answer was, "Not very pretty, not very clean. Sad, in fact." Because, you see, if the population continues to grow, the facilities to accommodate that population must grow, too. Thus we have more highways and fewer trees; more electricity and fewer undammed rivers; more cities and less clean air. Mankind has spread across the face of the earth like a great unthinking, unfeeling cancer. We have horribly disfigured this planet, ungrateful and shortsighted that we are. Our frontier spirit involves no reverence for any forms of life other than our own, and now we are even threatening ourselves with the ultimate disrespect of suicide.

If I had enough time, I'd try to get rich, become a philanthropist and endow a foundation. But I have less than 10 years; and so, for that matter, do you. This business of impending extinction is something that the so-called real and unreal worlds share. I can't eat a dollar bill; and Howard Hughes can't eat my diploma. The real and unreal worlds both have to become pragmatic on a grand scale, or there won't be any worlds left.

Political realities are clouding this issue of human survival every day. On the primary level there is the political reality that we simply can't go into a country and force it at gunpoint to adopt population control measures. On a secondary level there is the political reality that this situation is far less interesting to our government than the space program, anti-ballistic missiles, or even the size of print on cigarette packages. This conspicuous lack of interest may be due to the fact that there is hardly anybody, save a few individuals, lobbying to save the human race. And the absence of a lobby may be due to the fact that pushing to save the human race will turn no one an instant profit.

And, as of this moment, the problem seems vaguely unreal. Some of us have never gone hungry a day in our lives. Starvation is a remote concept. The shelves of grocery stores are still crammed with things to eat. Why should I believe that anything will happen to change that? You and I should believe that the famine can and will happen if for no other reason than we still may be able to do something. And doing something to save the human race has always been a fond dream of idealists—both over and under 30.

19

Reflections of a Non-Parent

STEWART R. MOTT
Philanthropist, political activist

I felt a distinct sense of satisfaction, on being informed in mid-July of 1973, that I had been selected as the "Non-Father of the Year" by a new organization for non-parents. This sense of satisfaction resulted not so much from the personal honor but from the fact that a Non-Parent's Day, in recognition of others such as I, had been established as well. Having a rather strongly developed sense of justice, it seemed to me most just and most appropriate that a special day had been set aside for all of us who formerly had to hang our heads when those traditional holidays, Mother's Day and Father's Day, rolled around. Non-Parent's Day, by the way, is August 1, and I am looking forward to its recurrence.

I was informed that I had been selected to receive this title in recognition of my "diverse and valuable efforts as a philanthropist and political activist which served the larger 'family' of community and society." Though I always have strong reasons for social and public interest projects in which I become involved, I had never thought of what I do in just those terms—i.e., serving the larger "family" of community and society.

Yet this is certainly my intention; and, on reflection, I realized that this motivation has probably played a role in my decision not to marry and have children. There may come a time when I will do one or both; but for the time being I am both a confirmed bachelor and a confirmed non-parent.

I might explain my feelings this way: it is my belief that when one undertakes anything in life, it should be with the in-

National Organization for Non-Parents *Newsletter,* December 1973

tention of discharging whatever is undertaken to the best of one's abilities. This necessarily means that responsible individuals must make choices about where they are going to direct their efforts.

Often, one cannot do two things well; specifically, often one cannot do justice to family life if one's predominant interests are elsewhere. I frankly reject the idea that "of course, one can have a family *too*"—as though having a successful family life were something that could be accomplished easily, almost as a sidelight, to one's primary focus. Probably I, personally, could combine family life in some way with my activities right now, because (as is often pointed out to me) I could afford hired help to care for a child or children.

But that is not the answer either. If a family is desired, one should be willing to devote the requisite *personal* time and energy to it. Thus, having a family means—or *should* mean—some sacrifice of self or other interests.

At this point in time, my outside interests are all-involving. I am concerned with the way in which this nation is governed, the way in which political morality can be established, and the ways in which constitutional freedoms can be guaranteed and kept alive. I am concerned both with the institutions and agencies of government, and with the quality of persons elected to office. My efforts were given, in 1972, to the campaign of a presidential candidate who, I felt, would lead our nation wisely. My efforts will doubtless be given to a similar candidate in our next presidential election. I am meanwhile involved in causes which range from campaign finance reform and restoration of respect for the presidency to investigative journalism and family planning.

To me, these present efforts seems not only more personally gratifying than paternity, but also more valuable to society in general. I am unconvinced that society has any urgent need for me to produce a child.

Perhaps my advantaged position has shielded me from some typical impolite attitudes faced by non-parents. In social situations I am usually accorded deferential treatment and I cannot recall even one instance of being asked to explain my motives for non-parenthood. Because I happen to have some degree of wealth, however, I am sometimes asked to whom I will leave my fortune if I have no biological inheritors. (It seems to be assumed that having a child to whom one can leave one's fortune is in itself sufficient *reason* to have a child.) I disagree with this line of thinking. Children make their parents no promises when they are born. Were I to have a child, I would have no guarantee that that child would devote the wealth he inherited to purposes of which I would approve. For that matter, children make no promises to carry on one's basic values or way of life. The idea that children are a guarantee of "immortality" is one that has never been explained to my satisfaction. I am pragmatic enough to think that anything of value must be earned—including immortality. And true immortality cannot be earned by so simple a means as reproduction. To my way of thinking, immortality is worth striving for if one defines it in terms of deeds: and calls to mind, as models, the poets and philosophers, scientists and scholars whose ideas and works and discoveries have survived them. To view immortality as a mere matter of biology is completely unsatisfactory.

But it seems to me that what most of us are striving for in life is not immortality—that may just be a convenient excuse for doing what is socially expected. It seems to me that what nearly every human being desires is a feeling of being accepted, respected, and admired by others. Here is where many fall into parenthood as an automatic, unthinking matter—since it seems an easy ticket to social approval.

Therefore, society ought to question its habit of congratulating new parents so effusively for their status. I have observed that new fathers automatically become the center of attention in any situation (even in political strategy meetings wherein decisions are made which could hold implications for decades to come). Columnist Nicholas von Hoffman has commented that new parents are greeted with only slightly less fervor and hysteria than are returning astronauts, and perhaps that's so. Parental status has been made to fit nicely in with commercialism as well, given the money which is spent on Mother's Day and Father's Day.

Until this traditional hoopla modifies itself, it is a good idea indeed to boost the morale of those non-parents such as I by suggesting that we, too, deserve a bit of praise and admiration. A Non-Parent's Day might seem, to some, a whimsical idea—but not to me. I take it quite seriously.

We are faced, in this nation, with indisputable evidence that our "universal parenthood" system just has not worked; (anyone who doubts that can just try to say the following simple sentences with a straight face: "All parents I know are happy. All children I know are happy.") We are also faced with sobering evidence of an overpopulation problem that is causing a frightening drain on our environmental resources.

These are two good reasons to celebrate non-parenthood. But there is a third reason, too. Non-parents have been ignored by our society, their interests and status either envied or derided.

A holiday for non-parents is a symbolic expression of the fact that we, too, are human beings of worth and value and deserve a special day of recognition to contemplate and celebrate our "childfree" status.

Happy Non-Parent's Day.

20

Changes in Views Toward Childlessness: 1965-1970

EDWARD POHLMAN
Director of the Birth Planning Research Program, University of the Pacific, Stockton, California

Between 1965 and 1970, there was a significant and strong drop in the number of children that seemingly comparable groups of college students said they wanted:

		More traditional college		*More avant-garde college*	
		1965	*1970*	*1965*	*1970*
Number of Children wanted:	0	0%	6%	10%	18%
	1	4%	1%	0%	7%
	2	27%	63%	39%	55%
	3 or more	68%	30%	52%	19%
Number of students sampled		96	95	54	110

Focus of the study was on intentional childlessness, with two major hypotheses: (1) that views about childlessness had become more permissive between 1965 and 1970, and (2) that the more "avant-garde" college students would have more permissive views. The first hypothesis was supported in both groups of students, and the second was supported in both years. All students were from the University of the Pacific, which had recently added new, small "cluster colleges," an innovation. Predictions of differences between students in these colleges and the larger and more traditional liberal arts colleges depended on several bases. The table shows consistent differences in desired family size in both years, and consistent 1965–1970 shifts among both kinds of students—

Summary of a preliminary report

with the modal family size dropping to two children. Not tabulated are the data for attitudes toward childlessness.

Respondents were asked "What is your opinion of married people who choose not to have children?" Two judges made ratings, "blind" where possible, of open-ended questions and answers, and inter-judge reliability was judged satisfactory. As predicted, both 1970 samples (contrasted with the parallel 1965 samples) were significantly more likely to mention that such couples were helping the population problem, significantly less likely to express pity for them ("Poor people, they are really missing a lot"), and showed significantly more positive distributions in a "positive-negative-neutral" rating.

21

Motivation of Childless Marriages

PAUL POPENOE

Institute of Family Relations, Los Angeles, California

The increasing proportion of childless marriages has been a striking feature in America as in other civilized countries. Figures show that the proportion of marriages in the United States that never produce a child is about 17 percent, while if consideration is limited to the educated part of the white population, the amount of childlessness is nearer one in five.

Some of this childlessness is voluntary, some involuntary, and there have been wide differences of opinion as to the proportions of the two kinds in the total. Analysis of childless marriages, in the data collected by Katherine Bement Davis, showed that three-fourths had wanted children and one-fourth were childless by preference. It is not certain, however, even when people are answering an anonymous and confidential questionnaire, that they will tell the whole truth in this connection. It is easy for them to rationalize their own feelings. In addition to the explanations of the childless couples themselves, there is need of a commentary from their close friends and relatives, whose interpretation of the reasons for a childless marriage might not wholly correspond with the interpretation given by the principals.

I therefore asked more than 100 adult students at the University College, University of Southern California, to list all the cases of permanent childlessness that they knew among their closest friends and relatives, selecting only such marriages as they felt sure would at no time in the future produce children, and only

The Journal of Heredity, vol. 27, 1936

those couples whom they knew so intimately that they felt no doubt as to the motivation of childlessness. The students contributed histories of 862 couples, which are nearly all from the educated part of the population, with an excess of professional people, particularly teachers. The findings might not apply to a wholly different socio-economic level of the population. How far they are typical of the white-collar population in other states than California is a matter of opinion and, I hope, of investigation by others in the same way.

These were divided as follows:

Voluntary	582	67%
Involuntary	280	33%
	862	100%

It will be noted that in only one-third of these marriages was childlessness undesired, as compared with three-fourths in K. B. Davis' study. One can not be sure that this percentage is representative. In the first place, my students may unconsciously have selected cases in which they knew the couple did not want children. In the second place, the percentage of biological sterility probably varies greatly in different parts of the United States and in different social strata. Personally, I do not believe that the finding of Dr. Davis (three-fourths of the childless marriages involuntary) is representative of the facts among educated people at the present day; but this is a question that deserves further study.

The causes of involuntary sterility can not be studied profitably by the method here used. Often the causes are not known even to the subjects themselves. Some childless marriages in this series are due to the advanced age of the wife at marriage. More than 10 percent are due to surgical operations performed on the wife (or occasionally the husband) which resulted either incidentally or intentionally in sterility. In another 20 percent of cases, some disease or other physical condition was thought to explain childlessness. But all these factors together leave nearly two-thirds of the cases in which my informants at least had no knowledge of the causation. It would not be profitable to analyze any further the cases of involuntary sterility in this series.

The detailed enumeration of presumed reasons for voluntary refusal to bear children was extremely interesting, but difficult to summarize satisfactorily. For the present purpose they may be classified as follows:

	Number	Percent
Self-centered	180	31
Wife's career	128	22
Economic pressure	96	16
Health	51	9
Dislike of all children	49	8
Miscellaneous	36	6
Eugenics	27	5
Marital discord	15	3
	582	100

1. "Self-centered" is a term I have used, for lack of anything better, to cover such comments as "social climbers," "wanted to be free to travel," and the like. Mr. and Mrs. *A*. are "too busy working and making money to bother with children." In the case of the *B.'s,* "wife wants to teach; husband wants to hunt and fish; each wants to follow own inclination and a child would disturb both of them." The history of the *C.'s* is a common type: "they wanted to save for a home and furniture first, but never reached the point where they were satisfied." The *D.'s* think an apartment is no place to bring up a child; and they simply couldn't consider living anywhere except in an apartment! Mrs. *E*. can't afford a maid, and she is certainly not going to let a child interfere with her club and social activities. Such histories are typical of a large number.

Perhaps a dozen of the wives have avoided pregnancy because, as they frankly told their friends, they feared the experience would spoil their looks or figures, and they did not want to make that supreme sacrifice. They are well matched by an equal number of men who insisted on sterility because they were afraid a child might take first place in the wife's affections, leaving them to "eat at the second table" of affection, without the amount of petting, mothering, and babying that they craved. Four couples had foregone parenthood, my students said, because this feeling was mutual: "they were so much in love with each other that they couldn't bear to think of children that might come between them and spoil the perfection of their romance." This is the much advertised Companionate Marriage raised to the *n*th degree!

2. "Wife's career" covers those cases in which the wife gave up maternity to work, not because she needed the money but because she preferred the outside occupation and did not want to interrupt it. This classification is large because so many of my students are teachers, social workers, and the like, and report the cases of their own friends in the professions.

Mrs. *F.* "doesn't like to stay at home," so she works instead. Mrs. *G.* has a little better excuse,—she has taught for 20 years and has not only "got the habit" but does not want to lose her retirement pay, which will soon be due her. Most of the stories under this heading are of a commonplace type: the wife was educated for a career, not for motherhood, and she wants her "freedom."

3. "Economic pressure" is a classification intended to take only those cases where husband and wife could not afford children,—not those in which they preferred to be childless and rationalized this emotional attitude by explaining that they didn't want to have a child until they were sure they could give him every advantage, etc., etc. Doubtless rationalization enters into a good many of the cases in this category; but some are at least plausible.

Some must support their parents; in other cases the husband has been out of employment, or sick, so much that the wife has had to stay close to the payroll. A tuberculous husband is mentioned in several instances. Others have been hit by the depression. Mrs. *H.* married a ready-made family, and didn't feel that she dared add one of her own to those her husband already had. Mrs. *I.* faces the same situation except that her husband is also paying alimony to a previous wife. Mrs. *J.* is slaving to support an imbecile sister and sacrifices her own possibility of motherhood to the care of this unfortunate.

4. "Health" may be a rationalization occasionally, but in many of these cases it is a grim reality. Even in this educated stratum of society, a number of the childless marriages give every evidence of being due to syphilis; others to tuberculosis, still others to glandular deficiency.

5. "Dislike of children," which includes "fear of childbearing," is to me the most interesting of all the groups, for the light it throws on the attitudes and educational background of supposedly intelligent people. Occasionally the fear of childbearing is to some extent justified, as with the woman whose pelvis is too narrow for normal delivery. Other women would be perfectly willing to take the risk of a Caesarean operation; but if a woman does not want to take this risk, she should not be compelled to. Most of the cases are purely neurotic, however. Was it Oswald Spengler who said that "The modern woman has neuroses instead of babies"? This little study shows that it is equally true of the modern man!

Mrs. *K.'s* mother died in childbirth; her sister also died giving birth to her first baby. With these examples ever in mind, Mrs.

K. will not take the risk. Mr. *L.*, on the other hand, lost his first wife in childbirth; he will not allow his second wife to jeopardize herself. Mr. *M.* did not even have that excuse; but "he adored his wife and did not want her to suffer or be disfigured."

Such cases, in which there is a fear of childbearing, shade insensibly into the cases of mere dislike of offspring. The latter cases shade insensibly into group 1, made up of persons who are so self-centered and infantile that they do not want to have to divide the spotlight with an offspring. I have tried to differentiate categories 1 and 5 by putting in the former those who did not dislike children but liked themselves better; in the latter those who, while doubtless not disliking themselves, had an active dislike or antagonism toward offspring.

Mrs. *N.* likes children but her husband is terribly annoyed by them—to the extent that they have gradually lost all their friends who have children. Mr. *O.* is like a number of others who were unhappy in childhood and will not bring children into the world to go through such an ordeal. Mrs. *P.* "can't stand to have a child around"; Mrs. *Q.* says children make her nervous; Mrs. *S.* had a particular aversion to children and died after an abortion. Mrs. *T.* is dominated by a neurotic mother, who doesn't like children (she ought to know). Mr. *U.* says it is hard enough to get along with a wife; he wouldn't want to undertake responsibility for a child as well. Mrs. *V.* has seen so many unhappy marriages where there are children that she doesn't want to add to the number. Mr. *W.*, who takes life seriously and children more so, was so upset by the news of his wife's pregnancy that he became violently ill and she consented to an abortion to save his life, so to speak. And so the story continues,—a striking commentary on present-day education.

6. Eugenics is, as the reader will note, invoked by only one couple in every twenty, among the voluntarily childless. In other words, the part that eugenic motivation plays in producing childlessness is virtually negligible. The cases in which it is invoked seem to be legitimate enough, mostly involving the existence of mental disease in the ancestry.

7. Finally, there are a few cases in which husband and wife are so inharmonious that they do not want children, perhaps thinking that the presence of offspring would complicate matters still further and also create difficulties in case of a divorce. Several of these are mixed marriages between a Protestant and a Catholic, in which the difference of religion is invoked as an explanation of childlessness,—though one would suppose that this explanation

could hardly be made by a Catholic in good standing with his church!

It will be remembered, in conclusion, that the causes here cited as leading to voluntary childlessness are not given by the couple themselves. As a fact, *their* explanations might be altogether different. This study has been made by asking the close friends and relatives of childless couples to tell what they, and not the couples themselves, think is the real motive for the childlessness. I suspect that in this way a more objective and accurate picture is obtained than if the husband and wife told their own story. At least, both methods of inquiry should be followed. The present method indicates that the great bulk of the voluntary childless marriages are motivated by individualism, competitive consumption economically, and an infantile, self-indulgent, frequently neurotic attitude toward life. It seems to me, therefore, to suggest several lines along which the education of young people might profitably be changed in the interest of society.

22

Correlates of Voluntary Childlessness in a Select Population

SUSAN O. GUSTAVUS and JAMES R. HENLEY, JR.

Department of Sociology, University of Utah, Salt Lake City, Utah; and Department of Sociology, Texas Christian University, Fort Worth, Texas

For several decades, social scientists and demographers interested in population processes have focused research efforts on the formation of attitudes toward childbearing. Many variables, including race, religious preference, social class, and social mobility have been found to be instrumental in the formation of these attitudes and in the subsequent fertility experienced by the couples. However, little data can be found on what factors predispose a couple to negative fertility attitudes, that is, to desire to have no children.

The lack of attention given to the voluntarily childless couple, and indeed to the childless couple in general, probably stems from several factors. Firstly, the phenomenon of childlessness, whether voluntary or involuntary, is increasingly rare. Table 1 shows the percent of ever-married women who were childless at selected ages and dates from 1940 to 1967. The total age group, as well as selected age categories within the total group, have experienced steady declines in childlessness. But to assume that this trend will continue may be an error. With increasingly effective means of contraception available, with abortion laws undergoing examination and change, and with increasing concern with, and publicity over, growing population, this trend may very well reverse itself.

Secondly, the neglect of the voluntarily childless couple may be a result of the tendency to view childlessness as just another quantitative state of parity. It would seem that there are important qualitative differences associated with childless and childed states,

Paper prepared for presentation at annual meetings Southwestern Sociological Association, March 25–27, 1971, Dallas, Texas

TABLE 1

PERCENT OF WOMEN CHILDLESS AT SELECTED AGES AND SELECTED DATES, NONINSTITUTIONAL POPULATION OF THE UNITED STATES

Age	*1967*	*1965*	*1962*	*1960*	*1957*	*1952*	*1950*	*1940*
15–44	13.3	14.2	14.4	15.0	15.9	20.7	22.8	26.5
20–24	28.0	28.0	23.4	24.2	26.9	30.9	33.3	39.9
30–34	6.4	7.2	9.9	10.4	11.3	14.7	17.3	23.3
40–44	8.9	11.0	12.8	14.1	14.1	19.8	20.0	17.4

SOURCE: Figures for 1967 taken from U.S. Bureau of the Census, 1969, Table 7. Figures for all other dates taken from U.S. Bureau of the Census, 1969, Table 1.

since those who are presently childless are in violation of the statistical and social norm to have children.

Finally, were the above problems to be ignored or deemed not prohibitive, the design of a systematic study of voluntarily childless couples is a formidable task. Where would such couples be found? How could the researcher be sure that the childlessness was voluntary?

Materials and Methods

In an attempt to bridge this research hiatus and to begin to cope with the difficult problems of sampling, this paper deals with the seventy-two childless couples who during the last two years applied to the Association for Voluntary Sterilization (AVS) for help in obtaining surgical sterilizations. Such couples, of course, are not representative of the total population of voluntary childless couples in the country. It might be maintained that these couples are more dedicated to the idea of remaining childless than other couples might be, since they are willing to take this frequently irreversible step.

Undoubtedly there are couples who have had such operations for the purpose of preventing conception without the aid of AVS. But the couples who come to AVS are sometimes from communities where it is difficult to obtain such operations. As one applicant stated rather bitterly: "I have tried to obtain a vasectomy locally but Puritanism is still strong in this part of the country and no consideration whatsoever is given to private individual judgments and wishes." If this is often the case, these couples may be the most flagrant norm violators of all.

They are described here, then, not as a representative or probability sample of all voluntarily childless couples. Instead they constitute an availability sample. In fact, they might best be treated as a separate population since there is little basis for estimating the degree to which even gross demographic characteristics of the national population of voluntarily childless couples are represented by these seventy-two couples. Nevertheless, it is hoped that detailed description of their characteristics will provide theoretical and research leads for further investigations of negative fertility attitudes.

Data and Results

Table 2 gives preliminary descriptive data on the applicants to AVS. The vast majority of these applicants are males, presumably since a vasectomy is a simpler operation than a tubal ligation would be. Most of them come from the northeastern region of the United States. Table 2 also shows that most of these couples come from large urban areas. Indeed, while 12% of them seem to come from very small communities this is probably an overstatement of the numbers actually from isolated small communities

TABLE 2

Percentage Distribution of Childless Applicants for Voluntary Sterilization by Selected Characteristics

Characteristic	%
Sex	
Male	95
Female	4
Nonresponse	1
Total	100
Residence	
Northeast	61
North Central	17
West	10
South	12
Total	100
Size of place	
Less than 2,500	12
2,500 to 10,000	17
10,000 to 50,000	25
50,000 to 100,000	6
More than 100,000	40
Total	100

Characteristic	%
Number of years married	
One or less	24
Two or three	25
Four or five	18
Six or seven	8
Eight or more	25
Total	100
X	5.2
Source of referral to AVS	
Other agency	20
TV or radio	19
Magazine	33
Newspaper	10
Friend or relative	4
Other	13
Nonresponse	1
Total	100

since some of the small places included in that category are in fact suburbs of very large metropolitan areas.

The mean number of years these couples have been married is 5.2, but half of them have been married for less than four years and two-thirds have been married for less than six years before applying to AVS for assistance. Finally, most of the couples heard about AVS through some form of mass media, including radio or TV, magazines, and newspapers. While most of the applicants for the actual operations were males, the magazines most frequently mentioned as sources of information about AVS were *McCall's, Redbook,* and other magazines traditionally thought of as women's publications.

Table 3 shows the age, religion, and socioeconomic status of both husbands and wives, as measured by their occupation, education, and income. Also shown are comparable data for the United States population at selected dates. This enables some comparison of these voluntarily childless couples with the general population on at least four of these characteristics.

The mean age of husbands in this sample is 32 and of wives 29—the traditional three-year difference in age found in most populations. Over 50% of both husbands and wives are less than 30. The decision to be sterilized in order to prevent conception is apparently an early one. However, 17% of the husbands and 10% of the wives are over 40, so that this decision is not exclusively confined to extremely young couples by any means.

Perhaps the most theoretically interesting finding concerning the characteristics of these couples is the disproportionate number among them who have no religion whatever. Forty percent of the husbands and 36% of the wives fall into this category, as opposed to 4% and 1% of U.S. males and females respectively. Catholics are under-represented among these couples in comparison with their proportion in the population, as might be expected given the prohibition against birth control and the value placed on children in this religion. But other religious groups are also under-represented among the childless couples, with two exceptions. Jewish men, who comprise 11% of the childless husbands, constitute only 4% of the general population. Secondly, both sexes in the "Other Protestant" category are somewhat over-represented among the 72 couples when compared to national proportions.

By any of the three measures of socioeconomic status shown in Table 3 these childless couples are clearly of higher status than the United States population in general. The occupational score used here is a measure computed by using standardized scores of income and education associated with each occupation in the United States. If we compare the husbands of the childless couples to the heads of U.S. families in 1960 (a not entirely comparable group) it can be seen that the childless husbands are much more likely to be in the highest status occupations (62%) than are the U.S. family heads (14%). Even the childless wives have higher occupations overall than do U.S. family heads.

The educational attainment comparison is even more striking. Fully 62% of the childless husbands have a college degree or more, while only 10% of the male U.S. population could claim such an educational attainment in 1960. It is only fair to point out, however, that since the childless couples are largely below 30, their

TABLE 3

PERCENTAGE DISTRIBUTION OF RELIGION, AGE, OCCUPATION, EDUCATION, AND INCOME OF CHILDLESS COUPLES REQUESTING VOLUNTARY STERILIZATION, AND OF THE UNITED STATES POPULATION AT SELECTED DATES

	Childless Couples		*United States*	
Characteristic	*Husbands*	*Wives*	*Male*	*Female*
Age				
25 or less	22	32		
26–30	29	33		
31–35	21	11		
36–40	7	10		
41 or more	17	10		
Nonresponse	4	4		
Total	100	100		
X	32	29		
Religion *				
Catholic	6	6	28	28
Jewish	11	4	4	4
Baptist	3	4	15	15
Methodist	6	7	13	14
Presbyterian	4	6	6	6
Other Protestant	30	37	28	30
No religion	40	36	4	1
Total	100	100		
Occupation †				
0–29 (low)	1	3	20	
30–59	15	14	41	
60–79	14	28	25	
80–99 (high)	62	28	14	
No occupation	8	27		
Total	100	100	100	
X	78	70		

TABLE 3 (*Con't*)

PERCENTAGE DISTRIBUTION OF RELIGION, AGE, OCCUPATION, EDUCATION, AND INCOME OF CHILDLESS COUPLES REQUESTING VOLUNTARY STERILIZATION, AND OF THE UNITED STATES POPULATION AT SELECTED DATES

	Childless Couples		*United States*	
Characteristics	*Husbands*	*Wives*	*Male*	*Female*
Education ‡				
Less than 8th grade			23 (17)	20 (14)
Some high school	6	3	37 (35)	37 (34)
High school graduate	19	28	21 (29)	28 (37)
Some college	12	28	9 (10)	9 (9)
College graduate	38	28	10 (9)	6 (6)
Graduate degree	24	9		
Nonresponse	1	4		
Total	100	100	100	100
Income §				
Less than $3,000	6	33	30	65
$ 3,000–5,999	18	22	24	26
$ 6,000–9,999	35	31	30	7
$10,000–14,999	29	10	11	1
$15,000 or more	7		5	1
Nonresponse	5	4		
Total	100	100	100	100
X	$8,860	$4,436	$6,159	$2,601

* For the United States as a whole, data from U.S. Bureau of the Census, 1957.

† For the United States as a whole, figures for Head of Family are listed under "Male." Data for 1960. U.S. Bureau of the Census, 1963.

‡ Figures for the United States for ages 25–34 are given in parentheses for comparison. Data for 1960. U.S. Bureau of the Census, 1960, Table 173.

§ For the United States, data from U.S. Bureau of the Census, 1967.

educational attainment is likely to be higher than that for the entire U.S. population. Table 3 also gives the educational attainment distribution for males and females age 25–34 years in the United States in 1960. Still, the voluntarily childless couples show a much higher educational attainment.

The distribution of income follows this same pattern. The mean income of the childless husbands is $8,860 while that same figure for U.S. males in 1967 was $6,159. Similarly with females there is nearly a $2,000 differential in the income of these childless wives and U.S. females in 1967.

Table 4 gives the contraceptive and pregnancy histories of these couples. The great majority of them (89%) were contracepting at the time they requested sterilization and had been doing so for a number of years. Eight percent had used some form of contraception previously but were not now doing so. Three percent of them had never contracepted.

Since most of the couples mentioned using various methods of contraception, the percentages in this column do not add to 100 and multiple responses are included. Oral contraceptives were by far the most frequent method of contraception used. Condoms and diaphragms were less frequently used by these couples, and other methods shown in Table 4 were not often mentioned.

The mean number of years these couples had been contracepting, by whatever method, is 4.3. The largest group of them had contracepted for five or more years, with one couple reporting they had been practicing birth control for 18 years. Apparently the decision to be sterilized is not often a quick one made in reaction to the inconvenience of contracepting. A disappointingly

TABLE 4

CONTRACEPTIVE AND PREGNANCY HISTORIES OF CHILDLESS COUPLES REQUESTING VOLUNTARY STERILIZATION

Use of contraception		Miscarriages and abortions	
Previously, not now	8	1 or more miscarriages	7
Previously and now	89	1 or more abortions	4
Never used	3	1 or more of both	2
		Neither	71
Total	100	Nonresponse	16
Methods used *		Total	100
Diaphragm	32		
Condom	42		
Suppository	3		
Jelly	18		
Oral	68		
Other	18		
How long contracepting			
Less than one year	4		
1 to 2 years	17		
3 to 4 years	19		
Five or more years	24		
Nonresponse	36		
Total	100		
X	4.3		

* The percentages here do not add to 100 since several couples mentioned using several different methods.

large percentage of these couples did not report these data, most probably due to the actual wording of the question, which asked them to specify when they began using contraceptives. It could be that they could not remember or that they did not feel these data were relevant to AVS.

Finally, Table 4 gives the pregnancy history of these couples. Apparently 71% of them have never been pregnant, since they are presently childless and have had neither miscarriages nor abortions. Another option exists—to bear a child and then give it up by adoption—and these data would not show how many couples have done so. Six percent of the couples have had abortions, and 9% have had miscarriages, which may or may not have been deliberately inflicted.

Table 5 shows the reasons these couples gave on their applications for wanting to be sterilized. Unfortunately, 24% of the applicants said simply that they did not wish to have any children—making them unusable for an analysis which tries to tap

TABLE 5

PERCENTAGE DISTRIBUTION OF THE FIRST REASONS GIVEN AND TOTAL REASONS GIVEN FOR WANTING TO BE STERILIZED BY CHILDLESS COUPLES

Reason	*First Mention*	*Total Mentions* *
Population concern	15	28
Health	16	25
Career	10	17
Too old	11	11
Dislike for children	7	12
Economic	3	12
Fear of pregnancy	1	8
World conditions		7
Intend to adopt	4	12
Don't want children	24	24
Other	8	22
Total	100	

* The percentages in this column do not add to 100 since respondents were permitted to cite multiple reasons and often did so.

reasons for not wanting children. Table 5 gives both the first reason given by the couples in making their application and the total reasons mentioned by the couples. The most common reason given by these couples was some concern for the world or national population problem. The theoretical question this finding raises is whether this is a true reason which motivates these couples or whether this is a socially acceptable reason they have seized upon with the advent of population propaganda in order to justify a decision they have already made. These data do not provide answers to questions of this sort.

Health reasons were also important in leading to this decision to seek sterilization. Included here were heart conditions, blood problems, or other physical conditions, particularly of the wives, which would make childbearing difficult at best. These are presumably conditions out of the direct control of these couples and might not qualify them as strictly voluntarily childless.

Several of the couples mentioned deep or time-consuming involvement with careers which would make child rearing inconvenient. Typical of this kind of comment, made by 17% of the sample, is the following:

> Before my wife and I were married seven years ago, we both expressed our desires to have no children, so that we could do justice to our work, unhindered. I am a writer. My wife is deeply involved in sculpturing. We both have jobs and come home at night to our hobbies.

Eleven percent of the sample simply stated that they were too old to begin their families now. In some cases these couples married late, but in others no reason is given for not starting the family at an earlier age.

A plain dislike for children was given as a reason for wanting to remain childless by 12% of the sample. Typical of this kind of response are the following:

> Both of us are too familiar with the smell of sour pablum, diaper pails, and baby "b.m.'s" and we find equally nauseating the sound of crying, screaming, and infant temper tantrums. These so called "joys of parenthood" are definitely not for us.

Or the couple who said:

> We are unable to tolerate the presence of children for any appreciable length of time and cannot imagine any circumstances in which either of us would ever want children of our own.

Some of the couples mentioned economic problems which they felt prohibited them from having children. Examples of these couples' comments include:

> We are unable to afford the expenses of pregnancy, child birth, child raising and subsequent family illnesses. . . . An accidental pregnancy now would keep us living in cheap apartments for the rest of our lives.

One of the wives wrote:

> Another reason we do not want children is our financial problems. My husband never finished school, and his low paying job doesn't really meet our needs, with the high cost of living. It pays the bills and there is none left over for saving. There is no real future in his job. . . . We live in a one bedroom 8′ by 31′ housetrailer and it's really too crowded for the two of us. It will be several years, if ever, before we can hope to do better. A new car must come first, as our 14 year old Chevrolet won't stand up much longer without falling apart.

Other reasons given by fairly small proportions of the sample include some mention of a preferred style of life, other than professional ambitions, which would be inhibited by children. Included here are couples who intend to travel or who enjoy solitude for its own sake. World conditions, other than overpopulation, were mentioned by 7% of this group. These respondents were concerned about war, pollution, crime, etc., and did not feel such a world was a good place to bring up children. Finally, nine of the couples intend to adopt children, which, of course, does not make them voluntarily childless at all.

Included in the category labeled "Other" reasons were a smattering of couples who were mentally retarded, who thought such an operation would improve their sexual life, or who said only that they were frankly untrusting of the birth-control methods available to them, for health or effectiveness reasons.

Summary and Conclusions

This has indeed been a cursory look at a select population of couples who, with the exception of nine potential adopters, intend to be permanently childless. With such limited data and given such a population, the most we can hope to do is pick up a few leads as to what sorts of characteristics persons with negative fertility attitudes are likely to have and what they perceive as some of the reasons behind this attitude. Our data show that an average couple in this group is likely to be living in a large metropolitan area and to have been married an average of about five years. They are likely to be about thirty years of age, to say they have no religion, and to be of generally high socioeconomic status. Most all of them have used some method of birth control, usually the pill, have been contracepting for a number of years, and are not likely to have had a miscarriage or abortion. Such a profile of the average person in our sample, of course, obscures as much as it enlightens.

Finally, in looking at the reasons for wanting to remain childless, population concerns and health considerations are the two most mentioned reasons and if truly a reflection of the couple's rationale are not "selfish" reasons which may be ascribed to childless couples by society in general. Reasons which might be more reasonably associated with hedonism include career commitments, style of life, or economic desires. Disliking children and fear of pregnancy might be classified as "hang-ups" which may or may not be associated with selfish pursuits.

In future research on the voluntarily childless couple, the strategy that might be taken in locating these couples is not clearly indicated by these data. It is clear from the small percentage of the population which they comprise that random samples of the population, unless quite large, are not likely to unearth sufficient numbers of them to do detailed tabulations. An availability sampling technique might be tried in large communities—with no hope of representativeness. These authors tried, prior to receiving these data from AVS, to search out such couples in several ways, including surveying couples in apartments known to be one-bedroom or smaller where the presence of children was unlikely. This method of course turns up mostly couples who are postponing their childbearing, a few single people, and several pregnant wives. Further, even among the couples found who claim to be permanently and voluntarily childless, some of them will no doubt experience an accidental pregnancy in the future and keep the child. It is possible to place ads in various newspapers and other community publications asking childless couples to volunteer to answer a questionnaire. Such a method is plagued by the usual problems associated with using volunteers in any research.

Nevertheless, these two methods in concert, used over a period of time in a large community, might yield another select population like the one discussed here. Certainly any additional data would be useful, since as mentioned above, the literature on these special couples with negative fertility attitudes is so sparse.

Acknowledgments

The authors wish to thank the Association for Voluntary Sterilization for their cooperation in furnishing us with these data. The analysis of the data was funded by the Research Committee of the University of Utah, to which the authors are indebted.

23

Voluntarily Childless Wives: An Exploratory Study

J. E. VEEVERS

Sociologist, University of Western Ontario, London, Ontario

Students of the family have generally tended to accept the dominant cultural values that married couples should have children, and should want to have them. As a result of this value bias, although parenthood (especially voluntary parenthood) has been extensively studied, the phenomenon of childlessness has been virtually ignored (Veevers, 1973a). This selective inattention is unfortunate, for to a large extent the social meanings of parenthood can be comprehensively described and analyzed only in terms of the parallel set of meanings which are assigned to non-parenthood (Veevers, 1973b). Although occasionally sociologists have discussed the theoretical relevance of voluntary childlessness, and have speculated regarding some empirical aspects of it (Pohlman, 1970), virtually no direct research has been conducted. As a preliminary step towards filling this gap in the sociological study of the family, an exploratory study of voluntarily childless wives was conducted. The present paper will not attempt to describe this research in its entirety, but rather will be concerned with brief discussions of four aspects of it: first, the career paths whereby women come to be voluntarily childless; second, the social pressures associated with that decision; third, the symbolic importance attributed to the possibility of adoption; and fourth, the relevance of supportive ideologies relating to concern with feminism and with population problems.

Paper presented at the annual meeting of the National Council on Family Relations held in Portland, Oregon, in November 1972; *Sociology and Social Research: An International Journal,* 1973

Selection and Nature of the Sample

Conventional sampling techniques cannot readily be applied to obtain large and representative samples of voluntarily childless couples (Gustavus and Henley, 1971). Only about five percent of all couples voluntarily forgo parenthood (Veevers, 1972b), and this small deviant minority is characterized by attitudes and behaviours which are both socially unacceptable and not readily visible. The present research, which is exploratory in nature, is based on depth interviews with a purposive sample of 52 voluntarily childless wives. Although the utilization of non-random samples without control groups is obviously not the ideal approach, and can yield only suggestive rather than definitive conclusions, in examining some kinds of social behaviours it is often the only alternative to abandoning the inquiry. In the present study, respondents were solicited by three separate articles appearing in newspapers in Toronto and in London, followed up by advertisements explicitly asking for volunteers. Of the 86 individuals who replied, 52 wives were selected. Three criteria were evoked in these selections. First, the wife must have stated clearly that her childlessness was due to choice rather than to biological accident. Second, she must either have been married for a minimum of five years, or have been of post-menopausal age, or have reported that either she or her husband had been voluntarily sterilized for contraceptive purposes. Third, she must have affirmed that she had never borne a child and had never assumed the social role of mother.

The interviews, which were unstructured, averaged about four hours in length, and included discussion of the woman's life history, considerable detail concerning her marriage and her husband, and attitudinal and evaluative aspects of her responses to the maternal role. Data are thus available on the characteristics of 104 voluntarily childless husbands and wives, whose demographic and social characteristics may be briefly summarized as follows. The average age of the sample is 29, with a range from 23 to 71 years. All are Caucasian and living in urban areas, most are middle class, and many are upwardly mobile. Although educational experience ranges from grade school to the post doctoral level, most have at least some university experience. With the exception of one housewife, all are either employed full time or attending university. Most individuals are either atheists or agnostics from Protestant backgrounds, and of the minority who do express some religious preference, almost all are inactive. Most individuals come from stable homes where the mother has been a full time housewife since her first child was born. The incidence of first born and only children is much higher than would be ordinarily expected. With the exception of two widows, all are presently involved in their first marriage. The average marriage duration is seven years, with a range from three to twenty-five years. Configurations of marital adjustment cover the entire continuum described by Cuber and Haroff (1965), ranging from conflict-habituated to total relationships, with many wives reporting vital or total involvements with their husbands. Most couples have relatively egalitarian relationships but still maintain conventional marriages and follow the traditional division of labour. All of the couples agree on the desirability of preventing pregnancy at least at the present time. Most of the wives had never been pregnant, but about a fifth had had at least one induced abortion, and most indicate they would seek an abortion if pregnant. More than half of the wives are presently on the pill. About a quarter of the husbands have obtained a vasectomy, and another quarter are seriously considering doing so. Many of the women express positive interest in tubal ligation, but only one, a girl of 23, has actually been sterilized.

The Nature of Childless Careers

In reviewing the processes whereby couples come to define themselves as voluntarily childless, two characteristic career paths are apparent. One route to childlessness involves the formulation by the couple, before they are even married, of a definite and explicitly stated intention never to become involved in parental roles; a second and more common route is less obvious, and involves the prolonged postponement of childbearing until such time as it is no longer considered desirable at all. These two alternatives will be briefly elaborated.

Nearly a third of the wives interviewed entered into their marriages with a childlessness clause clearly stated in their marriage contract. Generally these women made their negative decisions regarding the value of children during their early adolescence, before the possibility of marriage had ever been seriously considered. Childlessness was a firm condition of marriage, and they deliberately sought a future mate who, regardless of his other desirable qualities, would agree on this one dimension. Although these women consider their anti-natal attitudes to be of central importance to their self-image, and something on which they are unable to compromise, they are unable to clearly articulate the specific reasons or motivations involved in this stance. In contrast, a very few of the wives had indifferent or even vaguely positive attitudes towards childbearing until they met their future husbands. During their courtship and engagement, they gradually allowed themselves to be converted to the world view of voluntary childlessness, and by the time of their marriage were quite content to agree to never have children. Because these women have been forced to examine openly the desirability of children, they are better able to verbalize the content and the source of their negative orientations.

More than two thirds of the wives studied remained childless as a result of a series of decisions to postpone having children until some future time, a future which never came. Rather than explicitly rejecting motherhood prior to marriage, they repeatedly deferred procreation until a more convenient time. These temporary postponements provided time during which the evaluations of parenthood were gradually reassessed relative to other goals and possibilities. At the time of their marriages, most wives involved in the postponement model had devoted little serious thought to the question of having children, and had no strong feelings either for or against motherhood. Typically, they simply made the conventional assumption that like everyone else they would probably have one or two eventually. During the early years of marriage, they practiced birth control conscientiously and continuously.

Most couples involved in the postponement pattern move through four separate stages in their progression from wanting to not wanting children. The first stage involves postponement for a definite period of time. In this stage, the voluntarily childless are indistinguishable from conventional and conforming couples who will eventually become parents. In most groups, it is not necessarily desirable for the bride to conceive during her honeymoon. It is considered understandable that before starting a family a couple might want to achieve certain goals, such as graduating from school, travelling, buying a house, saving a nest egg, or simply getting adjusted to one another. The degree of specificity varies, but there is a clear commitment to have children as soon as conditions are right.

The second stage of this career involves a shift from postponement for a definite period of time to indefinite postponement. The couple remains committed to the idea of parenthood, but becomes increasingly vague about when the blessed event is going to take place. It may be when they can "afford it," or when "things are going better" or when they "feel more ready."

The third stage in the cycle involves another qualitative change in thinking, in that for the first time there is an open acknowledgment of the possibility that in the end the couple may remain permanently childless. The third stage is a critical one, in that the very fact of openly considering the pros and cons of having children may increase the probability of deciding not to. During this time, they have an opportunity to experience directly the many social, personal and economic advantages associated with being childless, and at the same time to compare their life styles with those of their peers who are raising children. It seems probable that the social-psychological factors involved in the initial decision to postpone having children may be quite disparate from the social-psychological factors involved in the inclination to remain childless and to continue with the advantages of life style to which one has become accustomed. At this stage in the career, the only definite decision is to postpone deciding until some vague and usually unspecified time in the future.

Finally, a fourth stage involves the definite conclusion that the couple are never going to have children, and that childlessness is a permanent rather than a transitory state. Occasionally this involves an explicit decision, usually precipitated by some crisis or change in the environment that focuses attention on the question of parenthood. However, for most couples, there is never a direct decision made to have or to avoid children. Rather, after a number of years of postponing pregnancy until some future date they gradually become aware that an implicit decision has been made to forgo parenthood. The process involved is one of recognizing an event which has already occurred, rather than of posing a question and then searching or negotiating for an answer. At first, it was 'obvious' that 'of course' they would eventually have children; now, it is equally 'obvious' that they will not. The couple are at a loss to explain exactly how or when this transition came about, but they both agree on their new implicit decision, and they are both contented with its implications.

Childlessness and Informal Sanctions

All of the wives interviewed feel that they are to some extent stigmatized by their unpopular decision to avoid having children, and that there exists a ubiquitous negative stereotype concerning the characteristics of a voluntarily childless woman, including such unfavourable traits as being abnormal, selfish, immoral, irresponsible, immature, unhappy, unfulfilled and non-feminine (Veevers, 1972a). In addition, these devaluating opinions are perceived to have behavioural consequences for their interaction with others, and to result in considerable social pressure to become mothers. Some of the sanctions reported are direct and obvious, including explicit and unsolicited comments advocating child-birth and presenting arguments relating to the importance of motherhood. Other pressures are more subtle and in many cases are perceived to be unintentional. For example, the childless frequently complain that whereas parents are never required to explain why they chose to have children, they are frequently required to account for their failure to do so. The responses of others depend to a large extent on the apparent reason for childlessness. The involuntarily childless couple are perceived to be unfortunate, rather than immoral, and the appropriate responses to them therefore involve sympathy and perhaps even pity. Some reasons for deliberate childlessness, such as delicate health or unemployment, are perceived to be more or less legitimate excuses from the obligation to procreate, but in most cases when the voluntarily childless do try to justify and to explain their unusual choice, their reasons and arguments are discounted and disbelieved.

Childlessness is of course not always a disapproved state. Couples are rewarded, not punished, for remaining childless for the first several months of marriage, and thereby negating the possibility that they were "forced" to get married. After the minimum of nine months has passed, there is a short period of time when the young couple is excused from not assuming all of their responsibilities, or are perceived as having been having intercourse for too short a period of time to guarantee conception. The definition of how long a period of time child bearing may be postponed and still meet with conventional expectations is difficult to determine, and apparently varies considerably from one group to another. In most groups, the first twelve months constitutes an acceptable period of time. After the first year, the pressure gradually but continually increases, reaching a peak during the third and fourth years of marriage. However, once a couple have been married for five or six years there appears to be some diminution of negative responses to them. Several factors are involved in this change: part may be attributable to the increased ability of the childless to avoid those who consistently sanction them; part may be attributable to the increased ability of the childless to cope with negative and hostile responses, making the early years only seem more difficult in retrospect; and part may reflect an actual change in the reactions of others, in that after five or six years one's family and friends give up the possibility of persuading the reluctant couple to procreate and resign themselves to the fact that intervention, at least in this case, is ineffective.

It is noteworthy that although all wives report considerable direct and indirect social pressures to become mothers, most are remarkably well defended against such sanctions. Although on specific occasions they may be either indignant or amused, in most instances they are indifferent to negative responses, and remain inner-directed, drawing constant support and reaffirmation from the consensual validation offered by their husbands. Many strategies are employed which 'discredit the discreditors' (Veevers, 1973c), and which enable the voluntarily childless to remain relatively impervious to the comments of critics and the wishes of reformers. One such strategy concerns the possibility of adoption.

The Symbolic Importance of Adoption

A recurrent theme in discussions with childless wives is that of adoption. Most wives mention that they have in the past considered adopting a child, and many indicate that they are still considering the possibility at some future date. However, in spite of such positive verbalizations, it is apparent that adoption is not seriously contemplated as a viable alternative and that their considerations are not likely to result in actually assuming maternal roles. The lack of serious thought about adoption as a real possibility is reflected in the fact that generally they have not considered even such elementary questions as whether they would prefer a boy or a girl, or whether they would prefer an infant or an older child. With few exceptions, none of the couples have made even preliminary inquiries regarding the legal processes involved in adoption. Those few that had made some effort to at least contact a child placement agency had failed to follow through on their initial contact. None had investigated the issue thoroughly enough to have considered the possibility that, should they decide to adopt, a suitable child might not be immediately available to them. For the voluntarily childless, the importance of the recurrent theme of adoption appears to lie in its symbolic value rather than in the real possibility of procuring a child by this means and thereby altering one's life style. This symbolic importance is twofold: the reaffirmation of normalcy; and the avoidance of irreversible decisions. A willingness to consider adoption as a possibility communicates to one's self and to others that in spite of being voluntarily childless, one is still a 'normal' and 'well-adjusted' person who does like children, and who is willing to assume the responsibilities of parenthood. It is an effective mechanism for denying the possibility of considerable psychological differences between parents and non-parents, and legitimates the claim of the childless to be just like parents in a number of important respects. The possibility of adoption at a later date is of symbolic value, in that it prevents the voluntarily childless from being committed to an irreversible state. One of the problems of opting for a postponement model is that eventually one must confront the fact that childbirth cannot be postponed indefinitely. The solution to this dilemma is to include possibility of adoption as a satisfactory 'out' should one be needed. The same strategy is employed by many couples who chose sterilization as a means of birth control, but who are not entirely comfortable with the absolute and irreversible solution. The theoretical possibility of adoption is also comforting when faced with the important but unanswerable question of how one will feel about being childless in one's old age.

The Relevance of Supportive Ideologies

The voluntarily childless appear to be in a state of pluralistic ignorance, in that they are unaware of the numbers of other individuals who share their world view. Although the deliberate decision to avoid parenthood is a relatively rare phenomenon, it is not nearly as rare as the childless themselves perceive it to be, especially among urban and well-educated middle class couples. A large proportion of wives indicated that until they read the article and/or advertisement asking for subjects for the present study, they had never seen the topic of voluntary childlessness discussed in the mass media. Many reported that they did not know any other couple who felt as they did about the prospect of parenthood, and many others reported having met only one or two like-minded people during the course of their marriage. Feelings of uniqueness and of isolation are somewhat mitigated by the explicit agreement of their husbands on the appropriateness of forgoing parental roles. However, regardless of how supportive the husband is in his reaffirmation of the legitimacy of childlessness, and how committed he is personally to avoiding fatherhood, he can only present a model of a voluntarily childless man, and as such does not share an entirely comparable situation. The childless wife often expresses the wish that, even though she is generally comfortable without having children, she would appreciate the opportunity to relate her own situation to that of other voluntarily childless wives who, unlike her husband, might have shared the same female experiences, might be truly able to empathize, and might provide a model for identification.

It is noteworthy that within the psychological world of the voluntarily childless, existing social movements concerned with population or with feminism have surprisingly little relevance, and provide relatively little intellectual or emotional support. The concern with population problems, especially as manifest in the Zero Population Growth movement, does provide a supportive rationale indicating that one is not necessarily being socially irresponsible and neglectful of one's civic obligations if one does not reproduce. However, although there is a clear statement that procreation is not necessary for all, most ZPG advocates are careful to indicate that it is not procreation *per se* they are opposed to, but rather excessive procreation. The slogan "Stop at Two" asserts that one should have no more than two children, but also implies that one perhaps should have at least one or two. Some of the childless wives are superficially involved in ZPG and sympathetic with its goals, but in all cases this identification is an *ex post facto* consideration, rather than a motivating force, and their satisfaction with being childless is related to concerns other than to their contribution to the population crisis.

It is sometimes suggested that an inclination to avoid motherhood is a logical extension of the new feminism. It is difficult to generalize about a social phenomenon as amorphous as the woman's liberation movement, a rubric which incorporates many diverse and even contradictory attitudes. However, "A significant feature of the woman's liberation movement is that, although its demands have been made on the basis of equity for women, it has not usually been anti-marriage or anti-children" (Commission for Population and the American Future, 1972:68). In fact, in many cases the ideologies expressed are actually pro-natal. Considerable concern is expressed with the problems involved in combining successful motherhood with comparable success in other careers. However, motherhood is not perceived as an unfulfilling and unrewarding experience; rather, it is perceived as a positive experience which, although desirable, is not sufficient in and of itself for maximum self-actualization. Rather than advising women to abandon motherhood careers, the new feminist literature advises them to consider other careers in addition to motherhood, and advocates changes in society which would make the motherhood role easier. For example, there is considerable stress on the provision of maternity leaves, on increased involvement of fathers in childcare, on accessability to adequate day care facilities. Although advocates of the new feminism may provide some support for the idea that motherhood is neither necessary nor sufficient for fulfillment, they do still advocate that normally it will be an important part of that fulfillment. Only a few of the voluntarily childless are at all concerned with women's liberation, and these few apparently came into the movement after their decision was made and their lifestyle was established.

Although none of the voluntarily childless are actively seeking group support for their life style, many would welcome the opportunity to become involved in a truly supportive social movement. The first example of such an association is the National Organization for Non-Parents (NON) * which was formed in California in 1971. Because of the state of pluralistic ignorance which surrounds voluntary childlessness, and because of the inadequacy of demographic and feminist movements in expressing the world view of the childless, such attempts to formulate a counter culture might be expected to be very successful.

Summary

The present research on a purposive sample of 52 voluntarily childless wives is exploratory in nature. Although it is not possible to make definitive statements regarding the nature of childless couples, several tentative conclusions are offered. It is suggested that couples come to be voluntarily childless by a number of diverse paths beginning both before and after marriage, and that considerable diversity might be expected between those who enter marriage only on the condition of a clear childlessness clause in the marriage contract, and those who remain childless after a series of postponements of parenthood. Although considerable social pressures are directed towards the childless, most of the individuals involved appear to be very well defended against such sanctions, and the mechanisms of re-defining situations and of protecting themselves are worthy of further study. One such mechanism appears to be the use of the possibility of adoption to deny the status of voluntary childlessness while not seriously threatening the accompanying life style. Finally, it is suggested that existing social movements do not provide much relevant support for the voluntarily childless, and that an explicit counter culture, such as the National Organization for Non-Parents, might be expected to meet with considerable success.

* The National Organization for Non-Parents now has national headquarters in Baltimore, Maryland.

24

Voluntary Childlessness: A Neglected Area of Family Study

J. E. VEEVERS

Sociologist, University of Western Ontario, London, Ontario

Studies of the family have tended to focus on some aspects of the institution to the exclusion of other pertinent topics. One area subject to such "selective inattention" is the phenomenon of childlessness, especially voluntary childlessness. Empirical research on childlessness would provide a necessary control group for analyses of motivations for parenthood, and of the effects of children on personal and marital adjustment. In addition, knowledge of the conditions under which voluntary childlessness constitutes a viable and satisfactory alternate life style would have wide reaching implications for more rational advice giving in marital counseling and for new alternatives for population control programs.

Ideally, the study of the family should be equally concerned with all phenomena which are relevant for a comprehensive and accurate description of the institution. In reality, the study of family behavior has focused upon some topics to the virtual exclusion of related aspects. Because social science is relatively young, and because the resources and facilities for research are limited, it is inevitable that some topics will not yet have been fully explored, and some relevant data will not yet have been collected. It is suggested, however, that although some omissions may be due simply to random oversight and error ". . . persistent avoidance by a group of scholars of *pertinent* topics is not purely or chiefly accidental." (Dexter, 1958, 176) The subjects selected for study in the field of marriage and the family reflect to a large extent the value preferences and biases of the social scientists involved. Instead of re-

The Family Coordinator, April 1973

searching with equal enthusiasm all questions which are theoretically interesting, they choose to focus the most extensive research on those questions which are congruent with the dominant norms, and which are supportive of their own value preferences. The present paper is concerned with the consequences of such "selective inattention" (Dexter, 1958) for the study of parenthood.[1]

The study of those aspects of the family pertaining to parenthood reflects systematic bias due to the pervasive influence of two important mores regarding procreation: one, the norm that married people should have children; and two, the norm that they should want to have them and should rejoice at the prospect of becoming parents. (Veevers, 1972a) In analyzing procreation, it is useful to classify all couples in a four-fold typology in terms of these two norms. Conforming couples who both want to have children and who actually have them do not pose a threat to conventional values, and consequently have been intensively studied. (LeMasters, 1970; Kellmer-Pringle, 1967) Some attention has been paid to those unfortunate couples who accidentally become parents of unplanned and unwanted children. (Osborn, 1963; Pohlman, 1969) In contrast, childless couples have either been completely ignored, or have received relatively little attention. Most family textbooks do not touch on the phenomenon of childlessness at all. (Kirkendall, 1968) When it is discussed, it is generally in terms of involuntary childlessness. Typically, an estimate of the incidence of childlessness is followed by a discussion of factors contributing to subfecundity and sterility, revealing an implicit assumption that fecundity problems are the only cause of childlessness, and that something should be done to help the childless couple. (Kephart, 1966; Landis and Landis, 1968; Landis, 1970) The phenomenon of voluntarily childless couples who are deviant from the dominant mores both in terms of their behavior and of their motivation has been virtually ignored.

"Significant advances in science have sometimes taken place when someone has realized that a problem hitherto neglected or excluded does in fact fit into the methods and techniques of his discipline." (Dexter, 1958, 176) It is suggested that the processes of selective inattention which have led to neglect of the topic of childlessness are unfortunate in that the study of childlessness is potentially of considerable import for the study of parenthood in general, and for the practical application of family study in counseling and policy making.

The study of the family is concerned with at least three related questions concerning parenthood. One, why do people assume parental roles? Two, what effect does parenthood have upon marital adjustment and the man-woman relationship? Three, what effect does parenthood have upon personal adjustment? In attempting to answer these questions, it is important to remember that one way of stimulating the imagination is by studying polar types. "Often you get the best insights by considering extremes—by thinking of the opposite of that with which you are directly concerned." (Mills, 1959, 214) In any attempt to systematically and empirically describe a phenomenon, some of the essential elements are drawn from contrasting that phenomenon with a comparable control group. In studying the impact of one element of family life on other elements, it is important to be able to hold other factors constant, and to manipulate only one aspect at a time. Sociological studies of the causes and effects of parenthood have generally failed to consider adequate control groups. How can one make definite assertions about the impact of children unless he has also examined a number of cases where the impact was not felt, and has observed concomitant variations? It is suggested that an intensive study of voluntarily childless couples would be an invaluable source of information about the reasons that people become parents, and the effects their parental roles have on their life adjustments.

Socialization for Parental Roles

Instinct versus Socialization

Some theorists have postulated the existence of a maternal instinct which provides the basic impetus for the bearing and raising of children. (Fletcher, 1968) Others have applied the same basic assumptions more broadly and have speculated on the influence of a more general parental instinct or impulse. (Kephart, 1966) The careful examination of voluntarily childless couples would provide an opportunity to assess the universality of such instincts, if they do exist, and the conditions under which they may be expected to be most compelling. Recently, social scientists have tended to discard the idea that parenthood is instinctive or inevitable or both and have postulated that individuals must be taught to aspire to parental roles. If such is the case, then the socialization processes involved are critically important for society. Unfortunately, little is known of the conditions under which such socialization is most successful. A comparison of the early family experience of individuals who did not learn to want children with the family experience of conforming individuals would provide vital cues as to the kinds of socialization most likely to produce a compelling desire to have and rear children.

Motivations for Parenthood

If desire for procreation is learned rather than instinctive, it becomes meaningful to examine systematically the plurality of reasons why people might want children. The basic value biases of researchers are reflected in their tendency to offer respondents their choice of reasons for wanting children, but not to inquire as to their reasons for wanting to avoid them. (Rabin and Greene, 1968) Parenthood implies a number of disadvantages as well as advantages and in many if not most cases the desire for children is somewhat ambivalent. (Kirkpatrick, 1963, 504–535) The only available description of the motivations of voluntarily childless couples is based on the perceptions of friends and relatives, rather than on interviews with the couples themselves. (Popenoe, 1936) Valid information concerning the motivations of voluntarily childless couples for not having children would give some insight into the dissatisfactions and resentments of those who do have them. (Jacoby, 1969; LeMasters, 1970)

The study of voluntary childlessness may be related to parental motivations in yet another way. A number of authors have observed that the stereotype of childlessness held by the general public depicts people without children in generally negative terms. (Pohlman, 1970; LeMasters, 1970) No empirical work has been done concerning the existence of a stereotype of childless couples. However, if, as many authors predict, such a stereotype does exist, it may be a significant factor in the motivation of people to have children. If the childless are believed to be unhappy, selfish, lonely, immature, and emotionally unstable, then perhaps some people have children in order to avoid such negative traits and/or negative images. (Pohlman, 1966)

Social Pressures Encouraging Fertility

In the early part of the century, Hollingworth (1916) outlined a number of social pressures exerted on women to have and to rear children. Similar social pressures still exist today and may have some influence in individual decisions regarding fertility. One method of identifying and analyzing the nature of such pressures would be to examine the numerous informal social sanctions directed toward childless couples. Although no conclusive evidence is available, informal interviews and testimonials in the popular press would seem to suggest that childless couples are subject to a considerable degree of social pressure to have children. (Balchin, 1965; Greene, 1963; Michels, 1970; Pohlman, 1970; Rollin, 1970; Peck, 1971) Such mechanisms of social control may be extreme examples of the kind of pressure exerted on parental couples to have a second, a third, or even a fourth child.

Desired Family Size

Demographers and sociologists have long been concerned with the differences between those people who desire relatively small families compared with those who want to have many children. The research in this area is somewhat biased by the fact that informants are asked: "How many children do you want to have?" rather than the equally relevant query: "Do you want to have *any* children?" The couple who choose to forego having children entirely can be heuristically viewed as the result of the many pressures toward small families carried to their logical extreme. It is possible that the factors which effect the choice of some-children or no-children may be directly related to factors which effect the preference for five or six children rather than two or three. Demographers implicitly acknowledge this similarity when they group individuals who want fewer than two children into a general category of low parity. (Westoff and Potvin, 1967) Knowledge about factors associated with a preference for childlessness may also be relevant to discussions of preference for other family sizes.

The Effect of Children on Marital Adjustment

Husband-Wife Dynamics

Although Feldman (1965) suggests that childless couples tend to enjoy more satisfactory marital relationships than their parental counterparts, on the basis of data from a number of contradictory studies it seems evident that the presence or absence of children *per se* is not consistently related to good or bad marital adjustment. (Udry, 1966) However, in addition to the overall evaluation of marital interaction, sociologists and marriage counselors are interested in the qualitative changes in patterns of adjustment and role-playing which accompany different stages in the life cycle. Since most couples do have children, it is difficult to determine which of the observed changes are due to the presence of children and which are simply due to the passage of time and increased exposure to and familiarity with each other. Experts such as Kirkpatrick (1963) can list the probable effects of childbirth on the family in a convincing and plausible way, but until one explicitly compares childless and parental couples controlling for length of marriage and other factors, such work is purely speculative.

Although the adjustment of childless couples may not be significantly better than the adjustment of their parental counterparts, it is still quite possible that the dynamics of husband-wife interaction are different for couples who are alone than for couples who share not only marriage but parenthood as well. Students of the family have always recognized the importance of comparing and contrasting dominant patterns of family organization with parallel patterns in other societies. Both the cross-cultural and the historical approaches are valued not only for the new information they provide but also for their comparative perspectives which make it possible to view the contemporary family in the context of other family forms. A great deal of research has been devoted to the description and explanation of conforming, conventional "normal" families, and of the life styles associated with them. The voluntarily childless couples who present *The Case Against Having Children* (Silverman and Silverman, 1971) or who offer warnings about *The Baby Trap* (Peck, 1971) are casting not only a "Vote Against Motherhood" (Greene, 1963) but also a vote for a different kind of life style. In a pluralistic society, it is of interest to examine and compare a variety of life styles including deviant and minority preferences as well as conforming and majority ones.

The Decision to Divorce

Although there is a clear relationship between childlessness and divorce, most experts agree that the correlation is a spurious rather than a causal one, reflecting the simple fact that most divorces occur in the early years of marriage before children are born in any case. (Udry, 1966; Williamson, 1966) The concern with divorce as a social problem has led to wide speculation regarding the factors involved in the decision to get a divorce. Marital happiness or unhappiness is recognized as only one of many variables. Do some couples remain together "for the sake of the children" as the folklore suggests? Do some childless couples seek divorce because they have not become parents? Are some divorces initiated because of the children? Are some kinds of people simply more divorce-prone than others? If one is to understand adequately the divorce decision it is necessary to compare unhappy couples who seek divorce with equally unhappy couples who decide to endure, controlling for as many variables as possible. One crucial variable is having or not having children.

The Effect of Children on Personal Adjustment

Parenthood and Maturity

Social scientists and laymen both make an implicit assumption that wanting and having children are necessary for development to full maturity. Childless people, especially the voluntarily childless, tend to be perceived as not quite mature and as lacking in full adult status. (Williamson, 1966) For example, Duvall (1962) lists "competency in bearing and raising children" as a necessary developmental task. Erikson considers "generativity" to be: "an essential state in the psychosexual as well as the psychosocial schedule." (1963, 267) Because of the limited research on childlessness, it has not been established whether or not people without children are more or less mature than parents. If such a relationship could be established, it would be interesting to then try to determine if the correlation reflected causation, and in what direction. Does the absence of children prevent people from reaching their full maturity, or do immature people express their immaturity by not having children?

Parenthood and Emotional Stability

The frequently expressed opinion that childlessness is associated with emotional instability and maladjustment has not been substantiated by research. (Pohlman, 1970) As with the issue of maturity, even if such a correlation could be established the direction of the relationship would remain unclear. Are parents relatively stable and adjusted because they have had children, or was their good adjustment an important factor in their decision to have children in the first place? Although family life experts occasionally do advise childlessness under some conditions (Womble, 1966; Blood, 1969; Lantz and Snyder, 1969; Landis, 1970; LeMasters, 1970) most implicitly endorse the folklore assumption that it is in the best interests of every married person to have at least one child. While parenthood may in fact be rewarding in many cases, it cannot automatically be assumed that having children necessarily maximizes the life chances of all individuals. If information were available concerning the circumstances under which voluntarily childless couples can achieve satisfactory social and psychological adjustment, perhaps psychologists and marriage counselors could offer more realistic guidelines regarding the kinds of individuals most likely to enjoy children and the kinds of situations most conducive to rewarding parent-child relationships.

Voluntary Childlessness and the Study of Population

Demographic Trends

Although there is a very high degree of consensus regarding the desirability of procreation, there still remains a deviant minority of individuals who deliberately do not become parents. Of all women who ever marry, at least one in twenty and perhaps as many as one in ten never become mothers. (Pohlman, 1970; Veevers, 1972c) Of these, approximately half are childless by choice. (Veevers, 1972c) Common sense would indicate that the incidence of childlessness in western society might be expected to increase. The changing status and role of women, the improvement in birth control technology, the persistent trends toward greater urbanization, and the growing awareness of population pressures could all be expected to influence more and more couples to decide not to have any children. In spite of these trends, exactly the reverse has happened. Since about 1940, there has been a steady and persistent decline in the incidence of childlessness, especially voluntary childlessness. (Whelpton, Campbell, and Patterson, 1966; Veevers, 1972c) [2] For example, a recent survey of more than 1600 married women in Toronto indicated that only 1.1 percent desired to remain childless. (Balakrishnan et al, 1972) The decline in rates of voluntary childlessness provides an unusual problem for students of human fertility. With the exception of race (Veevers, 1971a) childlessness tends to be influenced in the expected direction by the major socio-demographic determinants known to influence fertility in general. (Grabill and Glick, 1959; Veevers, 1971b, 1971c) Changes in the incidence of childlessness do not appear to be related to concurrent changes in the age at first marriage. (Veevers, 1972b) The paradoxical decline of rates of childlessness has not yet been adequately explained, and a complete examination of this problem must await further information on the nature and characteristics of voluntarily childless couples.

The Population Explosion

Growing concern with the problem of population has stimulated the search for a solution which will reduce the rate of population growth without seriously interfering with precious individual rights and freedoms. Meier argues very convincingly that: "The most feasible procedure for halting population growth and thereafter maintaining equilibrium (coincident with a policy of increasing the apparent freedom of choice in the society) would be to increase the social position of the infertile segment of the population." (1958, 175) Most approaches to the population crisis have involved persuading women to have fewer children and have not been spectacularly successful. The efficacy of such campaigns might be improved by a complimentary approach involving persuading some women to give up having children altogether, and rewarding rather than punishing them for that decision.

Summary and Conclusions

Although theoretically all aspects of the family are appropriate topics for sociological investigation, in practice sociologists have tended to focus upon those particular aspects which, because of their own values, they find especially interesting and to ignore other aspects which are equally pertinent to the discipline. The study of parenthood reflects such "selective inattention." In North American culture, two main mores regarding procreation specify that married couples should want children and should actually have them. Conforming couples do not pose a threat to conventional values and so have been the object of considerable interest and research. Couples who have had children accidentally, or who have wanted children but been unable to bear them, have received less extensive attention. Couples who deviate from both mores, who neither have children nor want to have them, have been virtually ignored. A comprehensive description and analysis of the characteristics of voluntarily childless couples would constitute a significant contribution to the study of the family, both as a deviant minority group of intrinsic interest, and as a basis for contrast and comparison with the conventional conforming majority.

A number of issues relevant to the study of parenthood have not yet been adequately resolved. Very little is known about the motivations for parenthood. Many aspects of this issue would be elucidated by deviant case analysis of individuals who do not wish to become parents. For example, what kinds of instinct or socialization lead to a strong desire for parenthood? What are the reasons for wanting or not wanting children? What kinds of incentives does the society offer to encourage people to accept parental roles? What determines the number of children people want? Given the world wide trend to smaller families, why is the incidence of childlessness decreasing rather than increasing? If there is concern about population pressures, is it feasible to encourage more people to remain childless?

Relatively little is known about the effects of children on individuals. In order to adequately test the available theories, it is necessary to compare individuals who have and who have not had children, controlling for as many other variables as possible. How can it be known whether or not children increase emotional maturity and stability if the personal adjustment of parents and nonparents have never been compared? How can the effects of children on marital adjustment be known unless childless husbands and wives are compared with mothers and fathers, and differences observed in their interaction patterns? The intensive study of voluntarily childless couples would provide a much needed control group for the study of parental couples and tell a great deal not only about those who are childless by choice, but about mothers and fathers as well. For those students of the family who are oriented toward active participation in family dynamics,. it would provide a more realistic and rational basis for the advice concerning parenthood which is dispensed to individuals, and for the general policies concerning procreation which are advocated to official control agencies.

Notes and References

Chapter 2

1. *Vital Statistics of the United States,* Vol. I-Natality, 1968, pp. 1–15. By January 1, 1969, women aged 35–39 had borne 3,124 children per 1,000 women. If it were possible to relate this cumulative cohort fertility to *ever-married* women only, we would find that births per ever-married women (what we think of as "family size") were considerably higher.

2. Tomas Frejka, "Reflections on the Demographic Conditions Needed to Establish a U.S. Stationary Population Growth," *Population Studies,* Vol. 22 (November 1968), pp. 379–397.

3. See, for example, Garrett Hardin, "The Tragedy of the Commons," *Science,* Vol. 162, pp.1243–1248; Paul R. Ehrlich and Anne H. Ehrlich, *Population, Resources, Environment* (San Francisco: W.H. Freeman & Co., 1970), pp. 254–256 and 272–274; and Kenneth Boulding, *The Meaning of the 20th Century* (New York: Harper and Row, 1964).

4. Frank W. Notestein, "Zero Population Growth," *Population Index,* Vol. 36 (October-December 1970), p. 448.

5. Conditional factors affecting rates are, for example, involuntary infecundity or the inability to find a mate because of an imbalance in the sex ratio due to migration. Conditional factors are those over which the individual has no control—his efforts cannot affect them, hence, his motives are not relevant to the outcome.

6. Ernest W. Burgess and Paul Wallin, "Idealization, Love, and Self-Esteem," reprinted in *Family Roles and Interaction,* Jerold Heiss (ed.), (Chicago: Rand McNally, 1969), pp. 121–122.

7. For a cross-culture analysis (based on almost 50 primitive and modern societies of sex-role differentiation, see Morris Zelditch, Jr., "Role Differentiation in the Nuclear Family: A Comparative Study," in Talcott Parsons and Robert F. Bales (eds.), *Family, Socialization and Interaction Process* (Glencoe, Illinois: The Free Press, 1955), pp. 309–351. For a discussion of contrasts between Europe and the United States, see, Judith Blake, "Demographic Science and the Redirection of Population Policy," in Mindel C. Sheps and Jeanne Clare Ridley, *Public Health and Population Change,* (Pittsburgh: University of Pittsburgh Press, 1965), pp. 41–69; and "Parental Control, Delayed Marriage, and Population Policy."

8. Robert W. Smuts, *Women and Work in America* (New York: Columbia University Press, 1959), pp. 110–155.

9. Betty R. Stirling, "The Interrelation of Changing Attitudes and Changing Conditions with Reference to the Labor Force Participation of Wives," unpublished Ph.D. dissertation, University of California, Berkeley, 1963, pp. 6–72.

10. *Ibid.*, pp. 73–81.

11. *Ibid.*, pp. 180–183.

12. National Manpower Council, *Womanpower* (New York: Columbia University Press, 1957), pp. 15–16.

13. Valerie K. Oppenheimer, "The Interaction of Demand and Supply and its Effect on the Female Labor Force in the United States," *Population Studies*, Vol. XXI (November 1967), pp. 239–259.

14. Smuts, *op. cit.*, p. 109.

15. See, for example, Dorothy Gies McGuigan, *A Dangerous Experiment. 100 Years of Women at the University of Michigan* (Ann Arbor: Center for Continuing Education of Women, 1970).

16. Mabel Newcomer, *A Century of Higher Education for American Women* (New York: Harper & Brothers, 1959), p. 210.

17. *Ibid.*, pp. 146–147.

18. *Ibid.*, p. 60.

19. Lynn White, Jr., *Educating our Daughters* (New York: Harper & Bros., 1950), pp. 46–48.

20. *Ibid.*, pp. 46–47.

21. William O'Neill, *Everyone Was Brave: The Rise and Fall of Feminism in America* (New York: Quadrangle Books, 1968), p. 37.

22. White, *op. cit.*, pp. 71–76.

23. *Ibid.*, p. 76.

24. *Ibid.*, pp. 93–96.

25. *Ibid.*, p. 101.

26. Mirra Komarovsky, *Women in the Modern World* (Boston: Little, Brown & Company, 1953), pp. 66–67.

27. *Ibid.*, pp. 68–69, 69–71, 72. The underlining is mine.

28. Rose K. Goldsen, Morris Rosenberg, Robin M. Williams, Jr., and Edward A. Suchman, *What College Students Think* (Princeton, New Jersey: Princeton University Press, 1960), pp. 46–47.

29. *Ibid.*, pp. 47–49.

30. *Ibid.*, p. 58.

31. *Ibid.*, pp. 58–59.

32. *Ibid.*, p. 90.

33. *Ibid.*, p. 48.

34. *Ibid.*, p. 53.

35. It should be noted that, as might be expected, the non-college sample of 18–24-year-olds is more pronatalist in its attitudes than the college group.

36. Betty Friedan, *The Feminine Mystique* (New York: Dell Publishing, 1963), pp. 381–382. Italics mine.

37. Alice S. Rossi, "Equality Between the Sexes: An Immodest Proposal," *Daedalus* (Spring, 1964), p. 610.

38. *Ibid.*, pp. 639–646.

39. Cynthia Fuchs Epstein, *Woman's Place* (Berkeley and Los Angeles: University of California Press, 1970), pp. 99–100.

40. See William H. Whyte, "The Wife Problem," *Life* (January 7, 1952), reprinted in Robert F. Winch, Robert McGinnis, and Herbert R. Baringer (eds.), *Selected Studies in Marriage and the Family* (New York: Holt, Rinehart, Winston, 1962), pp. 111–126.

41. Robert Kingsley, "What are the Proper Grounds for Granting Annulments?" *Law and Contemporary Problems* (Vol. 18, 1953), pp. 40–41.

42. For a discussion of American family law and the shift "from a patriarchal family structure to one in which the spouses are more nearly equal as between themselves but dominant in their legal relations with their children," see Herma H. Kay, "The Outside Substitute for the Family," reprinted in John N. Edwards (ed.), *The Family and Change* (New York: Knopf, 1969), pp. 261–269. Kay also documents indications that "the future path of legal development will be directed toward the emergence of thc child as a person in his own right." p. 266.

43. O'Neill, *op. cit.*, pp. 30–36.

44. Carl N. Degler, "Revolution Without Ideology: The Changing Place of Women in America," *Daedalus* (Spring, 1964), p. 668.

45. Dr. Clara Thompson, a psychiatrist writing in the 1940's, was one of the first to question systematically and objectively the Freudian description of female psychology. See her, "Cultural Pressures in the Psychology of Women," reprinted in Patrick Mullahy (ed.), *A Study of Interpersonal Relations* (New York: Hermitage Press, 1949), pp. 130–146. Mirra Komarovsky has also analyzed the effect of Freudianism on sex role definitions. In particular, she has noted the influence on the mass media of the Freudian characterization of the neurotic, unfulfilled career woman (the "Lady in the Dark") who loses by being successful. See Mirra Komarovsky, *Women in the Modern World* (Boston: Little, Brown, 1953), pp. 31–52. Philip Rieff also analyzed and criticized Freud's feminine psychology in *Freud: The Mind of the Moralist* (Garden City, New York: Doubleday, 1961), pp. 191–204. This book was first published in 1959. The woman's liberation movement of the 1960's has engaged in far more detailed criticisms of Freudian psychology. Among the more penetrating are those of Betty Friedan and Kate Millet. See, Betty Friedan, *The Feminine Mystique* (New York: Dell Publishing Co., 1963), Chapter 5; and Kate Millett, *Sexual Politics* (Garden City, New York: Doubleday, 1970), pp. 176–220.

46. See Sigmund Freud, *New Introductory Lectures on Psychoanalysis,* translated by J. H. Sprott, (New York: W. W. Norton & Co., Inc., 1933); *Three Contributions to the Theory of Sex,* translated by A. A. Brill, (New York and Washington, D.C.: Nervous and Mental Disease Publishing Company, 1920); Analysis Terminable and Interminable," *The International Journal of Psychoanalysis,* Vol. XVIII, October 1937,

pp. 373–405. "Some Psychological Consequences of the Anatomical Differences Between the Sexes," in *Collected Papers of Sigmund Freud,* Joan Riviere (ed.), (New York: Basic Books, 1959, Vol. IV); and "Female Sexuality," *Collected Papers,* Volume V. For post-Freudian works in the same vein of fulfillment-through-motherhood, see Helene Deutsch, *The Psychology of Women* (New York: Grune and Stratton, 1945, 2 volumes); and Erik H. Erikson, "Inner and Outer Space: Reflections on Womanhood" (*Daedalus,* 93, 1964), pp. 582–606.

47. The pro-motherhood bias in modern erotic literature has been noted by many. The unmistakable "message" of modern sexually uninhibited literature is that most women's problems can readily be solved by copulation and impregnation—a primal fix. For a discussion of Freud's influence on some important literary figures, see, Kate Millett, *Sexual Politics, op. cit.,* pp. 237–313 and Betty Friedan, *The Feminine Mystique, op. cit.,* pp. 174–196, and 247–270.

48. Philip Rieff, *Freud: The Mind of the Moralist* (Garden City, New York: Doubleday, 1961), p. xxi.

49. Talcott Parsons and Robert F. Bales, *Family, Socialization and Interaction Process* (Glencoe, Illinois: Free Press, 1955), pp. 21–22.

50. Theodore Lidz, "Family Organization and Personality Structure," reprinted in Norman W. Bell and Ezra F. Vogel (eds.), *A Modern Introduction to the Family,* revised edition (New York: Free Press, 1969). Underlining mine.

51. Irving Bieber, *Homosexuality. A Psychoanalytical Study* (New York: Vintage Books, 1962), p. 18.

52. Such as the Bieber study cited in the previous footnote.

53. See Bieber's discussion of the studies by Hooker, and Charles and Block. *Ibid.,* pp. 17–18, and 305–336. A recent study by Evans replicates the Bieber study using individuals who had never sought psychotherapy. See Ray B. Evans, "Childhood Parental Relationships of Homosexual Men," *Journal of Consulting and Clinical Psychology,* Vol. 33, 1969, pp. 129–135.

54. Alfred C. Kinsey *et al., Sexual Behavior in the Human Male* (Philadelphia: W. B. Saunders, 1948), and Clellan S. Ford and Frank A. Beach, *Patterns of Sexual Behavior* (New York: Harper, 1951).

55. Robert F. Bales and Philip E. Slater, "Role Differentiation in Small Decision-Making Groups," in Talcott Parsons and Robert F. Bales (eds.), *Family, Socialization and Interaction Process* (Glencoe, Illinois: "The Free Press, 1955), pp. 259–306.

56. Morris Zelditch, Jr., "Role Differentiation in the Nuclear Family: A Comparative Study," in Talcott Parsons and Robert F. Bales, *op. cit.,* pp. 309–351. Zelditch's data on the similarities of sex role differentiation are based on almost 50 primitive and modern societies.

57. See, for example, Melford E. Spiro, *Kibbutz, Venture in Utopia* (New York: Schoken Books, 1963), and, by the same author, *Children of the Kibbutz* (New York: Schoken Books, 1965) especially Chapters 4 and 5.

58. Talcott Parsons, "Age and Sex in the Social Structure of the

United States," in Talcott Parsons (ed.), *Essays in Sociological Theory Pure and Applied* (Glencoe, Illinois: The Free Press, 1949), pp. 218–232.

59. Talcott Parsons, "The American Family: Its Relations to Personality and to Social Structure," in Talcott Parsons and Robert F. Bales, *op. cit.*, pp. 14–15.

60. Parsons, *Ibid.*, p. 15.

61. Leo Kanowitz, *Women and the Law* (Albuquerque: University of New Mexico Press, 1969).

62. *Ibid.*, p. 3.

63. *Ibid.*, p. 152.

64. *Ibid.*, p. 153.

65. *Ibid.*, p. 154.

66. Mirra Komarovsky, "Cultural Contradictions and Sex Roles," reprinted in, Hyman Rodman (ed.) *Marriage, Family, and Society* (New York: Random House, 1965), p. 24.

67. *Ibid.*, pp. 27–28.

68. John P. McKee and Alex C. Sherriffs, "Men's and Women's Beliefs, Ideals, and Self-Concepts," *American Journal of Sociology*, Vol. LXIV (January 1959), pp. 356–363.

69. *Ibid.*, pp. 359–361.

70. J. P. McKee and A. C. Sherriffs, "The Differential Evaluation of Males and Females," *Journal of Personality*, Vol. XXV (1957), pp. 356–371; and, A. C. Sherriffs and J. P. McKee, "Qualitative Aspects of Beliefs about Men and Women," *Journal of Personality*, Vol. XXV (1957), pp. 451–464.

71. Paul Rosenkrantz, Helen Bee, Susan Vogel, Inge Broverman, and Donald Broverman, "Sex-Role Stereotypes and Self-Concepts in College Students," *Journal of Consulting and Clinical Psychology*, Vol. 32 (1968), pp. 287–293.

72. *Ibid.*, p. 291.

73. *Ibid.*, p. 293.

74. Inge K. Broverman, Donald M. Broverman, Frank E. Clarkson, Paul S. Rosenkrantz, and Susan R. Vogel, "Sex-Role Stereotypes and Clinical Judgments of Mental Health," *Journal of Consulting and Clinical Psychology*, Vol. 34 (1970) pp. 1–7.

75. *Ibid.*, pp. 4–5.

76. *Ibid.*, p. 5.

77. *Ibid.*, p. 6.

78. Paul H. Mussen, John J. Conger, and Jerome Kagan, *Child Development and Personality* (New York: Harper & Row, 1963), p. 261.

79. *Ibid.*, p. 263.

80. *Ibid.*, p. 263.

81. *Ibid.*, pp. 272–273, and pp. 370–372.

82. *Ibid.*, p. 372.

83. *Ibid.*, p. 372.

84. James S. Coleman, *The Adolescent Society* (New York: Free Press, 1961).

Chapter 3

Albrecht, Milton C. 1956. "Does Literature Reflect Common Values?" *American Sociological Review* 21:722–729.

Berelson, Bernard and Patricia J. Salter, 1946. "Majority and Minority Americans: An Analysis of Magazine Fiction," *Public Opinion Quarterly* 10:168–190.

Blake, Judith, 1969. "Population Policy for Americans: Is the Government Being Misled?" *Science* 164:522–529.

Clarkson, Frank E. et al., 1970. "Family Size and Sex Role Stereotypes," *Science* 167:390–392.

Davis, Kingley, 1967. "Population Policy: Will Current Programs Succeed?" *Science* 158:730–739.

Franzwa, Helen H., In Press. "Female Roles in Women's Magazine Fiction," in Rhoda Unger and Florence Denmark (eds.) *Woman: Dependent or Independent Variable,* Chicago: Aldine-Atherton.

Hoffman, Lois Wladis and Frederick Wyatt, 1960. "Social Change and Motivation for Having Larger Families," *Merrill-Palmer Quarterly* 6:235–244.

Hollingworth, Leta S., 1916. "Social Devices for Impelling Women to Bear and Rear Children," *American Journal of Sociology,* 22:10–29.

Johns-Heine, Patricke and Hans H. Gerth, 1949. "Values in Mass Periodical Fiction, 1921–1940," *Public Opinion Quarterly* 13:105–113.

Konsinski, Jerry, 1973. "Packaged Passion," *American Scholar* 42:193–204.

Leavitt, Susan, 1973. "The Image of Women in Women's Magazine Fiction, 1971–1972," Hunter College, unpublished paper.

Middleton, Russell, 1963. "Fertility Values in American Magazine Fiction, 1916–1956," *Public Opinion Quarterly* 24:356–371.

Peck, Ellen, 1971. *The Baby Trap*. New York: Pinnacle Books.

Ross, E. A., 1901. *Social Control: A Survey of the Foundations of Order*. New York: Macmillan.

Simmons, W. R. et al., 1963–1973. *Selective Markets and the Media Reaching Them*. New York: W. R. Simmons and Associates Research, Inc.

Warner, W. Lloyd and William E. Henry, 1948. "The Radio Day Time Serial: A Symbolic Analysis," *Genetic Psychology Monographs,* 37: 3–71.

Chapter 6

Chester, R., 1971a. The duration of marriage to divorce. *Br. J. Sociol.* **22,** 174.

Chester, R., 1971b. Contemporary trends in the stability of English marriage. *J. biosoc. Sci.* **3,** 389.

Chester, R., 1972a. Some characteristics of marriages of brief duration. *Med. Gynaecol. & Sociol.* **6,** 9.

Chester, R., 1972b. Current trends in marital breakdown. *Postgrad. med. J.* **48,** 529.

Day, L. H., 1964. Patterns of divorce in Australia and the United States. *Am. Sociol. Rev.* **29,** 509.
Dominian, J., 1968. *Marital Breakdown.* Penguin Books, Harmondsworth.
Farmer, M., 1970. *The Family.* Longmans, London.
Fletcher, R., 1966. *The Family and Marriage in Britain.* Penguin Books, Harmondsworth.
General Register Office, 1961. *Census.* Fertility Tables. HM Stationery Office, London.
General Register Office, 1964. *Registrar General's Statistical Review of England and Wales.* HM Stationery Office, London.
Hicks, M. W. & Platt, M., 1970. Marital happiness and stability: a review of research in the sixties. *J. Marriage and Fam.* **32,** 553.
Humphrey, M., 1969. *The Hostage Seekers.* Longmans, London.
Jacobson, P. H., 1950. Differentials in divorce by duration of marriage and size of family. *Am. Sociol. Rev.* **15,** 235.
Johns, E. A., 1965. *The Social Structure of Modern Britain.* Pergamon Press, Oxford.
Kephart, W. M., 1954. The duration of marriage. *Am. Sociol. Rev.* **19,** 287.
Kinsey, A. C., Pomeroy, W. B., Martin, C. E. & Gebhard, P.H., 1953. *Sexual Behavior in the Human Female.* Saunders, Philadelphia.
Klein, J., 1968. *Samples from English Cultures,* 2 vols. Routledge and Kegan Paul, London.
Marsden, D., 1969. *Mothers Alone.* Allen Lane, London.
McGregor, O. R., Blom-Cooper, L. & Gibson, C., 1970. *Separated Spouses.* Duckworth, London.
Monahan, T. P., 1952. How stable are remarriages? *Am. J. Sociol.* **58,** 280.
Monahan, T. P., 1955. Is childlessness related to family stability? *Am. Sociol. Rev.* **20,** 446.
Monahan, T. P., 1958. The changing nature and instability of remarriages. *Eugen. Q.* **5,** 73.
Rowntree, G. & Carrier, N., 1958. The resort to divorce in England and Wales 1858–1957. *Popul. Stud.* **11,** 188.
Schofield, M., 1965. *The Sexual Behaviour of Young People.* Longmans, London.
Slater, E. & Woodside, M., 1951. *Patterns of Marriage.* Cassell, London.
Turner, C., 1969. *Family and Kinship in Modern Britain.* Routledge and Kegan Paul, London.
Walker, K. & Whitney, O., 1965. *The Family and Marriage in a Changing World.* Gollancz, London.

Chapter 7

1. E. W. Burgess and L. S. Cottrell, Jr., *Predicting Success or Failure in Marriage,* Englewood Cliffs, New Jersey: Prentice-Hall, Inc., 1939, pp. 26–261.

2. J. T. Landis and M. G. Landis, *Building a Successful Marriage,* Englewood Cliffs, New Jersey: Prentice-Hall, Inc., fourth ed., 1963, pp. 466–468; P. H. Landis, *Making the Most of Marriage,* New York: Ap-

pleton-Century-Crofts, third ed., 1965, p. 599; H. R. Lantz and E. C. Synder, *Marriage,* New York: John Wiley and Sons, 1962, p. 299. See also earlier editions of the first two books and H. T. Christensen and R. E. Philbrick, "Family Size as a Factor in the Marital Adjustments of College Students," *American Sociological Review,* 17 (1952), pp. 306–307.

3. Burgess and Cottrell, *op. cit.,* p. 259.

4. R. O. Lang, *A Study of the Degree of Happiness or Unhappiness in Marriage as Rated by Acquaintances of the Married Couples,* unpublished master's thesis, University of Chicago, 1932, pp. 49–50.

5. Landis and Landis, *loc. cit.*

6. J. Bernard, "Developmental Tasks of the NCFR–1963–1988," *Journal of Marriage and the Family,* 26 (1964), pp. 29–38.

7. E. Pohlman, *The Psychology of Birth Planning,* Cambridge, Massachusetts: Schenkman, 1968.

8. Burgess and Cottrell, *op. cit.,* p. 247.

9. *Ibid.,* pp. 247, 260.

10. P. K. Whelpton, A. A. Campbell, and J. Patterson, *Fertility and Family Planning in the United States,* Princeton, New Jersey: Princeton University Press, 1966.

Chapter 10

Balchin, N., 1965. Children are a waste of time. *Sat. Eve. Post.,* October 9.

Beach, F. A., 1948. *Hormones and behavior.* New York: Hoeber.

Benedek, T., 1959. *Parenthood as a developmental phase. J. Am. Psychoanalytic Assn.,* 7. From Rabin, 1965b.

Berent, J., 1953. Relationship between family sizes of two successive generations. *Mil. Men. Fd. Quart.,* 31.

Bernard, J., 1964. Developmental tasks of the NCFR—1963–1988. *J. Marriage Fam.,* 26.

Blake, J., 1966. The Americanization of Catholic reproductive ideals. *Popul. Studies,* 20.

Blood, R. O., and Wolfe, D. M., 1960. *Husbands and wives: the dynamics of married living.* New York: Free Press of Glencoe.

Bossard, J. H. S., and Boll, E. S., 1956. *The large family system.* Philadelphia: Univ. of Pennsylvania Press.

Centers, R., and Blumberg, G. H., 1954. Social and psychological factors in human procreation: a survey approach. *J. soc. Psychol.,* 40.

Christophersen, V. A., and Walters, J., 1958. Responses of Protestants, Catholics, and Jews concerning marriage and family life. *Sociol. soc. Res.,* 43.

Clare, J. E., and Kiser, C. V., 1951. Preference for children of given sex in relation to fertility. In: Whelpton & Kiser (Eds.), 1946–1958.

Deutsch, H., 1945. *Psychology of women.* Vol. Two: *Motherhood.* New York: Grune & Stratton.

Duvall, E. M., 1962. *Family development.* (2nd Ed.) Philadelphia: Lippincott.

FGMA, 1961. Shorthand reference for the first Family Growth in Metropolitan America report, Westoff et. al., 1963.

FGMA, 1963. Shorthand reference for the second Family Growth in Metropolitan America report, Westoff et al., 1963.

Flanagan, J. C., 1942. A study of factors determining family size in a selected professional group. *Genetic Psychol. Monographs,* 25.

Flugel, J. S., 1947b. The psychology of birth control. In: *Men and their motives.* New York: International Universities Press.

GAF, 1959. Shorthand reference for the first Growth of American Families report, Freedman et al., 1959.

GAF, 1966. Shorthand reference for the second Growth of American Families report, Whelpton et al., 1966.

Greene, G., 1963. A vote against motherhood. *Sat. Eve. Post,* Jan. 20.

Gurin, G., Veroff, J., and Feld, S., 1960. *Americans view their mental health: a nationwide interview survey* (Joint Commission on Mental Illness and Health, Monograph series, no. 4). New York: Basic Books, O.P.

Hill, R., Stycos, J. M., and Back, K. W., 1959. *The family and population control: a Puerto Rican experiment in social change.* Chapel Hill, N.C.: Univ. of North Carolina Press.

Hoffman, L. W., and Wyatt, F., 1960. Social change and motivations for having larger families: some theoretical considerations. *Merrill-Palmer Quart.,* 6.

Indianapolis Study, 1946–1958. Abbreviated reference to Whelpton & Kiser (Eds.), 1946–1958.

Itkin, W., 1952. Some relationships between intra-family attitudes and pre-parental attitudes toward children. *J. genetic Psychol.,* 80.

Kantner, J. F., and Potter, R. G., Jr., 1954. The relationship of family size in two successive generations. In: Whelpton & Kiser (Eds.), 1946–1958.

Kroger, W. S., and Freed, S. C., 1962. *Psychosomatic gynecology.* Hollywood, Calif.: Wilshire. Reprinted "edition" of 1951 publication by Saunders, Philadelphia.

Landis, J. T., and Landis, M. G., 1963. *Building a successful marriage.* (4th Ed.) Englewood Cliffs, N.J.: Prentice-Hall.

Landis, J. T., Poffenberger, T., & Poffenberger, S., 1950. The effects of first pregnancy upon the sexual adjustment of 212 couples. *Am. Sociol. Rev.,* 15.

LeMasters, E. E., 1957. Parenthood as crisis. *Marriage Fam. Liv.* 19.

Lorimer, F., 1954. *Culture and human fertility.* Paris: UNESCO.

Mead, M., 1935. *Sex and temperament in three primitive societies.* New York: Morrow.

Mead, M., 1949. *Male and female.* New York: Morrow.

Mehlan, K. H., 1965. Legal abortions in Roumania. *J. Sex Res.,* 1.

Meier, G., 1961. The effect of unwanted pregnancies on a relief load: an exploratory study. *Eugen. Quart.* 8.

Meier, G., 1963. Unwanted pregnancies among a group of relief recipients: a follow-up report on a persisting problem. *Eugen. Quart.*, 10.

Meier, R. L., 1959. *Modern science and the human fertility problem.* New York: Wiley.

Newton, N., 1955. *Maternal emotions.* New York: Paul Hoeber. O.P. Reprinted: Jackson, Miss.: Phronia Craft.

Population Council, 1964b. Turkey: national survey on population. Studies Fam. Planning, No. 5.

Potter, R. G., Jr., and Kantner, J. F., 1955. The influence of siblings and friends on fertility. In: Whelpton & Kiser (Eds.), 1946–1958.

Pratt, L., and Whelpton, P. K., 1955. Interest in and liking for children in relation to fertility planning and size of planned family. In: Whelpton & Kiser (Eds.), 1946–1958.

Rabin, A. I., 1965b. Motivation for parenthood. *J. Projective Techs.*, 29.

Rainwater, L., assisted by Weinstein, K. K., 1960. *And the poor get children.* Chicago: Quadrangle.

Rainwater, L., 1965. *Family design: marital sexuality, family size, and family planning.* Chicago: Aldine.

Reed, R., 1923. Changing conception of the maternal instinct. *J. abnorm. soc. Psychol.*, 18.

Rock., J., 1963. *The time has come.* New York: Knopf.

Ryan, B., 1952. Institutional factors in Sinhalesefertility. *Mil. Mem. Fd. Quart.*, 30.

Sears, R. R., Maccoby, E. E., & Levin, H., 1957. *Patterns of child rearing.* Evanston, Ill.: Row, Peterson.

Seitz, P. F. D., 1958. The maternal instinct in animal subjects: *I Psychosom. Med.*, 20.

Sloman, S. S., 1948. Emotional problems in "planned for" children. *Am. J. Orthopsychiat.*, 18.

Soddy, K., 1964. The unwanted child. *J. Fam. Welfare*, 11.

Solomon, E. S., Clare, J. E., & Westoff, C. F., 1956. Fear of childlessness, desire to avoid an only child, and children's desires for siblings. In: Whelpton & Kiser (Eds.), 1946–1958.

Stycos, J. M., 1958. Some directions for research on fertility control. *Mil. Mem. Fd. Quart.*, 36.

Stycos, J. M., and Back, K. W., 1964. *The control of human fertility in Jamaica.* Ithaca, N.Y.: Cornell Univ. Press.

Swain, M. D., and Kiser, C. V., 1953. The interrelation of fertility, fertility planning, and ego-centered interest in children. In: Whelpton & Kiser (Eds.), 1946–1958.

Wengraf, F., 1953. *Psychosomatic approach to gynecology and obstetrics.* Springfield, Ill.: Thomas.

Westoff, C. F., and Borgatta, E. F., 1955. The prediction of planned fertility. In: Whelpton & Kiser (Eds.), 1946–1958.

Westoff, C. F., Potter, R. G., Jr., Sagi, P. C., and Mishler, E. G., 1961. Family growth in metropolitan America. Princeton N.J.: Princeton Univ. Press.

Westoff, C. F., Sagi, P. C., and Kelly, E. L., 1958. Fertility through twenty years of marriage: a study in predictive possibilities. *Am. Sociol. Rev.*, 23.

Chapter 13

1. See Thomas D. Eliot, "Bereavement: Inevitable, but Not Insurmountable," in *Family, Marriage, and Parenthood,* edited by Howard Becker and Reuben Hill, Boston: D.C. Heath and Company, Second Edition, 1955.

2. Willard Waller, *The Old Love and the New,* New York: Liveright, 1930.

3. Robert C. Angell, *The Family Encounters the Depression,* New York: Charles Scribner's Sons, 1936.

4. Mirra Komarovsky, *The Unemployed Man and His Family,* New York: Dryden Press, 1940.

5. Ruth Cavan and Katherine Ranck, *The Family and the Depression,* Chicago: University of Chicago Press, 1938.

6. E. L. Koos, *Families in Trouble,* New York: King's Crown Press, 1946.

7. Reuben Hill, *Families Under Stress,* New York: Harper and Brothers, 1949.

8. William J. Goode, *After Divorce,* Glencoe: The Free Press, 1956.

9. See Hill, *op. cit.,* for an excellent review of this research.

10. To some extent, the original idea for this study was derived from Hill's discussion. See *op. cit.,* ch. 2.

11. Webster's Collegiate Dictionary, Springfield: G. and C. Merriam Co., Second Edition, 1944, p. 240.

12. Koos, *op. cit.,* p. 9.

13. Hill, *op. cit.,* p. 51. See also his review of definitions in ch. 2.

14. Arnold W. Green, "The Middle-Class Male Child and Neurosis," *American Sociological Review,* 11 (February, 1946), pp. 31–41.

15. Ruth Benedict, "Continuities and Discontinuities in Cultural Conditioning," *Psychiatry,* 1 (May, 1939), pp. 161–67.

16. Gertrude Wilson and Gladys Ryland, *Social Group Work Practice,* Boston: Houghton Mifflin Company, 1949, p. 49.

17. *Ibid.*

18. Leopold von Wiese, *Systematic Sociology,* adapted and amplified by Howard Becker, New York: Wiley, 1939.

19. This is essentially the point of view in Robert J. Havighurst's analysis, *Human Development and Education,* New York: Longmans, Green, 1953.

Chapter 14

1. Further details about the sample and the significance of the demographic factors on the marriage are available in the research report, *The Development of the Husband-Wife Relationship.*

2. For a clear statement of role theory as it applies to marriage, see Hill, R., and Rodgers, R., "Developmental theory." In H. Christensen, *Handbook of Marriage and the Family*. Rand McNally, 1964.

3. For further information about the characteristics of the marital cycle phases, see Feldman, H., *Development of the Marital Relationship.*

4. The data were gathered with the active collaboration of the Maternity Center Association and the Midwife Nurse Training Center, Queens County Hospital, New York City. The Clara Elizabeth Maternity Center, Flint, Michigan, and the Tompkins County, New York, State Medical Association Obstetrics Department.

5. These hypotheses and findings are derived from a paper read at the American Psychological Association 1968 Annual Meeting in San Francisco, entitled "Correlates of Changes in Marital Satisfactions with the Birth of the First Child" by H. Feldman and M. Rogoff, Cornell University, 1969.

6. For the viewpoint of others about the controversy, see D. Hobbs, R. Ryder, J. D. Rossi, R. Dyer, and J. Meyerowitz.

7. Cottrell, L. S., Jr. *Roles and Marital Adjustment.* Publications of the American Soc. Society, May 1933, Vol. XXIII, #2, pp. 107–115.

Chapter 15

1. Helena Znaniecki Lopata, *Occupation: Housewife* (New York: Oxford University Press, 1971), pp. 182–223.

2. E. E. LeMasters, "Parenthood as Crisis," *Marriage and Family Living,* Vol. 19 (1957), pp. 352–355; Everett D. Dyer, "Parenthood as Crisis: A Restudy," *Marriage and Family Living,* Vol. 25 (1963), pp. 196–201; Daniel F. Hobbs, Jr., "Parenthood as Crisis: A Third Study," *Journal of Marriage and the Family,* Vol. 27 (1965), pp. 367–372.

3. Talcott Parsons, "Age and Sex in the Social Structure of the United States," *American Sociological Review,* Vol. 7 (1942), pp. 6–12.

4. G. H. Mead, "On Mind as the Product of Social Interaction," in Marcello Truzzi (ed.), *Sociology: The Classic Statements* (New York: Random House, 1972), p. 273.

5. Eli Ginzberg with Ivan E. Berg, et al., *Life Styles of Educated Women* (New York: Columbia University Press, 1966), p. 55.

6. Lopata, *op. cit.,* pp. 192–193.

7. Richard E. Dawson and Kenneth Prewitt, *Political Socialization* (Boston: Little, Brown and Company, 1969), p. 19.

8. Gabriel A. Almond and Sidney Verba, *The Civic Culture: Po-*

litical Attitudes and Democracy in Five Nations (Boston: Little, Brown and Company, 1965), p. 272.

9. R. R. Bell, *Marriage and Family Interaction,* Third Edition (Homewood, Illinois: The Dorsey Press, 1971), p. 433.

10. Linda Gordon, *Families* (Boston: The New England Free Press, 1970), pp. 1 and 3.

11. *Ibid.,* p. 16.

12. Alvin W. Gouldner, "Attitudes of 'Progressive' Trade Union Leaders," *American Journal of Sociology,* Vol. 52 (1947), pp. 389–392.

13. Paul Burstein, "Social Structure and Individual Political Participation in Five Countries," *American Journal of Sociology,* Vol. 77 (1972), pp. 1090–1091.

14. Angus Campbell, Philip E. Converse, Warren E. Miller, and Donald E. Stokes, *The American Voter* (New York: John Wiley and Sons, 1960), pp. 103–105 and 479–498; Robert Dahl, *Who Governs?* (New Haven: Yale University Press, 1961), pp. 286–293.

15. Campbell, et al., *op. cit.* pp. 103–105.

16. Giussepee DiPalma, *Apathy and Participation: Mass Politics in Western Societies* (New York: The Free Press, 1970), p. 50.

17. Campbell, et al., *op. cit.,* pp. 103–105.

18. This indicator seems to be the most stable of the four items in the political efficacy scale. For further elaboration, see Shanto Iyengar, "The Problem of Response Stability: Some Comparisons Between Items and Scales," paper delivered at the Midwest Political Science Association, Chicago, 1972.

19. Region, social class, rural-urban, labor force participation, income, and education have all been found to be related both to political participation and political efficacy. See Campbell, et al., *The American Voter,* Angus Campbell and Henry Valen, "Party Identification in Norway and the United States," *Public Opinion Quarterly,* Vol. 25 (Winter, 1961), pp. 505–525; Almond and Verba, The Civic Culture; Norman H. Nie, G. Bingham Powell, Dr., and Kenneth Prewitt, "Social Structure and Political Participation: Developmental Relationships II," *American Political Science Review,* Vol. 63 (September, 1969), p. 817.

20. Lopata, *op. cit.,* chapter three.

21. Lee Rainwater, Richard P. Coleman, and Gerald Handel, *Workingman's Wife: Her Personality, World, and Life Style* (New York: Oceana Publications, Inc., 1959), pp. 88–89.

22. Alice S. Rossi, "Equality Between the Sexes," *Daedalus,* Vol. 93 (1964), p. 615.

23. Harriet B. Presser, "The Timing of the First Birth, Female Roles and Black Fertility," *Milbank Memorial Fund Quarterly,* Vol. 49 (1971), p. 333, and Donald J. Bogue, *Principles of Demography* (New York: John Wiley and Sons, Inc., 1969), p. 687.

24. Edward Pohlman, "The Timing of First Births: A Review of Effects," *Eugenics Quarterly,* Vol. 15 (1968), p. 252; Campbell, et al., *The American Voter;* Seymour Martin Lipset, *Political Man* (Garden City, New

York: Doubleday and Company, 1960); Robert E. Lane, *Political Life* (New York: The Free Press, 1959).

25. Presser, *op. cit.,* pp. 336–338.

26. Burstein, *op. cit.,* pp. 1090–1097.

27. The mobility of this age group also mitigates against political participation, but in our sample the mean period of residence in Manhattan was five years, thus giving us a rather stable group. See Lipset, *Political Man;* Paul F. Lazarsfeld, Bernard Berelson, and Hazel Gaudet, *The People's Choice* (New York: Columbia University Press, 1968); Campbell, et al., *The American Voter.*

28. Campbell, et al., *op. cit.,* pp. 515–519; Dahl, *op. cit.,* pp. 286–293.

29. Afaf Fahmy Abdel Baki Ibrahim, "Self-Concept and Family Planning," *Dissertation Abstracts,* 1968, 29(6-A), p. 1953.

30. Robert Weller, "The Employment of Wives, Role Incompatibility and Fertility: A Study Among Lower-and-Middle-Class Residents of San Juan, Puerto Rico," *Milbank Memorial Fund Quarterly,* Vol. 46 (1968), pp. 507–526.

31. Lane, *op. cit.,* p. 235.

32. George Herbert Mead, *Mind, Self and Society,* Charles W. Morris, ed. (Chicago: University of Chicago Press, 1934); Elihu Katz and Paul F. Lazarsfeld, *Personal Influence* (Glencoe, Illinois: The Free Press, 1955).

33. Joseph Woelfel and Archibald O. Haller, "Significant Others, The Self-Reflexive Act and the Attitude Formation Process," *American Sociological Review,* Vol. 36 (1971), pp. 74–87.

34. Kenneth Prewitt, *The Recruitment of Political Leaders: A Study of Citizen Politicians* (Indianapolis: The Bobbs-Merrill Company, Inc., 1970), p. 10.

35. Lester W. Milbrath, *Political Participation* (Chicago: Rand McNally and Company, 1965), pp. 110–113.

36. Veronica Stolte Heiskanan, "Sex Roles, Social Class and Political Consciousness," *Acta Sociologica,* Vol. 14 (1971), p. 86.

37. Warren E. Miller, "The Political Behavior of the Electorate," in Edward C. Dreyer and Walter A. Rosenbaum (eds.), *Political Opinion and Electoral Behavior* (Belmont, California: Wadsworth Publishing Company, 1968), p. 180.

38. William Kornhauser, *The Politics of Mass Society* (Glencoe, Illinois: Free Press), esp. chapter four.

39. Almond and Verba, *op. cit.,* p. 244.

40. Kornhauser, *op. cit.,* p. 109.

41. Lane, *op. cit.,* p. 289; Nie, Powell, and Prewitt, *op. cit.,* p. 816.

42. Almond and Verba found that an almost equal number of men and women in the United States said that individuals had an obligation to participate actively in public affairs, *The Civic Culture,* p. 330.

43. Lane, *op. cit.,* p. 288.

44. Heiskanan, *op. cit.,* p. 90.

45. Lane, *op. cit.,* p. 288.

46. Almond and Verba, *op. cit.,* pp. 303–304; Milbrath, *op. cit.,* p. 45.

47. Almond and Verba, *op. cit.,* p. 304.

48. Elizabeth K. Nottingham, "Toward an Analysis of the Effects of Two World Wars on the Role and Status of Middle-Class Women," *American Sociological Review,* Vol. 12 (1947), pp. 666–675.

49. Lane, *op. cit.,* pp. 115–116.

Chapter 22

U.S. Bureau of the Census, 1958. *Current population reports, 1957.* Series P-20, No. 79. Government Printing Office, Washington, D.C.

———, 1963. *Methodology and scores of socio-economic status.* Working Paper 15. Government Printing Office, Washington, D.C.

———, 1963. *Eighteenth census of the United States,* 1960. Government Printing Office, Washington, D.C.

———, 1969. *Income in 1967 of persons in the United States.* Series P-60, No. 60. Government Printing Office, Washington, D.C.

———, 1969. *Marriage, fertility, and childspacing: June 1965.* Current Population Reports, Series P-20, No. 186. Government Printing Office, Washington, D.C.

———, 1971. *Previous and prospective fertility: 1967.* Current Population Reports, Series P-20, No. 211. Government Printing Office, Washington, D.C.

Chapter 23

Commission on Population Growth and the American Future, 1972. *Report.* Washington, D.C.: Commission on Population Growth and the American Future, 726 Jackson Place, N.W.

Cuber, John F., and Peggy B. Haroff., 1966. *Sex and the Significant Americans: A Study of Sexual Behavior Among the Affluent.* Baltimore, Maryland: Penguin Books.

Goffman, Erving, 1963. *Stigma.* Englewood Cliffs, New Jersey: Prentice-Hall.

Gustavus, Susan O., and James R. Henley, Jr., 1971. "Correlates of voluntary childlessness in a select population." *Social Biology* 18:277–284.

Harrington, Judith A., 1969. "Childlessness in Canada 1961." Unpublished Master's Thesis. London: University of Western Ontario, Department of Sociology.

Kiefert, Robert M., 1966. "The childless female: an unexplored topic." Unpublished M.S. Thesis. University of North Dakota Library.

Pohlman, Edward, 1970. "Childlessness, international and unintentional: psychological and social aspects." *The Journal of Nervous and Mental Disease* 151:2–12.

Veevers, J. E., 1972a. "The violation of fertility mores: voluntary childlessness as deviant behaviour." pp. 571–592 in C. Boydell et al. (eds.), *Deviant Behaviour and Societal Reaction in Canada.* Toronto: Holt, Rinehart and Winston.

———, 1972b. "Factors in the incidence of childlessness in Canada: an analysis of census data." *Social Biology* (in press).

———, 1972c. "Parenthood and suicide: an examination of a neglected variable." *Social Science and Medicine* (in press).

———, 1973a. "The study of voluntary childlessness: an example of 'selective inattention.'" *The Family Coordinator* (in press).

———, 1973b. "The social meanings of parenthood." *Psychiatry: Journal for the Study of Interpersonal Processes* (in press).

———, 1973c. "The moral careers of voluntarily childless wives: notes on the construction and defense of a deviant world view." Forthcoming in S. Parvez Wakil (ed.), *Marriage and the Family in Canada*. Toronto: Holt, Rinehart and Winston.

Chapter 24

Notes

1. It is suggested that the processes of selective inattention are also evident in the kinds of behaviors which family sociologists consider need to be explained, and in the kinds of motivations which they speculate may be associated with them. For example, in family textbooks, the reasons for falling in love, getting married, being faithful, and staying married are seen as "obvious" and generally have positive connotations; the reasons for falling out of love, remaining single, committing adultery, and getting divorced are seen as problematic, and generally have negative connotations. (Kirkendall, 1968)

2. Precise information on the most recent trends in the rates of childlessness will not be available until detailed analyses have been done of the 1970 American and the 1971 Canadian censuses.

References

Balakrishnan, T. R., John D. Allingham, and John F. Kantner, 1972. "Canadian Family Growth Study." London: University of Western Ontario, Department of Sociology, unpublished mimeographed manuscript.

Blood, Robert J., Jr., 1969. *Marriage*. New York: Free Press.

Balchin, Nigel, 1968. "Children Are a Waste of Time." *The Saturday Evening Post*, October 19, 10–11.

Dexter, Lewis Anthony, 1958. "A Note on Selective Inattention in Social Science." *Social Problems*, 6, 176–182.

Duvall, E., 1962. *Family Development*. New York: J. B. Lippincott.

Erickson, Erik K., 1963. *Childhood and Society*. New York: W. W. Norton.

Feldman, Harold, 1965. "The Development of the Husband-Wife Relationship." Ithaca, New York: Cornell University, Department of Child Development and Family Relationships, unpublished mimeographed report.

Fletcher, Ronald, 1968. *Instinct in Man*. London: Unwin University Books.

Greene, Gael, 1963. "A Vote Against Motherhood." *The Saturday Evening Post,* January, **26,** 10–12.

Grabill, W. and P. Glick, 1959. "Demographic and Social Aspects of Childlessness: Census Data," *Millbank Memorial Fund Quarterly,* **37,** 60–86.

Hollingworth, Leta S., 1916. "Social Devices for Impelling Women to Bear and Rear Children." *The American Journal of Sociology,* **22,** 19–29.

Jacoby, Arthur P., 1969. "Transition to Parenthood: A Reassessment." *Journal of Marriage and the Family,* **31,** 720–727.

Kellmer-Pringle, M. L., 1967. *Adoption Facts and Fallacies: A Review of Research in the United States, Canada, and Great Britain Between 1948 and 1965*. London: Longmans.

Kephart, W. M., 1966. *The Family, Society, and the Individual*. Boston: Houghton Mifflin.

Kirkendall, Lester A., 1968. *A Reading and Study Guide for Students in Marriage and Family Relations*. Dubuque, Iowa: William C. Brown Co.

Kirkpatrick, C., 1963. *The Family as Process and Institution*. New York: Ronald Press.

Landis, J. and M. Landis, 1968. *Building a Successful Marriage*. Englewood Cliffs, N.J.: Prentice-Hall.

Landis, Paul N., 1970. *Making the Most of Marriage*. New York: Appleton-Century-Crofts.

Lantz, H. and E. Snyder, 1969. *Marriage: An Examination of the Man-Woman Relationship*. New York: John Wiley.

LeMasters, E. E., 1970. *Parents in Modern America*. Homewood, Illinois: The Dorsey Press.

Meier, R. L., 1958. "Concerning Equilibrium in Human Population." *Social Problems,* **6,** 163–175.

Michels, Lynnell, 1970. "Why We Don't Want Children." *Redbook*. January, 10–14.

Mills, C. Wright, 1959. *The Sociological Imagination*. New York: Oxford.

Osborn, F., 1963. "Excess and Unwanted Fertility." *Eugenics Quarterly*. **9–10,** 59–71.

Peck, Ellen, 1971. *The Baby Trap*. New York: Bernard Geis Associates.

Pohlman, E., 1966. "Mobilizing Social Pressures Toward Small Families," *Eugenics Quarterly*. **13,** 122–127.

Pohlman, Edward, 1969. *The Psychology of Birth Planning*. Cambridge, Mass.: Schenkman.

Pohlman, Edward, 1970. "Childlessness, Intentional and Unintentional: Psychological and Social Aspects." *The Journal of Nervous and Mental Disease*. **151,** 2–12.

Popenoe, Paul, 1936. "Motivation of Childless Marriages." *Journal of Heredity,* **27,** 469–472.

Rollin, Betty, 1970. "Motherhood: Who Needs It?" *Look,* September 22, **34,** (19), 11–17.

Rabin, A. L. and R. J. Greene, 1968. "Assessing Motivation for Parenthood." *Journal of Psychology,* **69,** 39–46.

Silverman, Anna and Arnold Silverman, 1971. *The Case Against Having Children.* New York: David McKay.

Udry, R. J., 1966. *The Social Context of Marriage.* New York: J. B. Lippincott Co.

Veevers, J. E., 1971a. "Differential Childlessness by Color: A Further Examination." *Social Biology,* **18,** 285–291.

Veevers, J. E., 1971b. "Childlessness and Age at First Marriage." *Social Biology,* **18,** 292–295.

Veevers, J. E., 1971c. "Rural-Urban Variation in the Incidence of Childlessness." *Rural Sociology,* **36,** 547–553.

Veevers, J. E., 1972a. "The Violation of Fertility Mores: Voluntary Childlessness as Deviant Behavior." In C. Boydell et al. (Eds.) *Deviant Behavior and Societal Reaction.* Toronto: Holt, Rinehart and Winston.

Veevers, J. E., 1972b. "Declining Childlessness and Age at Marriage; A Test of a Hypothesis." *Social Biology.* September.

Veevers, J. E., 1972c. "Factors in the Incidence of Childlessness in Canada: An Analysis of Census Data." *Social Biology.* December.

Westoff, Charles and Raymond H. Potvin, 1967. *College Women and Fertility Values.* Princeton N.J.: Princeton University Press.

Whelpton, P., A. Campbell, and J. Patterson, 1966. *Fertility and Family Planning in the United States.* Princeton, N.J.: Princeton University Press.

Williamson, R., 1966. *Marriage and Family Relations.* New York: John Wiley.

Womble, D., 1966. *Foundations for Marriage and Family Relations.* New York: Macmillan.

For further information regarding topics discussed in *Pronatalism: The Myth of Mom & Apple Pie,* the following organizations can be contacted:

National Organization for Non-Parents
515 Madison Avenue
New York, New York 10022

National Organization for Women
1957 East 73rd Street
Chicago, Illinois 60649

Planned Parenthood-World Population
810 Seventh Avenue
New York, New York 10019

Zero Population Growth
1346 Connecticut Avenue N.W.
Washington, D.C. 20036